# BTEC
## NATIONAL
# Health and Social Care

Book 2

Layla Baker
Deborah Boys
Janet McAleavy
Val Michie

Nelso

D0490911

DELETON

## Web links in the book

Because Nelson Thornes is not responsible for third party content online, there may be some changes to this material that are beyond our control. In order for us to ensure that the links referred to in the book are as up-to-date and stable as possible, the web sites provided are usually homepages with supporting instructions on how to reach the relevant pages if necessary.

Please let us know at webadmin@nelsonthornes.com if you find a link that doesn't work and we will do our best to correct this at reprint, or to list an alternative site.

Published in 2008 by:
Nelson Thornes Ltd
Delta Place
27 Bath Road
CHELTENHAM
GL53 7TH
United Kingdom

08 09 10 11 / 10 9 8 7 6 5 4 3 2

A catalogue record for this book is available from the British Library

ISBN 978 0 7487 8172 0

Cover photograph/illustration by Digital Vision
Illustrations by Angela Knowles
Page make-up by Pantek Arts Ltd, Maidstone, Kent

Printed and bound in Slovenia by Korotan

# Contents

# Introduction

Health and social care workers work with diverse groups of vulnerable people including children, young adults, elderly people and people with mental health problems and learning difficulties. They work in a variety of settings such as hospitals, care homes and people's own homes. Now is an exciting time to be a care worker because reforms are creating new jobs and flexible ways of working, and there is a huge amount of opportunity for career progression. If you are committed to working in care and enthusiastic about training and development, you can be assured of a challenging and rewarding career. The BTEC National Diploma in Health and Social Care will get you off to a flying start by preparing you both for work in health and social care and for further study.

## How do you use this book?

Covering eight specialist units of the new 2007 specification and two specialist units, this book has everything you need if you are studying BTEC National Certificate or Diploma in Health and Social Care. Simple to use and understand, it is designed to provide you with the skills and knowledge you need to gain your qualification. We guide you step by step toward your qualification, through a range of features that are fully explained over the page.

## Which units do you need to complete?

*BTEC National Health and Social Care Book 2* provides coverage of eight specialist units for the BTEC National Diploma in Health and Social Care. To achieve the Diploma, you are required to complete eight core units plus specialist units that provide for a combined total of 1080 guided learning hours (GLH). *BTEC National Health and Social Care Book 2* provides you with the following:

### Specialist Units

Unit 12 **Public Health**

Unit 14 **Physiological Disorders**

Unit 20 **Health Education**

Unit 21 **Nutrition for Health and Social Care**

Unit 22 **Research Methodology for Health and Social Care**

Unit 26 **Caring for People with Additional Needs**

Unit 28 **Caring for Older People**

Unit 39 **Infection Prevention and Control**

Unit 13 **Physiology of Fluid Balance** and resources for Unit 44 **Vocational Experience for Health and Social Care** can be found online at www.nelsonthornes.com/btec. Together with *BTEC National Health and Social Care Books 1* and *2*, these provide coverage of enough Guided Learning Hours for the Diplomas in both Health and Social Care and the Health Studies pathway.

## Is there anything else you need to do?

1. Talk to people who use health and social care services. Find out how they want to be cared for and what sort of qualities they would like to see in their care workers.

2. Talk to people who work in the health and social care industry. Find out what qualifications, skills and experience they needed to get their job and what their work involves.

3. Get as much experience as you can in the care industry and be aware of what your experiences teach you.

4. Take responsibility for learning about service users and the health and social care industry. In addition to completing all the work your teacher or tutor sets, ask questions and watch, read and listen to anything that will improve your knowledge and understanding.

5. Never be afraid to ask for help when you need it

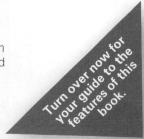
Turn over now for your guide to the features of this book.

*We hope you enjoy your BTEC course – Good Luck!*

# Features of this book

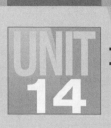

## UNIT 14

# Physiological Disorders

**This unit covers:**

- The nature of physiological disorders
- The processes involved in diagnosis of disorders
- The care strategies used to support individuals through the course of a disorder
- How individuals adapt to the presence of a disordey

Health and social care workers need to have an insight into the ways in which different physiological disorders present themselves and how the caring services diagnose, treat and care for patients.

 aims to give you a basic understanding of a variety of physiological disorders. It describes their causes, the body systems involved and associated signs and symptoms. It looks at the investigations and measurements involved in reaching a diagnosis, patient care and the roles of the people involved in delivering care. Finally, it explores how individuals cope with the difficulties caused by their disorder and how its progression could affect them in the future.

## Learning Objectives

At the beginning of each Unit there will be a bulleted list letting you know what material is going to be covered. They specifically relate to the learning objectives within the specification.

## Grading Criteria

The table of Grading Criteria at the beginning of each unit identifies achievement levels of pass, merit and distinction, as stated in the specification.

To achieve a **pass**, you must be able to match each of the 'P' criteria in turn.

To achieve **merit** or **distinction**, you must increase the level of evidence that you use in your work, using the 'M' and 'D' columns as reference. For example, to achieve a distinction you must fulfil all the criteria in the pass, merit and distinction columns. Each of the criteria provides a specific page number for easy reference.

| grading criteria | To achieve a **Pass** grade the evidence must show that the learner is able to: | To achieve a **Merit** grade the evidence must show that the learner is able to: | To achieve a **Distinction** grade the evidence must show that the learner is able to: |
| --- | --- | --- | --- |
| | **P1** describe the course of two different physiological disorders as experienced by two different individuals | | |
| | **P2** describe the physiology of each disorder and factors that may have influenced its development | **M1** explain the importance of the process of weaning | |
| | **P3** describe the clinical investigations carried out and measurements made to diagnose and monitor the disorder in each individual | **M2** explain possible difficulties involved in making a diagnosis from the signs and symptoms displayed by the individuals and the results of their investigations | |
| | **P4** describe the care processes experienced by each individual case and the roles of different people in supporting the care strategy | | **D1** evaluate the contributions made by different people in supporting the individuals with the disorders |
| | **P5** explain difficulties experienced by each individual in adjusting to the presence of the disorder and the care strategy | **M3** explain how the care strategies experienced by each individual have influenced the course of the disorder | **D2** evaluate alternative care strategies that might have been adopted for each individual |

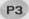

## Activities

are designed to help you understand the topics through answering questions or undertaking research, and are either *Group* or *Individual* work. They are linked to the Grading Criteria by application of the D, P, and M categories.

**activity**
**INDIVIDUAL WORK**

**P1**

Think about two people you know who are experiencing and receiving treatment for a physiological disorder. The disorders must be different in that they each affect a different body system eg CHD (circulatory system) and asthma (respiratory system).

Use both primary research methods eg interviews, and secondary research methods eg a literature search, to find out:

■ the signs and symptoms that are manifested by each disorder over time

■ how the disorders have affected and continue to affect your subjects.

## Case Studies

provide real life examples that relate to what is being discussed within the text. It provides an opportunity to demonstrate theory in practice.

*case study*

*14.1*

### The signs, symptoms and psychological effects of MS

Su is 35 years old. Although she has a boyfriend she chooses to live as a single mother with her two small children and elderly mother in their three storey terrace house. Her job requires her to drive extensively throughout the region in which she lives. She loves to work in her garden and, in order to keep costs down, has become quite a DIY expert at home.

Su has recently been diagnosed with MS. She has read the literature sent to her by the MS Society and is feeling devastated. Her family, friends and colleagues tell her that her feelings are quite natural and that given time, she will adapt to her situation. None of their comments is of any help.

An Activity that is linked to a Case Study helps you to apply your knowledge of the subject to real life situations.

**activity**

1. What signs and symptoms is Su likely to experience now and in the future?
2. How might having MS affect Su psychologically?
3. How might having MS affect Su's life?
4. How would you feel if you were in Su's shoes?

## Keywords

of specific importance are highlighted within the text, and then defined in a glossary at the end of the book.

The role of a health or social care worker is to advise about, not dictate, healthy lifestyle choices

One-to-one communication in a **health care setting** occurs, for example, when a doctor gives medical information to a patient. An example in a social care setting is when a councillor assists a client in therapy.

## Remember

boxes contain helpful hints, tips or advice.

**Professional Practice**

If you are involved in carrying out investigations and making measurements:

■ be aware of communication barriers and try to overcome them

■ make sure that any measurements you make are accurate

■ always follow your organisation's health and safety procedures

■ always follow your organisation's procedures for assessing risks.

## Professional Practice

boxes highlight any professional practice points relevant to the topic being covered.

**Link**

You will look more closely at diet in Unit 21.

## Links

direct you to other parts of the book that relate to the subject currently being covered.

*i*

The Multiple Sclerosis Society
www.mssociety.org.uk

## Information bars

point you towards resources for further reading and research (e.g. websites).

**Progress Check**

1. Describe the course of two physiological disorders, ie how the physical signs and symptoms, and emotional effects, change over time.
2. Describe the physiology of each disorder and the factors that may have influenced its development
3. Explain how the course of each disorder relates to its physiology.
4. Describe the investigations and measurements that are made to diagnose and monitor each disorder.
5. Explain why it might be difficult to make a diagnosis from signs and symptoms and investigation results.
6. Describe the care strategies used for each disorder
7. Compare and contrast the roles of the different people who provide care for individuals experiencing disorders.
8. Explain any difficulties that an individual might experience in adjusting to a disorder and the strategies used to care for them.

## Progress Checks

provide a list of quick questions at the end of each Unit, designed to ensure that you have understood the most important aspects of each subject area.

# Acknowledgements

Table Screening checks to detect normal and abnormal health and development from Ewles, L and Simnett I. Promoting Health a Practical Guide, 5th edition, Bailliere Tindall 2003. Reprinted with permission of Elsevier

Short quote from HPA Protection Agency Annual Lecture on Infectious Diseases, 29/3/07. Reprinted with permission of HPA

Tiny quote 'There is increasing evidence of serogroup W135...' © WHO from www.who.int

Incidence of Meningitis outbreaks figures. Reprinted with permission of HPA

Diagram of the Causes of Mortality in the Army in the East. The Royal Collection © 2005 Her Majesty Queen Elizabeth II

Use of quotes from www.nice.org.uk. Reprinted with permission

Table 'WHO: Causes of death by disease category (2002) © WHO

Percentages of all diagnoses of STIs and HIV that occurred in young adults (16–24) UK 2006. Reprinted with permission of HPA

'Cancer incidence rates in EU' from http://info.cancerresearchuk.org/cancerstats/geographic/canerineu/incidenceandmortality/?a=5441 December, 2007, Reprinted with permission of Cancer Research UK

Short extract re septic tanks and cesspools from www.dorsetforyou.com Reprinted with permission

Summary of theories: focus and key concepts, from 'Theory at a glance: A Guide for Health Promotion Practice' US Dept of Health and Human Services/ National Institutes of Health

Figure 'Tannahill's model of Health Promotion' from Tannahill 'What is health promotion?' Health Education Journal, 1985, Vol 44, issue 3, pp 167–168. Reprinted with permission of Sage Publications

'Dahlgren and Whitehead's model of factors affecting health' from Dahlgren, G., and Whitehead, M. 1991, Policies and Strategies to Promote Social Equity in Health. Reprinted with permission of Institute for Futures Studies, Swedenfigure

'The key milestones in WHO's history 1948–2004 © WHO

Table levels of community participation in planning healthwork from Ewles, L and Simnett I. Promoting Health a Practical Guide, 5th edition, Bailliere Tindall 2003. Reprinted with permission of ElsevierTable Principles of good practice from Ewles, L and Simnett I. Promoting Health a Practical Guide, 5th edition, Bailliere Tindall 2003. Reprinted with permission of ElsevierText

Definitions from WHO – 'Impairment' 'Disability' 'Handicap' © WHO from www.WHO.int

Extract from General Social Care Council Code of Practice. Www.gscc.org.uk

Crown Copyright materials reproduced with permission of the controller of the HMSO

## Picture credits

12.8 Florence Nightingale - Corbis; 12.9 The Royal Collection, Her Majesty Queen Elizabeth II; 12.10 William Henry Beveridge - Hulton-Deutsch Collection/Corbis; 12.12 Liam Donaldson - Touhig Sion/Corbis Sygma; 12.21 Needlestick injuries - Getty; 14.6 Asthma- Alamy/ Scott Camazine; 21.10 TV Dinner- Alamy/ Bubbles Photolibrary; 21.11 Undernutrition Alamy/ Sally & Richard Greenhill; 22.2 Questionnaire- Alamy/ Janine Wiedel; 22.3 - Fotolia; Man in a wheelchair – Almay; 22.4 Fotolia; 22.5 Secondary sources- Alamy/ Chris Stock Photography; 22.16 Using IT - IS985 (NT); 26.3 - Rex features; 26.11 - Fotolia; 28.15 Tai Chi- Alamy/ Philip Wolmuth; 28.15 Discussion- Alamy Photo Network; 39.4 Mumps- Science Photo Library; 39.6 Ringworm- Science Photo Library; 39.16 Putting the law into practice - istockphoto; All other photos from the NT Archive.

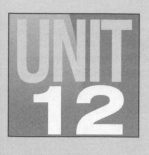

# Public Health

## This unit covers:

- Public health strategies in the UK and their origins
- The current patterns of ill health and factors affecting health in the UK
- The methods of promoting and protecting public health

Public health is concerned with the identification, protection and prevention of illness and disease within populations and communities. The study of the spread and incidence of infectious and non-infectious diseases is known as **epidemiology**. Within the National Health Service Framework the government has the National Infection Control and Health Protection Agency combining the existing functions of the Public Health Laboratory Service and three other national bodies the National Radiological Protection Board, the Centre for Applied Microbiology and Research, and the National Focus for Chemical Incidents nationally, regionally and locally to help co-ordinate and provide such information on the identification, spread and prevention of disease and ill health. This unit will examine how people's health is protected and promoted by looking at public health strategies, identifying current patterns of ill health and factors that contribute to ill health.

You will gain an understanding of how Public Health policy has been formulated in this country from the mid-1800s to the present day. We are fortunate in this country to be able to track the changes that have improved the quality of life and life expectancy of the general population. It is because of the radical organisation and understanding of the importance of public health and health services that we continue to have a health service that aims to protect the individual and the community at large.

## grading criteria

| To achieve a **Pass** grade the evidence must show that the learner is able to: | To achieve a **Merit** grade the evidence must show that, in addition to the pass criteria, the learner is able to: | To achieve a **Distinction** grade the evidence must show that, in addition to the pass and merit criteria, the learner is able to: |
| --- | --- | --- |
| **P1** describe key aspects of public health in the UK. Pg 9 | | |
| **P2** describe the origins of public health in the UK. Pg 20 | | |
| **P3** identify current patterns of ill health and inequality in the UK. Pg 25 | **M1** explain probable causes of the current patterns of ill health and inequality in the UK. Pg 25 | **D1** evaluate the role of factors that contribute to the current patterns of ill health and inequality in the UK. Pg 25 |

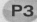

| To achieve a **Pass** grade the evidence must show that the learner is able to: | To achieve a **Merit** grade the evidence must show that, in addition to the pass criteria, the learner is able to: | To achieve a **Distinction** grade the evidence must show that, in addition to the pass and merit criteria, the learner is able to: |
|---|---|---|
| **P4** describe six factors that affect health status in the UK.  Pg 38 | | |
| **P5** describe methods of promoting and protecting public health.           Pg 44 | **M2** explain methods of promoting and protecting public health.           Pg 44 | |
| **P6** identify appropriate methods of prevention/control for a named **communicable disease** and a named non-communicable disease. Pg 48 | **M3** explain appropriate methods of prevention/control for a named communicable and a named non-communicable disease.           Pg 48 | **D2** evaluate the effectiveness of methods of promoting and protecting public health for the two named diseases.           Pg 48 |

# Public health strategies in the UK and their origins

## Key aspects of public health

### Health status of the community

In Great Britain the populace is made up of over 60 million individuals. Overall health is measured by quality of life, infant **mortality** rates and life expectancy. Incidence of disease and life threatening factors are collected at local level and this data is recorded so that a picture of the health of communities can be compared and measured throughout Great Britain. Some areas will have higher incidences of some diseases; some communities will reveal low incidences of diseases. The health status of the community is dependent on age, gender, socio-economic conditions, genetics and environmental factors.

In a community with a largely elderly population statistics would reveal that the most common illness might be influenza and the most common cause of death might be pneumonia. Awareness of this would lead to promotion and uptake of influenza vaccinations to reduce the incidence.

### Identifying health needs of the population

The health needs of the population are determined by the incidence of disease and trends identified. Nationally collated statistics may identify disease trends in the whole country. These statistics are used to determine how health can be improved or how areas of concern can be highlighted and effects of ill health reduced or prevented. It is the responsibility of health professionals to report the incidence of specific diseases and illnesses so that this information can be centrally collated and acted on.

Patterns of illness and disease may relate to several factors such as age, genetics, environment, lifestyle, education and take up of preventative measures, for example **immunisation**. The needs of the population are governed by social, financial and economic factors too. Some sectors of our society may be more susceptible to certain diseases and illnesses and these are highlighted in information found in the National

Statistics and social trends information that can be obtained online and is also published by the Department of Health. The health of the nation is measured by mortality (how long we live) and morbidity (what we die from) rates. Statistics show that we live longer than previous generations.

Figure 12.1 Life expectancy at age 65

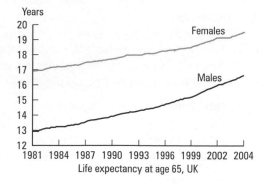

Life expectancy at age 65 in the United Kingdom has reached its highest level ever for both men and women. Men aged 65 could expect to live a further 16.6 years and women a further 19.4 years if mortality rates remained the same as they were in 2003–05.

However we cannot become complacent as there are still many diseases and illnesses that can have severe affects on our health. New strains of bacterial, protozoan, **fungal** and viral infections are discovered all the time.

## Developing programmes to reduce risk and screen for early disease

Health programmes are based on information that is gathered from epidemiologists working in Public Health departments. The Department of Health commissions a committee to write a Green Paper which proposes what the targets of health should be. Based on these findings the Government meet to decide how to implement the findings. From their findings a White Paper is commissioned that gives more details of how action should be taken. In the case of the White Paper for Health 'Our Healthy Nation' and 'Our Healthier Nation' (1999) reports were written. From these papers, for example national and local guidelines are produced to plan how to educate and protect the public. White Papers are produced to influence social changes in the health of the nation. Health Improvement Plans (HImPs) are devised for each local area based on the current needs of the local and national population. These are carried out at individual and group level by public health promotion specialists such as GPs, nurses, and health care workers.

Figure 12.2 Public Health Promotion Implementation Structure

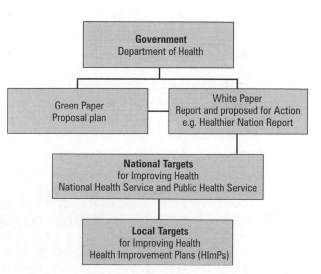

This might seem a lengthy process for new, emergent and dangerous diseases but the government has also put in place emergency action plans.

Public Health Programmes reduce the risks of disease by educating, providing and promoting health information, choices and active interventions.

Examples of Public Health Promotion programmes are:

### Five-a-day

People are encouraged to eat five portions of fruit and vegetables a day as this has been found to increase vitamin and mineral content in diets. This will improve fitness and well-being by providing natural ingredients that will support the immune system, help with bone and tissue repair and aid digestion.

### MMR immunisation programme

Parents are encouraged to have their children immunised with measles, mumps and rubella vaccines to reduce the incidence of contracting these diseases which can kill; and to reduce the spread of the disease for those people who are not able to be immunised. Notice the sharp rise in cases of mumps from 2002 to 2004.

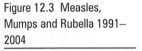

Figure 12.3 Measles, Mumps and Rubella 1991–2004

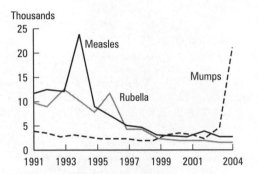

The number of cases of mumps recorded in the United Kingdom in 2004 was almost 21,000 – four and a half times the number recorded in 2003.

The Department of Health explains the rise as follows:

> 'The increase largely reflects lower immunity among older teenagers and young adults in their early 20s, particularly those born between 1983 and 1986 immediately before the introduction of routine vaccination in 1988. These young people would not have been exposed to mumps in childhood because of the swift success of the MMR (measles, mumps, rubella) vaccine in controlling the disease. Older adults were more likely to have had mumps when it was still a common childhood infection'.

Permission: Source: National Statistics website: www.statistics.gov.uk

The Department of Health presents information which may be given as a series of facts about diseases. These would then be accessed by health professionals to pass on or can be obtained by the public on the internet. An example of this could be about flu and how to know when to obtain vaccinations.

### Pandemic flu

Pandemic flu is a **virus** that spreads rapidly causing widespread **epidemics** around the world. Pandemic flu occurs when a new, highly infectious and dangerous strain of the influenza virus appears. In contrast to the 'ordinary' or 'seasonal' flu outbreaks which we see every winter in the UK, flu pandemics occur infrequently – usually every few decades. There were three last century. The most serious was in 1918, killing millions of people worldwide. Smaller pandemics happened in 1957 and 1968.

> 'The World Health Organization (WHO) has developed an alert system to help inform the world about the current threat of a pandemic emerging. The alert system has six phases, with Phase 1 having the lowest risk of human cases and Phase 6 posing the

greatest risk of pandemic. The world is presently in Phase 3 of the Pandemic Alert. This means that there is a new influenza virus subtype causing disease in humans, but is not yet spreading in an efficient (easily transmittable) and sustainable manner among humans.'

The Department of Health – Pandemic Flu
http://www.dh.gov.uk/PandemicFlu/

## Local NHS Stop Smoking Service

Following Government guidelines to educate people why smoking is harmful to health, local Stop Smoking Services are provided to offer practical face-to-face support to help people quit smoking. These may be based in health centres, community halls or local shopping centres.

Programmes to reduce the risk of disease are mainly based on the following models.

Figure 12.4  Public Health Campaign

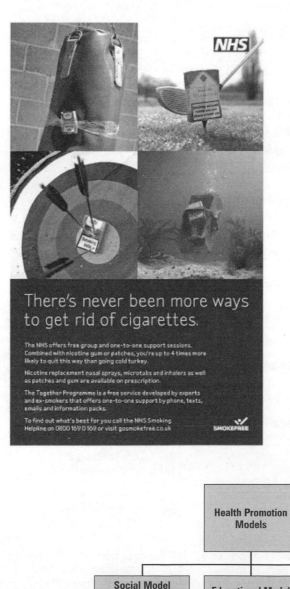

Figure 12.5  Health promotion models

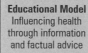

*The Social Model*
- Aims to improve health conditions for whole sectors of society.
- Aims to encompass the wider issues surrounding health, e.g. legislation to reduce smoking in public places.
- Choices are given but these may be restricted by economy, environment and timing.

*The Educational Model*
- Information is designed to inform and present health choices in a factual way.
- Factual, non-judgemental information is made available in various formats, e.g. advertisements, pamphlets, oral advice.
- People choose when, where and how they receive information.

*The Medical Model*
- Focus of care is mainly on intervention, prevention and treatment.
- The person receiving care is the patient.
- Procedures and practices are carried out to them.
- The patient may or may not have choice over decisions made about their care.
- Treatment is directed top-down.

Models of health also include other models such as client-centered, behaviour change approach and fear approach (Ewles and Simnett, 2003) which will be discussed in more detail in methods of promoting and protecting public health.

## Detecting disease – screening programmes

Disease and illness are caused by many factors. These may commonly be detected through screening to identify the agents responsible. Screening is the generic term used to test, examine and identify potential health problems. Prevention and treatment can then be given to reduce spread of infection or reduce potential health risks where possible.

Screening takes place at specified times across the whole population and starts throughout pregnancy, birth, childhood and adulthood. Checks are made of physical and mental health and well-being through examination by health care practitioners. Methods of screening may include the following:

Table 12.1  Screening checks to detect normal and abnormal health and development

| Screening method/Tests | Screening purpose | Screening to treat and detect illness/diseases |
| --- | --- | --- |
| Blood Urine Stool Cerebrospinal Fluid (CSF) Amniocentesis | To detect infectious, non-infectious, congenital illness/disease/syndromes/ normal and abnormal function of systems | Hepatitis, HIV, Leukaemia, Diabetes, Gastro-enteritis, Meningitis, Down's, Sickle Cell Anaemia, Cystic fibrosis |
| X-rays Ultrasounds CT Scans, EEGs EMI Scans | To detect skeletal problems, normal/ abnormal growth development, internal body functions, e.g. kidneys, liver, digestive system, brain | Broken bones, teeth and bone decay, foetal growth, brain structure and function, internal organ function, detect cancers, abnormal growth(s), haemorrhages |
| Cardiovascular Checks Blood Pressure, Pulse ECGs | To detect normal, abnormal functioning of heart and blood supply | Heart diseases: Angina, Myocardial Infarction, Vascular disease: Varicose veins, Deep Vein Thrombosis |

| Screening method/Tests | Screening purpose | Screening to treat and detect illness/diseases |
|---|---|---|
| Lung Function Tests | To detect normal, abnormal functioning of airway and lungs | Lung disease: Bronchitis, Asthma, Chronic Obstructive Airways Disease, Pneumonia |
| Physical Measurements, Height, Weight, BMI Centile Charts, Speech, Hearing, Sight Tests | To detect growth and development at expected age and stage of life span | Hyper/Hypo thyroidism, Obesity, Deafness, Visual difficulties |
| Family History/Genetic Screening | To detect family history of incidence of disease and illness | Haemophilia, Thalassaemia |
| Questionnaires Interviews Observations Consultations | To check for other factors which might contribute to illness and disease, e.g. environment, social well-being, intellectual well-being, emotional well-being | Work-related illness, e.g. Asbestosis, Deafness, Back injuries, Allergies |

## Controlling communicable disease

The prevention and control of infectious diseases is an important aspect of public health and is carried out using a variety of models and methods. Key aspects of this involve planning to include screening and early detection, isolation and treatment, containment, prevention and cure and eradication where possible.

Early detection of disease and illness is important as it will give details of cause and spread and highlight potential risk to individuals or groups of people. Some sections of the population are more vulnerable to illness and disease than others. These are the very young, babies and infants, because their immune systems are immature. The elderly population are also vulnerable because they have lower resistance to some diseases. People who have compromised immune systems are also at risk because they are not able to rely on their bodies to combat infectious disease, e.g. people who are receiving radiotherapy and chemotherapy for cancer; people who have AIDs.

Isolation of people who are infectious may not always be possible but it has been known to be effective in reducing the spread of disease. For highly infectious diseases, for example tuberculosis, isolation is essential and is carried out by hospital admission to the isolation unit. The person is 'barrier nursed' which means that they are nursed in a room with a double door entrance. The health care worker can walk from the ward into the first room to change and then into the patient's room once gowned and gloved. These clothes are removed before entering the main ward area again. This should occur every time the patient requires treatment during the infectious period. Other methods might be confinement to home surroundings. Think about when you have had an infection, e.g. tonsillitis, measles, flu. It is much better to stay away from crowds than to pass this on especially if you work in settings where people might be vulnerable as in childcare or elderly care.

Containment of the disease might happen at national and local levels. Once the source of the infection has been identified plans are put in place to reduce and prevent further occurrences. These may be short-, medium- and long-term measures. Short-term measures might be to reduce the amount of spread by limiting visiting, unnecessary travel, treatment and isolation. Medium- and long-term measures might include organising an immunisation programme or medical treatment as appropriate, educating people about risks and eradicating incidence of disease where possible. In the case of Salmonella poisoning it is known that it is a disease caught by eating raw eggs and undercooked meat such as chicken or pork. The medium- and long-term measures introduced should include education around cooking and hygiene methods. The short-term treatment and containment problem is to ensure that people who have sickness and diarrhoea receive treatment for potential dehydration problems and to ensure that soiled waste is disposed of correctly. Hands should be washed and toilet areas should be disinfected after use.

Eradication of disease is becoming more and more possible as scientific research advances. More is known about the causes of illness and disease due to the technology and knowledge about how disease organisms develop and spread. This is evidenced by the fact that we now live longer than our predecessors. The key aspects of public health that have made this possible are:

- Early detection and surveillance.
- Monitoring and screening.
- Treatment and immunisation programmes.
- Health education and promotion.
- Improved social reforms to ensure health is available for all.

## Promoting the health of the population

The health of the population is promoted locally and nationally by Health Promoters who are based in GP surgeries, drop-in centres, schools and via media sources such as TV, radio and magazines. Priorities are based on local need and availability of funding and resources. One of the ways that priorities are identified are from the number of reported incidences of disease and illness. If these are life threatening or cause long periods in hospital then these will be the main focus of health promotion. A good example of this is how the effects of being overweight can lead to physical diseases such as coronary heart disease and diabetes in later life. The health promoter's role would be to promote healthier diets, more exercise and ways for people to take control of their eating habits.

The health of the population is said to be healthy when there are fewer deaths and life threatening illnesses per population size and area. The cases that are reported are then mapped per region. This is why it is possible to say that some areas have a higher incidence of some diseases.

## Planning and evaluating the national provision of health and social care

The planning and evaluation of health and social care provision in the UK is government and National Health Service and Social Services led based on information given by health care and social care practitioners at local, regional and national levels.

The government have produced guidelines and information to state how they will tackle the problems of controlling and preventing infectious disease spread.

'The strategy sets out a series of proposed actions to create a modern system to prevent, investigate and control the infectious diseases threat and address health protection more widely. These include:

- a new National Infection Control and Health Protection Agency combining the existing functions of the Public Health Laboratory Service and three other national bodies (the National Radiological Protection Board, the Centre for Applied Microbiology and Research, and the National Focus for Chemical Incidents) to provide an integrated approach to protecting the health of the public against infectious diseases as well as chemical and radiological hazards.

- a local health protection service delivered by the new Agency, working with the NHS and local authorities to deliver specified functions relating to the prevention, investigation and control of infectious diseases as well as chemical and radiological hazards.

- a national expert panel to assess the threat from new and emerging infectious diseases.

- a strengthened and expanded system of infectious disease surveillance bringing in modern methods of data capture and integrating information from human infections with that from animals and from environmental monitoring.

- new action plans to address infectious disease priorities: tuberculosis, health care associated infection, antimicrobial resistance, blood-borne and sexually transmitted viruses and chronic diseases caused by micro-organisms.

- rationalisation of microbiology laboratories and introduction of standards for diagnosis and profiling of micro-organisms.

- a new Inspector of Microbiology post to ensure that laboratories meet their responsibilities for public health surveillance, to ensure compliance with standards and check that security is in place to reduce the risk of loss or misuse of microbiological agents.

- a programme of new vaccine development.

- strengthened clinical and preventive services for dealing with infection in childhood through the National Service Framework for Children.

- further development of plans to combat the threat to public health of deliberate release of biological, chemical or radiological agents.

- better public information and involvement on infectious diseases and their risks.

- stronger professional education and training programmes.

- a research and innovation programme.

- a review of the law on infection control to determine what changes are needed to underpin the strategy.'

Source: www.dh.gov.uk/en/Publicationsandstatistics/Publications/
PublicationsPolicyAndGuidance/Browsable/DH_4985569.

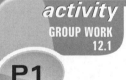

**activity**
**GROUP WORK**
**12.1**

**P1**

On a flipchart, take it in turns to write down a key aspect of public health in the UK. Now, going round the group, take turns to describe each aspect listed.

## Sources of information for determining patterns of health/ill health

Sources of health information on patterns of disease are available in a variety of formats which may include online resources, printed media such as pamphlets, news bulletins, letters, bound copies of statistics and health information.

### World Health Organization (WHO)

The World Health Organization is the United Nations' specialised agency for health. It was established on 7 April 1948. WHO's objective, as set out in its Constitution, is the attainment by all peoples of the highest possible level of health. Health is defined in WHO's Constitution as a state of complete physical, mental and social well-being and not merely the absence of disease or infirmity.

'The biggest enemy of health in the developing world is poverty.'

Kofi Annan

The World Health Organization provides information, medical aid, guidance and statistics on health in Third World and Developing countries. It tackles poverty through challenging the practices of governments and organisations so that money is spent on adequate health care for its population. An example of this might be to recommend improvements to roads and therefore access to health care; or to improve water and sanitation facilities; to implement immunisation programmes.

## Government, regional and local statistics and reports

This country has a much stronger public health system than many other countries. The Department of Health coordinates and provides guidance on, the prevention, investigation and control of infectious diseases in the population to ensure that it is addressed at national, regional and local level.

'Specialist agencies, notably the Public Health Laboratory Service and its Communicable Disease Surveillance Centre, provide expertise in informing policy, in co-coordinating surveillance activities and in the investigation of outbreaks and epidemics. A network of expert committees also provides advice.

At local level health authorities (through their Directors of Public Health and Consultants in Communicable Disease Control) work together with local authorities to address infectious disease problems in local communities. In hospitals, designated teams deal with hospital acquired infection.

Regional directors of public health have assumed overall responsibility for co-coordinating health protection activities in their regions. This has been particularly effective in the two recent emergencies – the foot and mouth outbreak (when measures had to be taken to protect human health as a result of disposal on a huge scale of animal carcasses) and the threat of terrorism.'

Source: Department of Health

Sources of information in this country are mainly obtained from Government reports and statistics which provide National, Regional and Local data on the incidence and spread of disease. The data for social health trends is collected from the National Census Surveys which are carried out every ten years. Current data for health, specific illnesses and diseases are passed regularly but this is not always standardised or coordinated across the whole country. This will sometimes account for health statistics that are not available in the previous or current year.

The main source of health information statistics and social trends in the UK are the Department of Health, Health Protection Agency and the Public Health Laboratory Services who produce information online and in media such as books, magazines and newsletters. These can be accessed through the internet, Public Library Services and some health and social care settings.

Here is an excerpt from a press release from the annual meeting of the Health Protection Agency in March 2007:

'Professor Trevor Jones CBE said "We are seeing the emergence ... or re-emergence... of a number of significant infectious diseases in both the developed and the developing world e.g. influenza, malaria, tuberculosis, HIVAIDS. The causes of this varies from neglect, poor health care infrastructure, poverty and the absence of funding to the development of resistance and the mutation of infectious **parasites** and micro-organisms. It is essential that we increase the amount of research and development for new medicines and vaccines in the continuing fight against these diseases.'

Up-to-date resources regarding **demographic** information may be found online. Legislation, policies, social trends and national statistics in the UK

www.statistics.gov.uk/

Publications and national statistics in the UK

www.dh.gov.uk/Publicationsandstatistics/

Local and Regional Health Protection Agency services work alongside the NHS providing specialist support in communicable disease and infection control, and emergency planning. They also oversee some laboratory services.

www.hpa.org.uk/lars_homepage.htm

Health and safety aspects of accident and health protection in the UK

www.hse.gov.uk/statistics/

Department of Health, Social Services and Public Safety for Northern Ireland – Health information and data

www.dhsspsni.gov.uk/index/stats_research/stats-pubs.htm

Information Services Division – Health information and data for Scotland

www.isdscotland.org/isd/

NHS Scotland-health information and statistics

www.show.scot.nhs.uk/

Health information and data for Wales

www.wales.nhs.uk/

Information on Health and Personal Social Services Statistics

www.performance.doh.gov.uk/HPSSS/

Information on community health profiles to include summaries and key aspects of health and social concerns for the area in which you live. Information is submitted on an annual basis from the Public Health Observatories.

www.communityhealthprofiles.info/

---

Local health information statistics can be obtained from Department of Health and Health Protection Agency online and publications by requesting county information. Alternatively some health authorities also publish local health statistics for each area in news bulletins.

Health information can also be obtained from charitable and private organisations that target specific health problems, e.g. MIND for mental welfare; RNIB for people with visual difficulties or who are blind.

---

World Health Organization (WHO)

www.who.int

European WHO

www.euro.who.int/

Médecins sans Frontières

www.msf.org

UNICEF

www.unicef.org

---

It is quicker to access information when you know which category, specific illness or disease you require information on. For example if we wanted to know how to find out the incidence of Meningitis worldwide we might look at the World Health Organization information statistics for infectious diseases, meningitis and choose which type of meningitis strain. If we then wanted to find figures for the UK we would look at the Department of Health Information statistics. If we wanted specific information about the area you live in then you might type in the county name or you might need to type in the local health authority area or look at Community Health profiles. A library search would also give you similar access to results but as stated not necessarily the most current figures in published versions.

Here is an information search for the incidence of Meningitis broken down into global, national and local researches.

■ Incidence of Meningitis outbreaks globally (worldwide)

'There is increasing evidence of serogroup W135 being associated with outbreaks of considerable size. In 2000 and 2001 several hundred pilgrims attending the Hajj in Saudia Arabia were infected with N. meningitidis W135. Then in 2002, W135 emerged in Burkina Faso, striking 13,000 people and killing 1,500.'

www.who.int/mediacentre/factsheets/fs141/en

■ Incidence of Meningitis outbreaks in UK (nationally)

'Latest figures from the Public Health Laboratory Service show that in the 15 to 17 year old group, in the last 12 weeks, six cases of Meningitis C were reported compared with 26 in the same period in 1999. Additionally, in children under one year old, there was only one case reported in this period compared with 19 in 1999. The total number of cases in the immunised age groups was therefore only seven, compared with 45 in 1999.'

'High immunisation uptake levels (85 per cent) for the meningococcal C conjugate vaccine (MCC) in target age groups (between 12 months to 17 years of age) resulted in an 80 per cent reduction in the incidence of meningococcal meningitis group C in these groups within the first 18 months of the start of the immunisation programme.'

www.dh.gov.uk/en/Publicationsandstatistics/Pressreleases/DH_4004941

■ Incidence of Meningitis outbreaks in your area (locally)

The UK was the first country in the world in 1999 to introduce Group C meningococcal disease vaccine. Cases of Group C disease in the South West since 1998 are as follows: 1998 – 59 cases, 1999 – 65, 2000 – 42, 2001 – 27, 2002 – 19, 2003 – 4 cases.

www.hpa.org.uk/southwest/press/040603_meningococcal.htm

The above information highlights the incidence of Meningitis and how immunisation programmes have been effective in helping to reduce the incidence of the disease. This survey can be carried out for most infectious diseases or illnesses.

## Epidemiological studies

The study of the incidence and pattern of disease spread is known as epidemiology. The study of diseases prevention is known as **immunology**. Sources of information about disease spread and incidence is based on facts gathered from detection and treatment of illness and causes of ill health. Sources of health information are only effective if information is passed on.

## Demographic data

Demographic data provides information on people and their lifestyles nationally in each region and local areas. Data gathered from demographic studies of the population include size, growth, density, and distribution, as well as statistics regarding birth, marriage, disease and death.

This can help in health promotion because realistic targets and deadlines can be set that will be more effective and relevant because they will be aimed at individuals and specific groups. Some areas are affected by higher incidences of disease and illness due to environmental factors such as location, the local economy and the availability of jobs and suitable housing. Data will also contain information about social class and lifestyles of communities.

Figure 12.6  NHS article for Department of Health advice on avian flu

> **Q&A**
> **Flu immunisation programme for people who work in close proximity to poultry**
> The Department of Health is offering free flu vaccination this winter to all those who work in close contact with poultry. This is being done as a precautionary public health measure and does not mean that workers are at any higher risk of getting flu this winter than usual. Nor does it mean that there is an increased risk of an outbreak of bird flu in the UK as this risk remains low. Nevertheless, experts have recommended that this precautionary measure be taken now for the reasons …
>
> Produced by COI for Department of Health 2006

## Public health observatories

Public health observatories undertake epidemiological surveillance, investigation and research of communicable disease and produces independent advice on the prevention and control of communicable disease. They have now merged with Communicable Disease Surveillance Centres also known as Health Protection Units (HPUs) and work with the NHS to identify and prevent disease. The following paragraph gives an overview of the valuable work carried out to protect the public.

## Health Protection Agency

Local and Regional Health Protection Agency services work alongside the NHS providing specialist support in communicable disease and infection control and emergency planning. They also oversee some laboratory services.

There are 39 Health Protection Units (HPUs), each covering an area broadly corresponding to a county or police boundary. Each unit consists of a director, consultants, nurses and other staff with specialist health protection skills. They have access to expert advice from the other HPA divisions.

The task of each HPU is to work directly with the NHS primary care trusts (PCTs), acute hospital trusts and local authorities in their area and agree with them how health protection should be delivered locally. Functions include local disease surveillance, laboratory services, alert systems, investigation and management of the full range of health protection incidents and outbreaks, and ensuring local delivery and monitoring of national action plans for infectious diseases.

# Historical perspectives of the Public Health System

Public health has developed over the years and in each period priorities of the time have reflected the main concerns of that era to produce the Public Health System we have today. Early reformers of social and economic conditions played a huge part in balancing the health status of the nation so that everyone had a chance to benefit. As medical knowledge increased with regard to how diseases were spread, advances were made in helping to reduce the incidence of infectious diseases that killed many people.

Many of the reforms that have taken place are due to awareness raising by individuals and groups to encourage the government to act on these findings by passing laws that are designed to influence the overall health and well-being of the nation.

## The nineteenth century

### The 'Poor Law Act' (1834)

The 'Poor Law Act' of 1834 was an act of Parliament made under Lord Earl Grey that reformed the country's poverty relief system. This hadn't been changed since 1601 and arose as a result of the findings of the social reformers Edwin Chadwick, George Nichols and Nassau William Senior who had been commissioned in 1832 to look at the 'Operation of the Poor Laws'. Judgments or means testing people under these laws had previously meant that people went to the work house if they were unable to support themselves. Many people died due to harsh working and living conditions and poor health.

## case study 12.1

# Legionnaire's disease: one person dies

'One man has died as a result of an outbreak of Legionnaire's disease which is said to have occurred at a work place in the South. Four people were admitted to hospital with suspected Legionnaires disease but were released following health screening checks for the bacillus and were allowed to go home.

The disease cannot be passed from person to person. The likely cause of the incident was thought to be caused by a faulty thermostat in a shower area which is used by workers following night shift work. The water in the heating tanks was found to be insufficiently heated over the weekend period causing a build up of bacteria. The disease is contracted through inhalation of aerosols from an infected water source.

Outbreaks are commonly caused by poorly maintained cooling towers; hot and cold water systems and spa pools. There are around 300 cases each year in England. Most are single cases with no specific source identified as a cause. Early treatment will limit deterioration or major illness.

Health care staffs, including GPs, have also been warned to look out for patients developing systems. Theses incidents have been passed on to the director of public health for the area concerned, who said that appropriate precautions have been taken to ensure that the spread f the disease is contained.

All people who have used the shower area in the last week have been contacted however if people think they have any of the symptoms then please contact their GP or NHS direct.'

Reporter: George Brown, The Daily Spa

## activity
### INDIVIDUAL WORK

Re-read the article and identify who was involved in the process of information sharing and prevention in this instance. Don't forget the role of the media!

### The Public Health Act (1848)

In 1848 The Public Health Act was made to ensure that adequate sanitary conditions were provided to ensure water, drainage, sewerage and clean pavements in populated areas in towns and cities in the UK (although London at the time had its own Sewer Commissioners). This Act brought about 'The General Board of Health' which was instrumental in ensuring that public health policies were administered and carried out. Edwin Chadwick was the first Commissioner of this board and the Public Health Act is strongly associated with him and his proposed reforms.

### Edwin Chadwick (1800–1890)

Edwin Chadwick, an English social reformer was particularly noted for his work on reforming The Poor Laws of the time. With Nassau William Senior he drafted a report in 1834 to create a centralised system of public health and to improve sanitation services for the general public. In 1842 he wrote 'The Sanitary Report of the Laboring Population' which promoted safe disposal of human waste and rubbish.

### John Snow (1813–1858)

John Snow, a British physician became known as one of the founding fathers of epidemiology in this country. He was a respected anesthetist and was a strong advocate of hygienic practices and cleanliness.

It was John Snow in 1854 who traced the source of the cholera outbreak in London to contaminated water. The practice in those days was for waste to be disposed of underneath the houses which drained into cesspits and then drained into the Thames. The water pump was situated near one of these cesspits where it was discovered to have leaking faecal waste draining into it.

In Snow's own words (in a letter to the Editor of the *Medical Times* and *Gazette in 1854*):

'On proceeding to the spot, I found that nearly all the deaths had taken place within a short distance of the [Broad Street] pump. There were only ten deaths in houses situated decidedly nearer to another street-pump. In five of these cases the families of the deceased persons informed me that they always sent to the pump in Broad Street, as they preferred the water to that of the pumps which were nearer. In three other cases, the deceased were children who went to school near the pump in Broad Street...

With regard to the deaths occurring in the locality belonging to the pump, there were 61 instances in which I was informed that the deceased persons used to drink the pump water from Broad Street, either constantly or occasionally...'

'The result of the inquiry, then, is that there has been no particular outbreak or prevalence of cholera in this part of London except among the persons who were in the habit of drinking the water of the above-mentioned pump well.

'I had an interview with the Board of Guardians of St James's parish, on the evening of the 7th inst [Sept 7], and represented the above circumstances to them. In consequence of what I said, the handle of the pump was removed on the following day.'

### Joseph Lister (1827–1912)

The link between hygiene and cross infection did not become widely known until Joseph Lister discovered antiseptics in 1865 based on the work of Louis Pasteur.

He insisted on regular hand washing, cleaning instruments and wards with carbolic and started the use of gloves. He was a founder of the aseptic technique' which promotes hygiene linked to keeping wounds and surgical instruments and equipment free from **bacteria** as much as possible, creating what we call today a sterile environment.

Figure 12.7  Joseph Lister

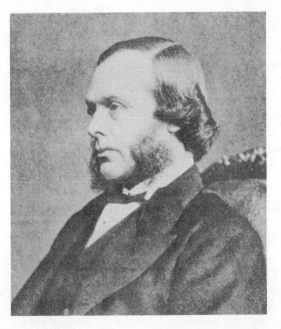

### Florence Nightingale (1820–1910)

Florence Nightingale was famous for her contribution to health care and the links she made between poor hygiene and sanitation and the welfare of patients. In the Crimean War where she was asked to train nursing staff to look after wounded soldiers she noted that the soldiers were not improving but dying. She collated statistics on incidence of death and it was later discovered that in addition to extremely poor sanitary conditions, diet and nutrition contributed to poor recovery. Once these conditions were improved through safe disposal of waste, better hygiene practices, and attention to diet, the chances of survival increased.

Figure 12.8  Florence Nightingale 1854: Nursing soldiers on the front line in a typical field hospital ward

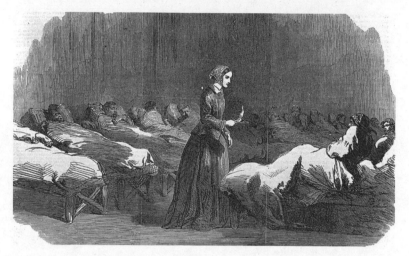

Figure 12.9  The causes of mortality in the Army in the East (April 1854 to 1855)

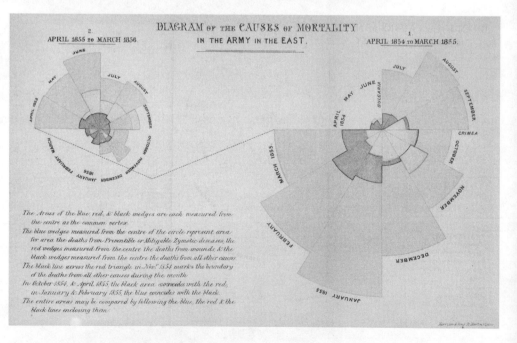

Florence Nightingale produced this diagram which indicates the number of deaths that occurred from preventable diseases (in blue), those that were the results of wounds (in red), and those due to other causes (in black). In her own words the legend reads:

'The Areas of the blue, red, & black wedges are each measured from the centre as the common vertex. The blue wedges measured from the centre of the circle represent area for area the deaths from Preventable or Mitigable **Zymotic diseases**, the red wedges measured from the centre the deaths from wounds, & the black wedges measured from the centre the deaths from all other causes. The black line across the red triangle in Nov. 1854 marks the boundary of the deaths from all other causes during the month. In October 1854, & April 1855, the black area coincides with the red, in January & February 1855, the blue coincides with the black. The entire areas may be compared by following the blue, the red, & the black lines enclosing them.

This "Diagram of the causes of mortality in the army in the East" was published in *Notes on Matters Affecting the Health, Efficiency, and Hospital Administration of the British Army* and sent to Queen Victoria in 1858.'

## The twentieth century

### William Henry Beveridge (1879–1963)

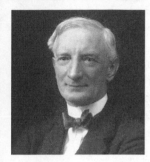

Figure 12.10  William Henry Beveridge

Lord Beveridge was a social reformer and economist. He wrote 'Social Insurance and Allied Services' in 1942 which became better known as 'The Beveridge Report'. The report became the basis of a series of reforms after the Second World War and was instrumental in the introduction of The Welfare State and the emergence of The National Health Service which started in 1949.

The main tenets of The Beveridge Report were summarised as three guiding principles of recommendations. These called for security and relief to tackle what he refers to as 'the five giants on the road to reconstruction', namely to tackle 'Want, Disease, Ignorance, Squalor and Idleness'

Here is an excerpt from 'Social Insurance and Allied Services' – The Beveridge Report (1942):

> 'The most important of the provisional rates is the rate of 40/- a week for a man and wife in unemployment and disability and after the transition in addition to allowances for children at an average of 8/- per head per week. These amounts represent a large addition to existing benefits. They will mean that in unemployment and disability a man and wife if she is not working, with two children, will receive 56/- a week without means test so long as unemployment or disability lasts, as compared with the 33/- in unemployment and the 15/- or 7/6 in sickness, with additional benefit in some Approved Societies, which they were getting before the war. For married women gainfully occupied, there will be a maternity benefit at the rate of 36/- a week for 13 weeks, in addition to the maternity grant of £4 available for all married women.'

One shilling equals 5p today (but not allowing for inflation). Money did go a bit further in 1942 but what might seem like a small amount today was helpful to families of the time – especially when financial assistance was hard to come by. Means testing meant that people were tested on what they could and could not do and what they could and could not afford. It was an imbalanced system and was dependent on the generosity of the means testing team. A lot of people treated themselves or died if they could not afford medical care.

### The National Health Service

The National Health Service of 1948, like today, treated every citizen regardless and more fairly without means testing which was the case previously. The National Health Service has provided health care and has helped many people over the years. It is something we can justifiably be proud of. However, 'postcode lottery' availability of assessment and treatment for some kinds of illnesses and diseases like cancer and dementia have caused tension.

### The Acheson Report (1998)

In 1998 a government health report was commissioned to look at 'Inequalities in Health'. Sir Donald Acheson's report identified and made the link between health and mortality. His evidence suggested that social class and deprivation were factors in early death rates. The report highlighted the widening class 'health' divide between people who have high incomes and those who do not. Statistics revealed that people in Social Class V (partly skilled workers and unskilled workers) were more likely to die from coronary and lung related illnesses due to lifestyle choices such as smoking, drinking and inadequate or poorly nutritious diets than people in Social Class 1 (professional/managerial workers such as doctors and lawyers).

Figure 12.11  Social Class
'Health' Divide (1998)

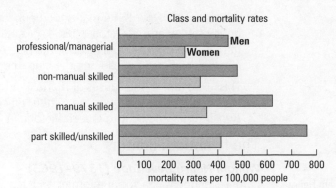

Sir Donald Acheson's report was the most influential social policy paper written since 'The Black Report' by Sir Donald Black in 1980 which had previously made the link between poor health and poverty.

The report made 75 recommendations in 39 categories which proposed that all government policies should address the impact of health inequalities so that they favoured 'the less well off'. The Acheson Report recommended that priority should be given to families with children and to women who are pregnant because therein lies the future of the next generations. His expectation based on the findings of this report were that life should be improved for all social classes and, importantly, reduce the higher death rates occurring in the poor sectors of our society.

### Our Healthy Nation (1997)
This was the Green Paper based on Sir Donald Acheson's report and it tackled inequalities of health and set out aims and objectives to improve the health of the nation by addressing the social determinants of ill health.

### Our Healthier Nation (1999)
The government introduced the White Paper 'Saving Lives: Our Healthier Nation' which specifically aims to address the major causes of ill health and death in this country by the year 2010. Following on from the Green Paper 'Our Healthy Nation', targets were specific to maintain the emphasis on the killer diseases and related factors. These are:

- Cancer: to reduce the death rate in people under 75 by at least a fifth

- Coronary heart disease and stroke: to reduce the death rate in people under 75 by at least two fifths

- Accidents: to reduce the death rate by at least a fifth and serious injury by at least a tenth

- Mental illness: to reduce the death rate from suicide and undetermined injury by at least a fifth.

The government in its public health policy acknowledges previous findings and links and it states that 'Health inequality is widespread: the most disadvantaged have suffered most from poor health. The Government is addressing **inequality** with a range of initiatives on education, welfare-to-work, housing, neighbourhoods, transport and the environment which will help improve health'. These issues are being addressed through the following proposals and reforms:

'Local authorities will work in partnership with the NHS to plan for health improvement:

- health action zones will break down barriers in providing services

- healthy living centres will provide help for better health.

For partnership to work, public health will need high standards, and for public health to be improved, it will need success measures. On standards, we will:

- establish a new Health Development Agency, a statutory body charged with raising the standards and quality of public health provision

- increase education and training for health, with a new skills audit and workforce development plan, and specific measures for nurses, midwives, health visitors, school nurses and others

- review public health information, establish public health observatories in each NHS region, set up disease registers, and promote research

- establish a new *Public Health Development Fund*.'

Figure 12.12 The Chief Medical Officer, Liam Donaldson

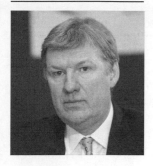

The Chief Medical Officer, Liam Donaldson advised the following tips for improving health.

Ten Tips For Better Health

1. Don't smoke. If you can, stop. If you can't, cut down.
2. Follow a balanced diet with plenty of fruit and vegetables.
3. Keep physically active.
4. Manage stress by, for example, talking things through and making time to relax.
5. If you drink alcohol, do so in moderation.
6. Cover up in the sun, and protect children from sunburn.
7. Practise safer sex.
8. Take up cancer screening opportunities.
9. Be safe on the roads: follow the Highway Code.
10. Learn the First Aid ABC – airways, breathing, circulation.

The initiatives to promote better health in this country are to be co-ordinated by the Health Development Agency. Guidelines for what the expectations are were set out in the Healthier Nations White Paper as follows.

In advising and supporting the Secretary of State for Health, the new Agency's key functions will include:

- maintaining an up-to-date map of the evidence base for public health and health improvement

- commissioning such research and evaluation as is necessary to support and strengthen the evidence base in areas where action programmes are required to improve health and tackle inequality, within an agreed framework governed by the Secretary of State's overall research strategy for health

- in the light of the evidence, advising on the setting of standards for public health and health promotion practice, and on the implementation of those standards by a range of organisations at national and local level

- in particular, providing advice on targeting health promotion most effectively on the worst off and narrowing the health gap

- through regular bulletins, guidance and advice, disseminating information on effectiveness and good practice in an authoritative, timely and effective manner to those working in the public health/health promotion field

- commissioning and carrying out evidence-based national health promotion programmes and campaigns which are integrated with the Department of Health's overall communications strategy and linked with regional and local activity

- advising on the capacity and capability of the public health workforce to deliver Ministers' strategy in these areas to the agreed standards, and on the education and training needs of the workforce, ensuring throughout that such advice is informed by research evidence and the appropriate quality standards

- organising public health policies and advising the health of the nation is an ongoing process which will evolve to help address the inequalities in social conditions and thus influence the effects of ill health. The pioneers of public health, social reform and epidemiology have paved the way to tackle the main determinants of health which today are:

- Crime and Health
- Education
- Employment
- Environment
- Housing
- Income.

To find out how health education campaigns are implemented see Unit 20, page 113.

## The twenty-first century

The Government set out a ten-year programme of reforms in a White Paper called 'The New NHS'. This was put into action as The NHS Plan in July 2000. The main points included the creation of:

- Approximately 500 Primary Care Groups – teams of GPs and community nurses, covering populations of about 100,000 – to take control of most of the NHS budget from April 1999. These Primary Care Trusts will provide all the normal GP services, as well as taking over the running of local community hospitals.

- NHS Direct – a 24-hour telephone hotline staffed by nurses to help reduce pressure on hospitals and GPs by giving on-the-spot health advice.

- NHSnet – a computer network allowing patients to get quicker test results and specialist advice in the local surgery, and book appointments.

- A guarantee that all patients with suspected cancer will see a specialist within two weeks.

- Two new national bodies, the National Institute for Clinical Excellence and the Commission for Health Improvement – to issue guidelines on best practice, monitor the extent to which they are followed, and sort out problems.

- Health Action Zones which will operate particularly in deprived areas and which will overcome barriers between different authorities and professions so that they work together and improve their services to patients.

---

**activity**
**INDIVIDUAL WORK 12.2**
**P2**

Draw a time line or table to describe the origins of public health in the UK. Describe key policies and actions that have influenced how people's health has been influenced by these.

---

**'Choosing Health: Making Healthy Choices Easier' (2004)**

The government continues to tackle current health problems and states how they are addressing these in the White Paper released in 2004: 'Choosing Health: Making Healthy Choices Easier'. The main focus of this reform is to enable and empower people to make healthier lifestyle choices. The report highlights the key determinants of health at this time and points out that our health is affected by lifestyle choices, education and the environment we live in.

In summary, public health is organised and protected through the following departments and agencies. Co-ordination and communication is gradually occurring across the country where in previous years many of the organisations worked independently.

- Department of Health
- National Infection Control and Health Protection Agency
- Local Health Protection Units
- NHS Epidemiology and Microbiology Departments
- Medical Staff, e.g. GPs, nurses.

Guidelines and policies regarding implementation of policies and procedures are provided for by Medical and Educational Training and Awarding bodies for example:

- National Institute for Health and Clinical Excellence (NICE)
- Royal College of Physicians and Surgeons
- Royal College of Nursing
- Independent and voluntary organisations

## Target setting

Target setting is founded on advice by the Government based on reports of incidence of disease and illness collected from health care providers such as GPs. Priorities as discussed previously are then based on local need and available resources and funding. Some areas may have a higher incidence of elderly deaths in winter for example. Health promoters would then focus on advertising how important it is to wrap up well, eat regular meals, and to keep the heating on. For some elderly people this might prove difficult so advice might include wearing layers of clothing; receiving discounts of gas or electric bills. Another example might be to encourage people to take up the influenza vaccine to reduce the incidence of flu over the winter period.

Target setting will almost always identify cause of disease and ill health and aim to reduce the ill-effects of the factors that cause these by promoting healthier options.

Figure 12.13 Choosing Health: Making Healthy Choices Easier (2004)

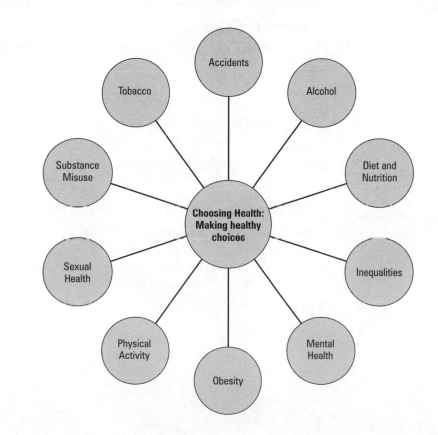

# Key groups in influencing public health policy

In this country, health and social reformers have tackled and highlighted public health issues.

Other key groups and individuals have also made contributions to the health of the nation and influenced health policy.

## Pressure groups

Pressure groups such as Greenpeace and Friends of the Earth have drawn our attention to treatment of the environment to reduce **pesticides**, over fishing and farming and banning toxic chemical substances that are harmful to our ecology, including nuclear waste. They have lobbied industry to reduce the amount and output of carbon, nuclear and fossil fuels that are burnt in our atmosphere.

Recent research has shown that there is not a significantly higher increase of cancers in people living near nuclear power plants. However pressure groups say that when power plants explode or have accidents, or when container ships or vehicles carrying nuclear fuels or waste leak or sustain damage, the cost to people and the environment is unacceptable.

Our environment is important to health and it is therefore necessary for any health and social reforms to protect public health and take this into consideration. Current influences have attempted to reduce the 'carbon footprint' we produce through flying, to use non-leaded fuels, to recycle plastics, paper and wood; to eat 'red meat' in moderation; and to decrease packaging of food products.

In 2006, a UK government advisory panel, the Sustainable Development Commission, concluded that if the UK's existing nuclear capacity were doubled, it would provide an 8% decrease in total UK $CO_2$ emissions by 2035. This can be compared to the country's goal to reduce greenhouse gas emissions by 60% by 2050.

## International groups

International groups such as the World Health Organization (WHO), United Nations (UN) and United Nations International Children's Fund (UNICEF) continue to strive to improve the health of global populations in reducing the incidence of disease and promoting immunisation and sustainable health programmes.

## National Groups UK

There are individual organisations dedicated to the control and eradication of disease in this country and include organisations that help promote health and well-being connected to social, physiological and mental health. Some of these are of charity status and rely on donations to help fund research, provide information and develop support group networks. For example, Cancer Research UK.

### Health Protection Agency (HPA)

The Health Protection Agency was formed in 2003. The functions of the Agency are 'to protect the community (or any part of the community) against infectious diseases and other dangers to health' (HPA Act 2004). The HPA describes itself as:

'an independent body that protects the health and well-being of the population. The Agency plays a critical role in protecting people from infectious diseases and in preventing harm when hazards involving chemicals, poisons or radiation occur.

We also prepare for new and emerging threats, such as a bio-terrorist attack or virulent new strain of disease.'

Figure 12.14 The structure of the Health Protection Agency

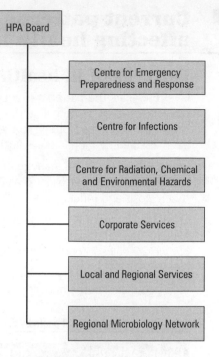

In addition to the Agency's role in reducing the dangers to health from infections and chemical and radiation hazards, it also provides support to and works in partnership with others who have health protection responsibilities, and advises, through the Department of Health, all government departments and administrations throughout the UK.

### National Institute for Clinical Health and Excellence (NICE)

NICE is an independent organisation responsible for providing national guidance on promoting good health and preventing and treating ill health.

NICE's role was set out in the 2004 White Paper 'Choosing health: making healthier choices easier'. In it the government set out key principles for helping people make healthier and more informed choices about their health. The government wants NICE to bring together knowledge and guidance on ways of promoting good health and treating ill health.

NICE was preceded by the National Institute for Clinical Excellence, which was set up in 1999 and also known as NICE. The functions of another NHS organisation, the Health Development Agency (HDA), were transferred to NICE on 1 April 2005.

NICE produces guidance in three areas of health:

- public health – guidance on the promotion of good health and the prevention of ill health for those working in the NHS, local authorities and the wider public and voluntary sector.

- health technologies – guidance on the use of new and existing medicines, treatments and procedures within the NHS.

- clinical practice – guidance on the appropriate treatment and care of people with specific diseases and conditions within the NHS.

Source: www.nice.org.uk/

# Current patterns of ill health and factors affecting health in the UK

## Patterns of ill health

Over the years the patterns of ill health in the UK have been influenced by social, environmental and improving awareness and knowledge of disease cause and spread. These have varied according to the economic and social status of the country and have been affected by global issues such as war, famine, incidence and spread of disease.

In the 1800s poor and inadequate sanitation, overcrowded social conditions and poverty led to infectious diseases such as cholera, typhoid, measles, whooping cough (pertussis), tuberculosis and influenza.

The introduction of immunisation programmes, treatment with antibiotics and improved hygiene and sanitation practices have helped to reduce these diseases to some extent but we are still susceptible to disease.

In 2002, the World Health Organization in its annual report produced a list of the recorded main causes of death for the global population by disease category.

Table 12.2  WHO: Causes of death by disease category (2002)

| Causes of death | No. deaths | % population |
|---|---|---|
| Cardiovascular diseases | 16,733,000 | 27% |
| Infectious and parasitic diseases | 10,904,000 | 19% |
| Malignant neoplasms | 7,121,000 | 13% |
| Respiratory infections | 3,963,000 | 7% |
| Respiratory diseases | 3,702,000 | 7% |
| Unintentional injuries | 3,551,000 | 6% |
| Perinatal conditions | 2,462,000 | 4% |
| Digestive diseases | 1,968,000 | 4% |
| Intentional injuries | 1,618,000 | 3% |
| Neuropsychiatric disorders | 1,112,000 | 2% |
| Diabetes mellitus | 988,000 | 2% |
| Diseases of the genitourinary system | 848,000 | 2% |
| Maternal conditions | 510,000 | 1% |
| Congenital abnormalities | 493,000 | 1% |
| Nutritional deficiencies | 485,000 | 1% |
| Nutritional/endocrine disorders | 485,000 | 1% |

Source: World Health Organisation, 2002

Note that the second highest cause of death globally was from infectious and parasitic diseases.

Current patterns of ill health in this country are linked to age-related disorders and lifestyles. Social class and environment statistics reveal that there are still inequalities in health and that these are linked to the determinants of health.

In the UK, infectious diseases caused deaths in mainly the over 75 year age group. This statistic reveals improved living conditions but that age, wear and tear can still be compromised.

Table 12.3 National mortality rates statistics for England and Wales in 2004

| Cause of death | Males Total deaths | Females Total deaths | Highest rate per age group |
|---|---|---|---|
| Certain infectious and parasitic diseases | 2,197 | 2,795 | 75+ years |
| Intestinal infectious diseases | 471 | 888 | 75+ years |
| Respiratory tuberculosis | 144 | 85 | 75+ years |
| Other tuberculosis | 44 | 62 | 65–74 years |
| Viral hepatitis | 128 | 69 | 45–54 years |
| Human immunodeficiency virus [HIV] disease | 117 | 73 | 35-44 years |
| Meningococcal infection | 32 | 43 | 1–4 years |

Source: Social Trends (2004)

Other common infectious diseases in this country are:

HCAIs (Health Care Associated Infections), e.g. MRSA, clostridium difficile and sexually transmitted diseases such as chlamydia, herpes, gonnorrhoea, syphillis and warts.

Figure 12.15  Sexually transmitted disease by age group, UK, 2005

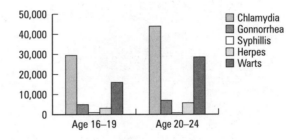

The Black Report (1980), The Acheson Report (1998), Our Healthier Nation (1999), Tackling Health Inequalities (2003) and Choosing Health (2004) reports have been produced to tackle ill health and the determinants of health. When these issues are addressed across the country then patterns of disease and the quality of life for all communities will improve. Public health departments and organisations have a huge task in communicating and implementing guidance and policies through educating and raising awareness of these health concerns and issues.

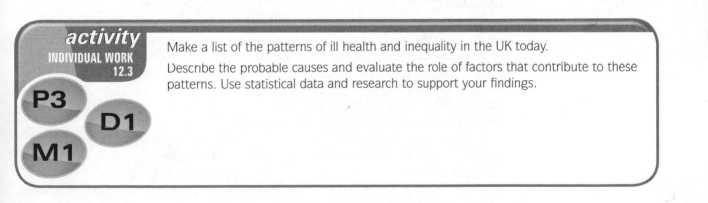

*activity*
INDIVIDUAL WORK
12.3

P3  D1
M1

Make a list of the patterns of ill health and inequality in the UK today.

Describe the probable causes and evaluate the role of factors that contribute to these patterns. Use statistical data and research to support your findings.

# Factors affecting health

## Socio-economic

Factors that affect health are linked to social circumstances such as housing, employment, support networks, class, health, education and are based on economic factors such as income, national economy, and demographics or transport for example. Generally, but not always, if you have achieved in education you are more likely to get a job that will enable you to fund a lifestyle that will provide more choices in terms of housing, where you live and quality of life. This isn't always the case but the higher earning potential a person has the more likely that health and well-being will be enhanced. Governments in the UK try to even the balance of this by providing social support, opportunities to improve living conditions, a wider access to education and improved health services for people who are less able to help themselves.

Figure 12.16 Socio-economic determinants of health

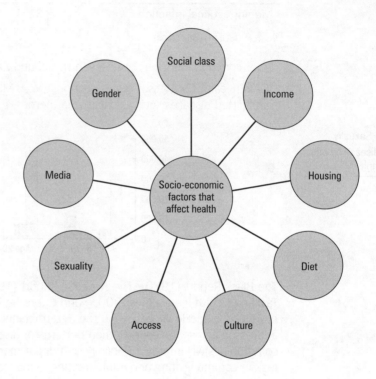

## Education

Recent studies have shown that early education, e.g. in pre-school, can lead to better choices as standards of literacy and numeracy improve and reduce crime. In this country programmes to ensure that skills are improved have been aimed at parents with young children through a national framework of schemes such as the Sure Start Programmes and the National Numeracy and Literacy curriculums being used in schools. Raising the standard of education will help to narrow the divide by providing opportunities for everyone to improve their future career prospects.

Other initiatives include the Healthy Schools Programme, which is a joint initiative between the Department for Education and Skills (DfES) and the Department of Health (DH), the aim of which is 'to create a health ethos within schools; improve the health and self-esteem of the school community; and enable children to make healthier choices and improve their educational achievement'.

## Employment status

Employment is vital to support and maintain our standard of living. There are not many people in this country who do not need to work for a living. However there are sections of our society who are not able to work due to age, ability, disability and opportunity.

Unemployed people are found to have:

- Lower levels of psychological well-being which may range from symptoms of depression and anxiety through to self harm and suicide.
- Higher rates of morbidity – such as limiting long-term illness.
- Higher rates of premature mortality, in particular for coronary heart disease and injuries and poisoning including suicide.

There is also the fact that poor health will affect people's employment opportunities. This can lead to social deprivation as well as poverty.

People in employment may also have poor health due to the nature of their work. It is not unusual for people to work longer hours, travel long distances and be subject to quite high stress levels within a competitive work environment. Although legislation and the work of the Health and Safety Executive and Trade Unions have done much to improve working conditions in this country the highest reported cause for time off work is due to back problems (musculo-skeletal disorders), stress-related problems, skin problems, hazards due to slips, trips and falls and occupational asthma.

The HSC (Health and Safety Committee) plan released in 2005 has been designed to link up to the government White Paper 'Choosing Health: Make healthier choices easier' (2004). In its own words it is a:

'"Fit for Work, Fit for Life, Fit for Tomorrow" Strategic Delivery Programme'.

The 'Fit3' Strategic Delivery Programme is based on analysis of injury and ill health generation across known hazard and sector hotspots in businesses, large and small.

## Housing

Poor housing environments contribute to ill health through poor amenities, shared facilities and overcrowding, inadequate heating or energy inefficiency. The highest risks to health in housing are attached to cold, damp and mouldy conditions. In addition, those in very poor housing, such as homeless hostels and bedsits, are more likely to suffer from poor mental and physical health than those whose housing is of higher quality. Damp conditions are associated with higher incidence sickness and diarrhoea in the young and with respiratory disorders in the young and elderly (Platt S, Martin C and Hunt S, 1989).

Rates of long-term illness among homeless people are also 2.5 times higher than among the general population (Victor CR, 1993).

## Income

The London Health Observatory summarises in their report for London the relationship between health and low income that exists across almost all health indicators. This may also be applied nationally. Some of the most obvious effects of health inequality are seen in:

- Premature mortality and morbidity: Strongly related to indicators of low income (Eames et al, 1993). Even at a borough level in London, premature mortality rates (i.e. before age 65) in the most deprived boroughs are nearly double those in the least deprived. There is evidence that this gap in health between the most and least well-off areas is increasing (Bardsley & Morgan, 1996).
- Infant mortality rates: Tend to be higher in the more deprived communities. These will cover stillbirths, neonatal deaths and infant mortality.

- Low birthweight: Inappropriate nourishment or smoking can reduce infant and pre-natal development. Slow early growth is associated with a range of health problems in later life.

- Poor nutrition: Consequent poor physical development can affect cognitive development in children.

- Mental health problems: Stress and depression reduce parents' stimulation of the child and disrupt emotional attachment.

- Health-related behaviours: Smoking, poor diet and lack of exercise (for example) can be more common in lower income social groups. Increasing the opportunities for healthier lifestyles is one way to achieve significant long-term health gains.

- Emergency admissions to hospital: Much higher in the most deprived areas of London.

- Accidents and injury to children: Tend to be more common in low income groups and there is some evidence of an increasing divide between social classes.

- Communicable diseases: Including respiratory and gastrointestinal disease tend to be higher amongst families in poor quality housing.

- Low income reduces a person's ability to make healthy choices and is linked to inequalities in health and social class.

## Social class

Inequalities in health are linked to health determinants and social class. Research in this country reveals that there is a health gap between the social classes. Social policy and health policies stress that improving health for all is the main priority.

Societal groupings were formulated to help categorise groups of people into a class structure which would identify them by the jobs they did. A major flaw in this was that it was taken from what the male occupant in a household did for a living. Today females are house owners and have full-time jobs other than child-rearing, which was assumed not to be the case when classifications were first used.

The best known of these classifications is the Registrar General's social classes, first used in 1911 and with virtually no changes in format from 1921 until 2000. From 1991 to 2000, the Standard Occupational Classification for the 1991 census was used to derive people's social class from their occupation and employment status. The armed forces and people who could not be classified formed three residual groups, which were usually combined in published analyses. In some analyses, the classes are collated into non-manual classes, Social Classes I, II, IIIN and the manual classes, Social Classes IIIM, IV, V.

In the General Household Survey and some other surveys, a different classification of occupations into socio-economic groups, was used up to 2000. In 2001, these two classifications were replaced by a new classification, the National Statistics Socio-economic Classification (NS-SEC).

Table 12.4 Operational categories of the NS-SEC linked to social class

| Social class | | NS-SEC operational categories |
|---|---|---|
| I | Professional, etc. occupations | 3.1, 3.3 |
| II | Managerial and technical occupations | 1, 2, 3.2, 3.4, 4.1, 4.3, 5, 7.3, 8.1, 8.2, 9.2 |
| III N | Skilled occupations – non-manual | 4.2, 4.4, 6, 7.1, 7.2, 12.1, 12.6 |
| III M | Skilled occupations – manual | 7.4, 9.1, 10, 11.1, 12.3, 13.3 |
| IV | Partly skilled occupations | 11.2, 12.2, 12.4, 12.5, 12.7, 13.1, 13.2, 13.5 |
| V | Unskilled occupations | 13.4 |

Source: Social trends

From the 1960s onwards, techniques have been developed for grouping together small areas, such as electoral wards, which have similar characteristics. These either use cluster analysis or aggregate variables based on factors such as low owner occupancy, high proportions of manual workers and high unemployment to derive scores or 'deprivation indices'. Three indices, the Jarman index, the Townsend index and the 'Depcat' or 'Carstairs index' were developed in the early 1990s, using data from the 1991 census. Towards the end of the 1990s, indices drawing on a much wider range of data were constructed in each of the four countries of the UK.

When classifying children by social class, decisions have to be made about which parent's occupational information should be collected and used, at least in those cases where a choice is available. In most official surveys undertaken up to 2000, the socio-economic group used in tabulations and analyses was that of the 'head of household', defined as the member of the household responsible for the accommodation or the husband of that person or, if responsibility was shared between members of the same sex, the older of the two. From 2000 onwards, this was replaced by the 'household reference person', defined as the member of the household responsible for accommodation, or if responsibility was joint, the person with the highest income and where this involved two people with equal incomes, the older of the two. The NS-SEC was used from 2001 onwards.

The survey for the decade 1990 to 2000 carried out by the Office for National Statistics in 2004 to look at the health of children and families by socio-economic status revealed several social class differences.

The percentage of low birth weight was lower for babies with fathers in non-manual occupations and their mean birth weight was higher compared with babies with fathers in manual occupations. These differences persisted throughout the decade. Birth weight distributions differed between ethnic groups. Babies with mothers born in the 'New Commonwealth' had higher rates of low birth weight than others and those whose mothers were born in West Africa or the Caribbean Commonwealth were more likely than others to be of very low birth weight. Babies from black and Asian ethnic groups were more likely to be of low birth weight and their mean birth weights were lower.

The reported prevalence of long-term illness rose marginally among children aged 0 to 15 years in Great Britain during the decade. In most years, long-term illness and limiting long-term illness was more common among children from manual households than in non-manual households.

Prevalence of longstanding illness was higher among boys than girls. It was much less common in children from Indian, Pakistani, Bangladeshi and Chinese groups than in the general population in England.

No sex or class differences were observed in reported acute sickness and there was no change during the decade. Bangladeshi and Chinese boys and Indian, Pakistani, Bangladeshi and Chinese girls were less likely to report acute sickness than children in the general population.

In the late 1990s, children from manual social groups in Great Britain were more likely than those from non-manual groups to consult a general practitioner. Indian and Pakistani boys and Indian girls were more likely to consult a GP compared with other minority ethnic groups and with the general population.

Social class differences in both breastfeeding and smoking during pregnancy persisted through the decade, despite the increase in the initiation of breastfeeding in the late 1990s and the decline in smoking since the 1980s. Children from Indian, Pakistani and Bangladeshi households were unlikely to have ever smoked.

People in lower socio-economic groups are more likely to work in places where they will be exposed to second-hand smoke.

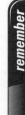

## Gender

Research figures suggest that men die on average about five years younger than women and are three times as likely to take their own lives. They are twice as likely as women to develop and die from the 10 most common cancers affecting both sexes, and have higher rates of heart disease. Yet men are far less likely to access health services. Men aged 16–45 are half as likely to go to see their GP as their female counterparts. The Equal Opportunities Commission as well as audit bodies such as the Healthcare Commission will be policing the rest of the NHS' compliance with new Gender Equality Duty.

Lung cancer is the most common cause of death from cancer in the EU with more than 230,000 deaths in 2000, which is one in five of all deaths from cancer. Most lung cancer deaths occur in men. Breast cancer is the most common cause of death from cancer in women.

Figure 12.17 Number of deaths from cancer in the EU

|  |  |
| --- | --- |
| Lung | 231,500 |
| Bowel | 138,400 |
| Breast | 91,000 |
| Stomach | 78,100 |
| Prostate | 66,500 |
| Pancreas | 54,300 |
| Liver | 40,200 |
| Bladder | 37,100 |
| Leukaemia | 35,300 |
| NHL | 28,900 |
| Ovary | 28,100 |
| Kidney | 27,900 |
| Oesophagus | 27,300 |
| Oral | 26,100 |
| Brain and CNS | 25,800 |
| Multiple myeloma | 16,400 |
| Cervix | 15,600 |
| Larynx | 14,900 |
| Uterus | 11,700 |
| Melanoma | 10,800 |
| Thyroid | 4,000 |
| Hodgkin's | 3,700 |
| Testis | 1,100 |
| Other | 141,200 |

Among males the highest cancer incidence and mortality rates are in Hungary, largely due to the high incidence of lung cancer in Hungarian men. The lowest male cancer incidence rates are in Greece and Cyprus while the lowest male cancer mortality rates are in Sweden (Figure 12.18).

The male incidence and mortality rates in the UK are significantly lower than the overall EU rate: UK male incidence rates rank 19th in the EU, and UK male mortality rates rank 17th.

Among females the highest cancer incidence and mortality rates are in Denmark. The high incidence reflects the fact that they have one of the highest incidences for female breast and ovarian cancer in the EU. The lowest female cancer incidence and mortality rates are in Cyprus and Greece. The female incidence and mortality rates in the UK are significantly higher than the overall EU rate: UK female incidence rates rank 7th in the EU, and UK female mortality rates rank 3rd.

## Access to services

Access to services is restricted for many sectors of the community. The reasons for this, in addition to financial and social care reasons are various, ranging from difficulty attending during working hours, inadequate and inconvenient opening times and availability of social and health care services, and limited transport to name a few.

Urban and rural living presents its own problems in terms of access to health and social care services. When services are available they are sometimes difficult to access due to waiting times and lists or there is a reluctance to 'bother' the staff.

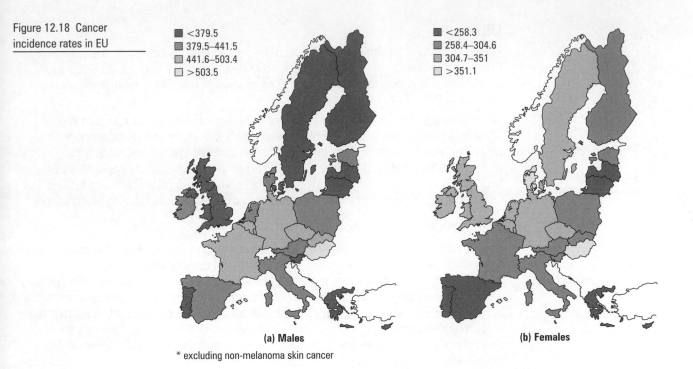

Figure 12.18 Cancer incidence rates in EU

(a) Males        (b) Females
* excluding non-melanoma skin cancer

Administration and paperwork can make access to services laborious and time consuming and in some cases appears to be designed to deter almost all ex cept the most determined. For people with social, physical, emotional and intellectual health problems there is help available but demand can exceed supply and consequently some people fail to gain access.

## Crime

Crime is associated with social disorganisation, low social capital, relative deprivation and health inequalities. The same social and environmental factors that predict geographic variation in crime rates may also be relevant to explaining community variations in health and well-being. This is prevalent in large inner city environments where affordable housing is harder to come by or has been overtaken by commercial interests at the expense of the local communities who find it difficult to locate work.

## Culture

Culture is the belief systems and values embraced by people from different areas and places around the world. It can consist of a global culture such as African or Indian or British, for example, or local cultures such as Liverpudlian, Glaswegian, London. Culture can be many things such as country of origin, place, and religion or group identity.

Ivan Illich (1976) makes links to the relationship between culture and health by saying that each culture gives shape to a unique **gestalt** of health and to a unique conformation of attitudes towards, pain, disease, impairment and death, each of which designates a class of that human performance that has been called the art of suffering.

This means that, in terms of public health and factors that may be influenced by culture, individual differences need to be considered and addressed with regard to how health information is shared and disseminated. For example studies in America (Collins O. Airhihenbuwa, 1995) have shown that a verbal one-to-one conversation is more likely to influence health practices in some cultures than others because of oral traditions and passing on information over time. In this country poverty and culture are linked with people from different countries more likely to have poor health status. This is not a uniquely cultural factor in that it will also be related to income, housing and employment opportunities.

## Diet

Health is linked to healthy diets. The recommendations for good health are linked to the recommended calorific intake (2,500–3,000 kJ for males and 2,000–2,500 kJ for females). The recommendations for consumption of daily food groups are shown in Figure 12.19.

Healthy eating and exercise will reduce the incidence of obesity which in turn reduces diseases linked to being overweight such as heart, lung, liver and musculo-skeletal problems. Public health departments and organisations have worked to continue promoting the benefits of healthy diets and exercise through campaigns such as 5-a-day (fruit and vegetables); recommendations for alcohol consumption; reducing fat and salt intake and other measures such as taking more exercise, e.g. walking to work, school.

## Peer pressure

Peer pressure is known to influence people's beliefs and ideas especially in the younger age groups where individual identity is emerging and developing. It is important for individuals to feel part of a group but unfortunately this can be unhealthy if the 'group' carries out risky behaviours. Family influences also play a part in an individual's healthy lifestyle choices and it can be difficult to break away from habits and attitudes that have been formed in early childhood. Examples of this can be linked to uptake of smoking and drinking, poor dietary choices and attitudes to exercise. Healthy role modelling will help influence healthy living style choices.

## Media

The media through TV, film, radio and advertisements greatly influence people's attitudes and beliefs concerning health. Current trends and practices dictate what is 'cool' and trendy and these to a large extent are emulated. Health can be promoted in a positive or negative way. Links to glamorous lifestyles through popular culture such as sport, music, film and political representatives are promoted through repetition and re-enforcement in newspapers, magazines, television programmes, films, posters and books. We may like to think that health choices are individual but unfortunately they do become influenced by current trends, availability and the general population as a whole, e.g. immunisation, alcohol, appearance, smoking, drug taking, whether we like it or not.

Figure 12.19 Food pyramid with daily recommendations for health diets

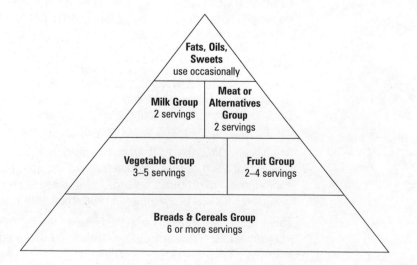

## Discrimination

Discrimination linked to public health in this country should be against the law due to legislation and good practice that aims to ensure that people are not discriminated against with regard to health. Everyone has access to health services providing they are living or work here. Visitors to this country have access to health services but may have to pay for some services.

Discrimination may be said to occur however if linked to availability of services in some areas. Health care is not always immediately available in some parts of the country. More needs to be done to ensure fair access, reduced waiting times for operations and equal availability of expensive medications. Is it discrimination if a drug is offered for treatment in one part of the country but not in another due to prohibitive costs?

## Environmental

Environmental factors that may affect health may include some of the following: urban (living in a town or city) or rural (living in a village, hamlet or solitary dwelling); the quality of services such as waste management, water supply, sanitation; affordable housing; energy sources; pollution; access to health and social care amenities and services; and access to leisure and recreational activities.

### *Rural and urban living*

Rural living is described as being in the country with open access to green fields, hills, lakes or the seaside and beaches with little or few facilities. Communities are concentrated around a small town or may be near a city. Whereas urban living may be characterised as being in an area surrounded by buildings, industry, roads, urban transport systems with limited or no access to fields, lakes or beaches but with an abundance of facilities.

Each area has its own individual health-related problems. Living in a rural area may cause health problems associated with environmental conditions linked to farming and production; isolation, access to hospitals, information, poverty. Living in urban areas may cause health-related problems linked to lifestyle, transport, pollution, overcrowding, transient or migrating populations.

Figure 12.20 Environmental determinants of health

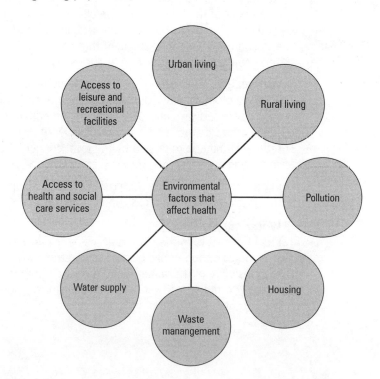

Access to leisure facilities may or may not be abundant for both rural and urban living. The opportunities for exercise and sport will be based on demand and funding. Some areas have a range of facilities available due to natural resources, e.g. rivers, lakes, parks, hills; other areas have facilities such as sports complexes, stadiums, swimming pools. Schools, colleges and sports clubs play a large part in promoting exercise by providing and promoting opportunities to widen participation.

Environmental and public health departments work to improve conditions for the general public and these are implemented by local government, environmental agencies, town and city councils. Rates and taxes go towards funding some of these services.

### Waste management

Waste management, which consists of disposal, recycling and processing, may be broken down into several areas: waste management linked to disposal of human bodily excrement (urine, faeces, etc.) generally known as sanitation (sewerage) services; waste management linked to what we consume and discard during daily living activities known as 'rubbish' and in some instances 'recycling'; and waste management linked to industrial waste from manufacture, mining and reprocessing.

Disposal of all types of human waste has cause for concern as populations increase and the potential harm this may have on our environment and subsequently to our health. Availability of waste disposal sites is becoming limited and sanitation services are stretched.

Currently rubbish is picked up by refuse collectors who may also offer recycling services too. Some councils employ their own designated staff and others sub-contract the work out to independent companies. Waste is disposed of in landfill sites, incinerated or recycled. Recycling is positively encouraged to reduce the need for landfill sites and unnecessary manufacture of products.

Health concerns have been raised about the proximity of landfill sites to housing and the safe disposal of toxic waste from manufacturing and farming. Gases and chemicals that seep into the earth can have detrimental effects on health although research shows that it is more likely when this occurs in confined spaces. Over-exposure to some of the gases can cause nausea, headaches and vomiting. Combustion or gas explosions produced as a result of the build up and breaking down of the by-products of waste disposal, e.g. methane, can occur but are quite rare in this country. Monitoring and evaluation of gas and chemical emissions is one of the main responsibilities of waste disposal companies and environmental protection agencies involved in waste management.

With regard to sanitation, individuals have responsibility for effluent flowing through wastage pipes directly connected to the house if they are home owners. Pipes that are under roadways and paths may in some instances be the responsibility of the local water-board or the council or both. Sewerage works which process human body waste (effluent) may be managed by the local council or contracted out to independent sanitation services.

Information about correct disposal of waste is supplied by local councils. An example of this is given concerning cess pools. See the box on page 35.

### Water supply

Each household in the UK has access to clean water. This service is paid for by individuals and in public places by governmental or private companies. It is the responsibility of the water management companies and the Environmental Protection Agency to monitor the standard and 'fit for purpose' consumption and quality of the water that is supplied and processed.

**Information given about management of cesspit**

*Septic tanks and cesspools*

In rural areas it is not uncommon for properties to be too remote to be connected to the mains drainage system. In these circumstances properties have to rely upon a private drainage system such as a cesspool or septic tank.

A cesspool is a sealed tank connected to a property by a series of drains. It collects the waste foul water from a property and when it is full it has to be emptied and the waste water taken away by tanker to a proper disposal point.

A septic tank is similarly connected to a property by a series of drains and it provides a very basic level of treatment of the foul waste. The septic tank collects the solid waste and allows the liquid waste to flow into a soakaway in the ground. Soakaways have to be carefully constructed to ensure that the liquid waste does not contaminate the surface of the ground, ditches or watercourses.

All new soakaways or improvements to existing soakaways require the prior consent of the Environment Agency.

Responsibility for the regular emptying of private cesspools and septic tanks rests with the property owner. Contractors who provide this service can be found under 'septic tanks' or 'waste disposal services' in Yellow Pages.

Source: Dorset County Council, 2006

The Environment Agency uses a variety of standards and targets to help protect and improve water quality thus counteracting any potential impacts of industry and agriculture. Water quality is protected by imposing directives, monitoring and acting on findings. The aim of the Environment Agency is carried out by:

- controlling risks to the quality of water abstracted for supply to our homes or used to irrigate crops
- making sure that our enjoyment of things like bathing, angling and boating are as safe as possible
- protecting wildlife and nature.

Most standards and directives are directly linked to European Directives on how water should be managed.

Excellent access to safe and hygienic water supplies has reduced risks of water consumption associated with human disease in this country, for example, cholera or typhoid.

### Pollution

Air Quality: A variety of air pollutants have known or suspected harmful effects on human health and the environment. In most areas of Europe, these pollutants are principally the products of combustion from space heating, power generation or from motor vehicle traffic. Pollutants from these sources may not only prove a problem in the immediate vicinity of these sources but can travel long distances, chemically reacting in the atmosphere to produce secondary pollutants such as acid rain or ozone.

DEFRA (Department for Environment, Food and Rural Affairs) have produced an information guide on what to do when air quality is affected by pollutants above the usual range. Table 12.6 on page 36 describes the health effects that sensitive individuals might experience at very high levels of these pollutants.

With the exception of carbon monoxide, very high levels of all these pollutants can irritate the lungs and cause inflammation. People with lung diseases, especially the elderly, may feel less well than usual. In some cases their symptoms may increase to such an extent that they need a change in treatment, or admission to hospital.

Table 12.5  Where does air pollution come from?

| Higher pollution | Lower pollution |
| --- | --- |
| Cities/towns in deep valleys. | Cities/towns on hills. |
| In summer, during sunny, still weather. | Windy or wet weather at any time of year particularly ozone in suburban and rural areas. |
| In winter, in cold, still foggy weather. | Rural areas away from major roads and particularly vehicle pollutants in large factories (for most pollutants except cities ozone). |
| Busy roads with heavy traffic next to high buildings and busy road junctions. | Residential roads with light traffic. |
| High levels of solid fuel, for example coal and wood, used for heating in the local area. | Smoke control area or areas with high levels of gas or electric used for heating. |

Source: Department of Health, 2006

DEFRA publishes information on daily outdoor levels of pollution, mostly from outdoor sources. Different sources are responsible for different pollutants. Road transport is the main source of nitrogen dioxide and carbon monoxide. Power stations and other industrial sources also produce nitrogen dioxide. Industry is the main source of sulphur dioxide. Particles come from many sources, including road transport, power stations and other industry. The burning of wood or coal for home heating can also be an important source of sulphur dioxide and particles. Ground level ozone is not emitted directly from any source. Instead it is formed when sunlight acts on nitrogen dioxide and other atmospheric substances close to the ground.

Table 12.6  Pollutant health effects at very high levels

| Nitrogen dioxide Ozone Sulphur dioxide | These gases irritate the airways of the lungs, increasing the symptoms of those suffering from lung diseases. |
| --- | --- |
| Particles | Fine particles can be carried deep into the lungs where they can cause inflammation and a worsening of heart and lung diseases. |
| Carbon monoxide | This gas prevents the normal transport of oxygen by the blood. This can lead to a significant reduction in the supply of oxygen to the heart, particularly in people suffering from heart disease. |

Source: Department for Environment, Food and Rural Affairs and air quality issues in England:http://www.defra.gov.uk/environment/airquality

## Genetic

Diseases that are inherited from one or both parents are known as genetic diseases. They may be carried in the DNA on a dominant or recessive gene which means that each child will have the disease or the disease may skip a generation or affect only one child in four.

Inherited diseases that are apparent in this country are:

- Cystic fibrosis
- Sickle cell anaemia
- Thalassaemia
- Huntington's disease
- Tay-Sach's disease

More details will be given about these diseases in the communicable diseases table (Table 12.11, page 45).

Screening for these diseases is offered alongside genetic counselling. Some people may be the carrier of the 'defective' gene and may or may not choose to have a family – especially if the partner also carries the genetic propensity for the same disease. Difficult decisions may have to be made. Specialist counselling will help people in these circumstances.

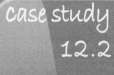

## Antonio Hayward

Antonio Hayward, aged 12, has sickle cell anaemia which was diagnosed from birth after screening his blood for this condition. Antonio has this condition as a result of inheriting two defective haemoglobin genes. The haemoglobin can take on an abnormal shape, distorting the shape of the red blood cell. The cells change from a normal round, doughnut shape to the elongated shape of a sickle, or the shape of the letter 'C'.

Unlike normal red blood cells, which move easily through small blood vessels, sickle cells are stiff and pointed. The sickle shape means that they have a tendency to get stuck in narrow blood vessels and block the flow of blood. This can cause episodes of pain and can also lead to organ damage because the cells aren't getting enough oxygen.

Antonio is generally a healthy young man but he is aware that he needs to take care of himself as he can be more susceptible to infections. His grandfather tells him that he is very lucky. Antibiotics, immunisations and pain killers that are available today help prevent the more serious effects of sickle cell anaemia that occur and more is known about the disease today. In his time many people suffered great pain and in some cases people died. Antonio had to have antibiotics in his early years to reduce these risks. His immunisations were carried out for the same reasons.

Antonio's mother has been given advice when to call the doctor. In spite of great advances in the treatment of sickle cell anaemia, Antonio could still be at risk if the following symptoms occur:

- fever of 38°C (101°F) or higher
- pain that isn't relieved by oral medication
- chest pain
- shortness of breath or trouble breathing
- severe headaches or dizziness
- severe stomach pain or swelling
- jaundice or extreme paleness
- painful erection in males
- sudden change in vision
- seizures
- weakness or inability to move any part of the body
- loss of consciousness.

### activity
**INDIVIDUAL WORK**

Who else might find this information useful?

Antonio would like to tell people at his school about his condition; what advice would you give and where can he find further information?

If Antonio had a sickle cell crisis at school what are the priorities in caring for him?

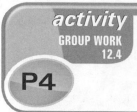

Split into two groups. Each group names three factors that affect health status in the UK.

**P4**

# Methods of promoting and protecting public health

## Aims

The aim of promoting public health is to improve the health of the nation and to reduce health inequalities. These are achieved through health promotion activities that are based on models of health and may be social, medical and/or educational. Health promotion can be further divided within these categories to include changing attitudes and behaviour, individual person-centred therapy through counselling and cognitive behavioural therapy approaches.

The Health Promotion Agency in Northern Ireland have summarised theories and models of health promotion as follows:

Table 12.7  Summary of theories: focus and key concepts

| | Theory | Focus | Key concepts |
|---|---|---|---|
| Individual level | Stages of change model | Individual's readiness to change or attempt to change toward healthy behaviours | Precontemplation<br>Contemplation<br>Decision/determination<br>Action<br>Maintenance |
| | Health belief model | Person's perception of the threat of a health problem and the appraisal of recommended behaviour(s) for preventing or managing the problem | Perceived susceptibility<br>Perceived severity<br>Perceived benefits of action<br>Cues to action<br>Self-efficacy |
| Interpersonal level | Social learning theory | Behaviour is explained via a 3-way, dynamic reciprocal theory in which personal factors, environmental influences and behaviour continually interact | Behaviour capability<br>Reciprocal determinism<br>Expectations<br>Self-efficacy<br>Observational learning<br>Reinforcement |
| Community level | Community organisation theories | Emphasises active participation and development of communities that can better evaluate and solve health and social problems | Empowerment<br>Community competence<br>Participation and relevance<br>Issue selection<br>Critical consciousness |
| | Organisational change theory | Concerns processes and strategies for increasing the chances that healthy policies and programmes will be adopted and maintained in formal organisations | Problem definition (awareness stage)<br>Initiation of action (adoption stage)<br>Implementation of change<br>Institutionalisation of change |
| | Diffusion of innovations theory | Addresses how new ideas, products and social practices spread within a society or from one society to another | Relative advantage<br>Compatibility<br>Complexity<br>Trialability<br>Observation |

Source: Health Promotion Agency, Northern Ireland

Models and theories of health promotion are useful in that they are designed to act as a guide to how individual behaviour and lifestyle needs to be taken into consideration when promoting individual and group health. What might work for some people might not be effective for others. The aim of health promotion is to empower people to take responsibility for their own health care with support from health and social care professionals.

Methods of promoting public health involve disseminating information in a variety of ways and formats so that access to health care and choice is available for everyone.

Health promotion methods might include some or a combination of the following:

- Providing information and facts
- Education and training
- Policies to advise staff on current practice
- Legislation
- Isolation procedures
- Personal protective clothing and equipment
- Safe disposal of waste products
- Correct hygiene and cleanliness procedures
- Reporting and recording incidence of disease
- Regular audits and target-setting to reduce the incidence and spread of disease.

The Department of Health in its paper: 'Better information, better choices, better health: Putting information at the centre of health' (2004) reveals a commitment to address the communication gaps and barriers that can occur due to limited information sharing. They say that 'Greater diversity is needed in how information is made available to people. Everyone should have the opportunity to access generic health information through ways that are personally acceptable. The way information is written, presented and made available should take into account diversity in ethnicity, culture, religion, language, gender, age, disability, socio-economic status and literacy levels'. They hope to achieve this by:

- Introducing a national translation and interpretation service.
- Providing community-based support for people accessing information.
- Making high quality information available nationally to the public and health professionals.
- Making health information available in a wider range of media, such as NHS Direct Interactive.
- Making it easy for people to access their own health care records.

The social model of health promotion methods use social policy, legislation and 'people power' to influence health nationally. Within the social model of health promotion a person would be prevented from carrying out anti-social activities that are harmful to their health and the health of others, e.g. smoking in public places. The social model of health has legislated that smoking is not permissible in restaurants. Raising the age that people can buy cigarettes is also a health promotion strategy within the social model of health.

The educational model of health promotion uses methods such as providing factual, non-judgemental information so that people can make their own choices regarding health care. Information may be given in a variety of ways such as spoken, written, visual imagery or a combination of all of these such as in media advertising and public health films.

The medical model of health's main method of promotion is usually one of intervention and treatment followed by education and information. When a person is receiving health promotion under the medical model they are usually suffering from the illness and disease and so will require active treatment. People will also require information on how to reduce the risks of re-occurrence.

## case study 12.3 — Chloe Jackson

Chloe Jackson is a 22 year old woman who is pregnant with twins. She smokes 30 cigarettes a day and drinks more than 14 units of alcohol a week. She has two jobs and regularly works more than 40 hours a week in her local pub. She lives with her boyfriend in his flat which they share. When she goes to see her GP he tells her that she must give up smoking and drinking as this will affect her health and the health of her unborn children.

A health plan is devised for her to follow. She will have nicotine replacement therapy to help her give up smoking and has been requested to join a 'Quit Smoking' Group organised by the Practice Nurse. Chloe has been given some leaflets about having a healthy pregnancy and food and drink items to avoid.

Chloe has been asked to consider changing her job as she is in an unhealthy environment due to past passive smoking, and the availability of alcohol which isn't helping her. However, legislation banning smoking in public places will prove helpful.

### activity
**INDIVIDUAL WORK**

1. Discuss which model of health is the main focus of health promotion for Chloe.
2. Highlight which aspects relate to the Medical, Social and Educational models of health promotion.
3. How might the other models of health influence Chloe's choices?

## Health promoting activities/Health education

The main focus of national health promotion activities today are connected to the White Paper: 'Choosing Health: Making Healthy Choices Easier' and have built on previous white papers to address the main causes of concern in this country.

Information on health education, treatment and advice may be presented or given in a variety of ways.

- Person to person(s) – talking, counselling, group work
- Media – TV, magazine articles, pamphlets, posters, radio, advertising, leaflets, factsheets
- Therapy – hypnotherapy, behavioural programmes, acupuncture
- Internet – websites which provide information, quizzes, advice, further help.

For health information to be passed on to many people, health promotion campaigns which target groups of people using a variety of media are used.

Table 12.8 Health promotion campaigns

| Health promotion target | Health promotion activity | Health promotion campaign examples |
|---|---|---|
| Accident prevention | Reduce accidents to young people | Mobile phones 'don't talk and walk' |
| Alcohol abuse | Alcohol awareness of harmful effects of drinking<br><br>Follow guidelines: 14 units (females); 21 units (males) | 'Binge drinking' |
| Healthy diet and nutrition | Promoting benefits of fruit, vegetables and minerals to families and children | '5-a-day'<br>'School dinners'<br>'drink milk' |

| Health promotion target | Health promotion activity | Health promotion campaign examples |
|---|---|---|
| Obesity | Awareness of causes and to reduce fat and salt intake and increase exercise levels | 'Small change; BIG difference' |
| Mental health problems | Standard One of the National Service Framework for Mental Health requires health and social services to promote mental health for all, working with individuals and communities, to combat discrimination against individuals and groups with mental health problems, and promote their social inclusion. It recognises the need for local health and social care communities to identify programmes for particularly vulnerable individuals and groups based on an assessment of local need | 'mind out for mental health' campaign combating stigma and discrimination surrounding mental health<br>'Don't be a bully...'<br>'Labels are for boxes... not people'<br>Mental Health Awareness Week |
| Physical activity | Improving exercise levels<br>Exercise 30 minutes x 5 a week | Walk to school<br>Healthy schools, colleges, workplaces |
| Sexual health | Raise awareness of spread of STIs | 'Don't play the sex lottery – use a condom'<br>HIV/AIDs Day |
| Substance misuse | Raising awareness of harmful effects of drugs | 'Talk to Frank' |
| Tobacco | Helping people to give up smoking | 'Easier ways to become unhooked'<br>'Quit', No Smoking Day |

## Specific protection

Specific protection to reduce the incidence and spread of infectious diseases and incidence of disease are centred around surveillance, protection advice, treatment and isolation. Public policy and guidance is issued by the Department of Health which is then passed on to health protection agencies and people working with and for public health such as GPs, nurses, carers and specialist health promotion specialists and advisors.

Overall public health is monitored and evaluated to include specific protection strategies which may involve:

- Information and guidance through public health policies
- Immunisation programmes
- Risk assessment and hazard reduction
- Promoting hygiene and infection control protocols
- Safe disposal of hazardous waste
- Training and education for public health staff
- Education and advice for members of the public
- Encouraging take up and use of health advice .

Information and guidance can be obtained from health centres, online, magazines and by talking to health care professionals such as Health Visitors, Counsellors, Support and advice workers.

## Screening and monitoring

Screening and monitoring for healthy development and reducing the risk of disease and illness occurs throughout life but is most intensive during pregnancy and until a child reaches school age.

The list below describes routine screening checks that are made to ensure healthy development. These are usually carried out by the GP, midwife, health visitor and/or specialist nursing staff at regular intervals, e.g. asthma nurse.

Screening tests include:

- hearing test at birth
- blood tests for conditions which could cause health problems
- checks of baby's hips
- checks of baby's heart
- checks of baby's eyes.

Other checks or reviews include:

- weight
- undescended testicles
- eye checks
- dental checks.

Developmental health checks are carried out at specific ages such as 3 months, 12 months, 18 months, 2 years, 3 years and 4½ years. After this checks are carried out at the request of parents, guardians or health specialists if required.

## Immunisation

Immunisation programmes in this country advise a programme of vaccinations for children from the age of 3 months to protect against diseases such as measles, mumps, rubella, poliomyelitis, Haemophillus influenzae bacteria (HIB), whooping cough, diphtheria, tetanus and TB. The reason why immunisation starts at 3 months of age is due to the immunity the baby receives passed on through breast milk. Immunisations are carried out to specifically treat these diseases up to adulthood and are also given to vulnerable sections of the community such as the elderly.

Immunisation protects the individual by helping the body to form antibodies which will attack the bacterial or viral invasion. Immunity can be acquired naturally (by contracting disease); actively (via live vaccination); passively naturally (via mother's breast milk) or passively actively (via ready made antibodies in immunisation). Children may still get these diseases but they will have sufficient protection to survive whereas without immunisation they might not.

## Risk assessment

Risk assessment and hazard reduction involves checking for possible harm as a result of working with chemicals, equipment or in areas where there are higher risks of accidents occurring, for example, building and construction sites, factories, farms. Health and Safety at Work regulations, COSHH (Control of Substances Hazardous to Health) assessment, First Aid regulations and RIDDOR (Reporting Incidence Disease Dangerous Occurrence Regulations) have helped to protect people but awareness of risks and hazards will further promote health in potentially dangerous environments.

## Disease surveillance

The most effective way of reducing the spread and incidence of disease after immunisation and isolation is to ensure that correct procedures and protocols are used to ensure strict hygiene standards are maintained. It is important to wash hands after contact with any bodily waste products and between different clients/patients, to ensure that personal protective clothing is also worn, e.g. gloves, aprons, masks as appropriate.

## Environmental

### Waste disposal

Safe disposal of hazardous waste and bodily products to protect health care workers and the general public is important. Provision of appropriate coloured bags for infected waste or waste for incineration (red/yellow/black). Yellow hazardous waste sharps boxes for safe disposal of needles and small glass vials.

The Royal College of Nursing Advice for Hand Hygiene recommends the following:

- Hands that are visibly dirty or potentially grossly contaminated must be washed with soap and water and dried thoroughly. Hand preparation increases the effectiveness of decontamination. You should:
  - keep nails short, clean and polish free
  - avoid wearing wrist watches and jewellery, especially rings with ridges or stones
- Artificial nails must not be worn
- Any cuts and abrasions should be covered with a waterproof dressing.

### Waste treatment

Sharps include needles, scalpels, stitch cutters, glass ampoules and any sharp instrument. The main hazards of a sharps injury are hepatitis B, hepatitis C and HIV.

Second only to back injuries as a cause of occupational injuries amongst health care workers, between July 1997 and June 2002, there were 1,550 reports of blood-borne virus exposures in health care workers – of which 42 per cent were sustained by nurses or midwives.

## Supply of safe water

### Pollution Control

Education and advice for the general public who may be at risk will involve: not sharing needles or razors; washing hands after using toilet facilities to avoid ingesting E.coli and other gut or faecal bacteria or parasites; advice against unprotected sex i.e. wearing a condom to protect against sexually transmitted infections; ensuring food is cooked and stored at correct temperatures to avoid bacterial poisoning; washing hands after stroking animals or pets to protect against infestations and parasites; wearing appropriate sun block and covering up to reduce risk of skin cancers.

## Diet and nutrition

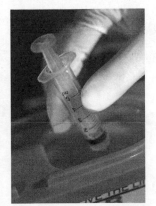

Figure 12.21 Reduce risk of needlestick injuries

Eating at least five portions of a variety of fruit and vegetables a day could lead to an estimated reduction of up to 20 per cent in overall deaths from chronic diseases, such as heart disease, stroke and cancer.

Breastfed infants are five times less likely to be admitted to hospital with infections, such as gastro-enteritis or respiratory infections, during their first year of life and are less likely to become obese in later childhood. Mothers who breastfeed are less likely to develop pre-menopausal breast cancer and are more likely to return to their pre-pregnancy weight.

## Sexual health

Chlamydia is the most common STI and affects an estimated one in ten sexually active young women. Because there are few symptoms it can be left undetected. If left untreated it can lead to pelvic inflammatory disease, ectopic pregnancy and infertility. Wearing a condom will prevent this occurring. Regular check ups and antibiotic treatment can cure this sexually transmitted disease.

Table 12.9  Reasons for using a condom: by sex and age, 2004/05

| | Percentages | | | | |
|---|---|---|---|---|---|
| | 16–19 | 20–24 | 25–34 | 35–44 | 45–49 |
| **Men** | | | | | |
| Prevent pregnancy | 25 | 39 | 44 | 70 | 73 |
| Prevent infection | 8 | 4 | 9 | 5 | 6 |
| Both reasons | 63 | 57 | 44 | 23 | 19 |
| Other reason | 4 | – | 3 | 2 | 1 |
| All aged 16–49 | 100 | 100 | 100 | 100 | 100 |
| **Women** | | | | | |
| Prevent pregnancy | 29 | 31 | 59 | 65 | 60 |
| Prevent infection | 2 | 6 | 7 | 6 | 12 |
| Both reasons | 68 | 62 | 33 | 25 | 22 |
| Other reason | – | – | 1 | 4 | 5 |
| All aged 16–49 | 100 | 100 | 100 | 100 | 100 |

Source: Omnibus Survey, Office for National Statistics

## Hospital Associated Infections (HAIs)

Due to the nature of hospitals there is a multitude of potential causes of viral and bacterial risks associated with admission and long-term stays in hospital.

### *Clostridium difficile*

Clostridium difficile infection is the most common cause of hospital-acquired diarrhoea. Clostridium difficile is an anaerobic bacterium that is present in the gut of up to 3% of healthy adults and 66% of infants. However, Clostridium difficile rarely causes problems in children or healthy adults, as it is kept in check by the normal bacterial population of the intestine. When certain antibiotics disturb the balance of bacteria in the gut, Clostridium difficile can multiply rapidly and produce toxins which cause illness.

The effectiveness of measures of health promotion success will be seen in statistics and information that shows that there is a drop in the number of new cases of disease or illness reported. Public health awareness is also a reasonable indicator of the success or failure of a health campaign. Noticeable evidence in lifestyle habits will also denote early signs of possible success. In future years it will be interesting to see if banning smoking from public places has been effective or not. Information might take a number of years to reveal signs of improvement and the success of health promotion strategies. This might later be evidenced in results from household surveys, independent health surveys and information returned to the Health Protection Agency by public health workers.

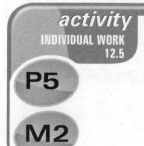

**activity**
INDIVIDUAL WORK
12.5

P5

M2

List as many methods as you can, that promote and protect public health.

Explain each one.

## Communicable diseases

Communicable diseases are diseases that are passed on to people in various ways which will be explained. People develop these diseases if they are not immune or are susceptible to them. Having contact with a disease causes the body to produce antibodies which counteract future attacks of the disease. Immunisation against a disease has a similar effect. However if the disease mutates or changes slightly a person's resistance may still be affected. A good example of a communicable disease is the common cold which has many strains and which is difficult to provide one form of immunity for because there are so many variations (strains).

Diseases are caused by micro-organisms that may be categorised into the following groups:

- Bacterial
- Viral
- Fungal
- Protozoan
- Parasitic.

They spread and multiply according to their specific pathogenic makeup. Most **pathogens** are spread through the following ways. See Table 12.11.

Table 12.10  Methods of spread of disease

| | |
|---|---|
| Direct contact | Skin to skin, touch, sexual intercourse |
| Indirect contact | Surfaces, clothes, animal hair, fur, soil |
| Droplet infection | Coughs, sneezes, saliva |
| Injected | Insect bites, needles, thorns |
| Ingested | Swallowed in contaminated food, water |

Table 12.11 Infectious diseases

| Infectious diseases | Signs and symptoms | Incubation/transmission | Treatment/prevention |
|---|---|---|---|
| Athlete's foot (Tinea pedis) | Itchy, scaly rash usually between toes; inflammation and soreness | Fungal Initially 1–10 days | Fungal cream. Dry between toes. Wash regularly. Change socks daily. Change shoes if causing excessive sweating. See doctor if problem persists. |
| Chlamydia | Purulent discharge. Lower abdominal pain. Urethritis. Sometimes no symptoms reported. | Direct sexual contact with infected partner | Antibiotics. Regular screening especially for people in under 25 year age group. Wear a condom. |
| Conjunctivitis | Itching and pain in eyes; may be discharge. | Viral or bacterial | Doctor. Medication. Isolation as appropriate. Use separate towel, flannel. |
| Food poisoning | Vomiting, diarrhoea, abdominal pain | ½ hour – 36 hours Indirect; infected food or drink | Fluids only for 24 hours, doctor if no better |
| Gastroenteritis | Vomiting, diarrhoea, dehydration | Bacterial: 7–14 days Viral: ½ hour – 36 hours Direct contact, indirect – infected food and drink | Fluids, water. Urgent medical aid in vulnerable, e.g. infants, children, elderly people. |

| Infectious diseases | Signs and symptoms | Incubation/transmission | Treatment/prevention |
|---|---|---|---|
| Measles. Measles is a highly contagious, viral infection that is most common in children. Treatment is supportive. | It is characterised by fever, cough, cold, conjunctivitis, (Koplik's spots) on the buccal or labial mucosa, and a maculopapular rash that spreads from head to toe (cephalocaudal). | 7–14 days Droplet infection | Vaccination is highly effective. Diagnosis is usually clinical. |
| Meningitis | Severe headache, neck stiffness, fever, vomiting, drowsiness or confusion, dislike of bright lights. Sometimes tiny red/purple spots or bruises | 2–10 days Bacteria or virus Droplet infection | Hospital. Antibiotics. |
| Mumps. Mumps is an acute, contagious, systemic viral disease. Diagnosis is usually clinical. | Painful enlargement of the salivary glands, most commonly the parotids. Complications may include orchitis, meningo-encephalitis, and pancreatitis. | 14–24 days Droplet infection | Treatment is supportive. Vaccination is highly effective. |
| Poliomyelitis (also known as Infantile Paralysis) | Can be asymptomatic (no obvious signs) but if enters central nervous system can lead to paralysis | Viral infection Water or airborne but commonly oral-faecal route. | Treat symptoms. Vaccination is effective in preventing incidence. Dispose faecal waste carefully. |
| Pneumonia *Streptococcus pneumoniae, Haemophilus influenzae*, and atypical organisms (i.e. *Chlamydia pneumoniae*) | Fever, cough, difficulty breathing, rapid breathing, and tachycardia (raised heart rate). | 14–21 days Droplet infection | Diagnosis is based on clinical presentation and chest x-ray. Treatment is usually antibiotic once cause identified if bacterial. |
| Rubella (German Measles) | Slight cold, sore throat, slight fever, enlarged glands behind ears, pains in small joints 1st day: sweat-like rash, bright pink; starts at roots of hair, may last 2–24 hours | 14–21 days Viral infection Direct contact Droplets | Rest if necessary. Fluids. Analgesia as required. |
| Syphilis | Primary: Ulcer type lesion in the genitor-anal area. Secondary: Possible neuro-muscular problems; blindness. | Bacteria Direct sexual contact with infected partner | Antibiotics e.g. doxycline. Screening/monitoring. Wear a condom. |
| Tapeworm | Nocturnal peri-anal itching causing inflammation and possible infection. Loss of weight in extreme cases. Bloating, abdominal pain and flatulence. | Parasitic Ingesting raw meat or fish Ingesting eggs found in soil, sandpits Contact with some animals | Medication. Cook meat/fish. |

## Non-infectious diseases

Non-infectious diseases are illnesses that are not usually passed on by direct contact unless they are genetic in origin. For some illnesses there are no known reasons at present why some people are susceptible to them more than others.

Table 12.12 Non-infectious diseases

| Non-infectious diseases | Signs and symptoms | Incubation/ transmission | Treatment/prevention |
| --- | --- | --- | --- |
| Asthma | Shortness of breath, wheezing, attacks vary in intensity. | Allergy – often to house dust, animals, pollen, extremes of temperature. | Doctor for acute attacks and ongoing treatment. Medication to reduce irritation in airways. |
| Cystic fibrosis Cystic fibrosis is an inherited disease of the exocrine glands affecting primarily the GI and respiratory systems. It leads to COPD, exocrine pancreatic insufficiency, and abnormally high sweat electrolytes. | Fifty percent of patients present with pulmonary manifestations, often beginning in infancy. Recurrent or chronic infections manifested by cough and wheezing are common. Cough is the most troublesome complaint, often accompanied by sputum, gagging, vomiting, and disturbed sleep. Intercostal retractions, use of accessory muscles of respiration, a barrel-chest deformity, digital clubbing, and cyanosis occur with disease progression. | Inherited disease | Diagnosis is by sweat test or identification of 2 cystic fibrosis mutations in patients with characteristic symptoms. Treatment is supportive through aggressive interdisciplinary care to involve physiotherapy, antibiotics and food supplements. Air/oxygen therapy may also be required. |
| Huntington's disease | Problems with movement, e.g. jaw clenching, balance; cognitive function, e.g. memory, recognition of objects and people; and neurological, e.g. depression, psychosis. | Inherited | No known cure; treatment based on support and reducing potential complications. |
| Sickle-cell anaemia caused by homozygous inheritance of Hb S. Sickle-shaped red blood cells (RBCs) clog capillaries, causing organs to have limited or reduced blood supply. | Acute pain (crises) may develop frequently. Infection, bone marrow aplasia, or lung involvement (acute chest syndrome) can develop acutely and be fatal. | Inherited disease | Crises are treated with analgesics and other supportive measures. Transfusions are occasionally required. Vaccines against bacterial infections, prophylactic antibiotics, and aggressive treatment of infections prolong survival. |
| Tay-Sach's disease. A degenerative disease of the nervous system. | May appear at the age of 6 months where baby loses ability to smile, crawl or turn over. This leads to blindness and unawareness of surroundings. Life span is usually short. | Inherited disease | No known cure; child's symptoms treated as appropriate. |
| Tetanus is an acute poisoning from a neurotoxin produced by *Clostridium tetani*. Symptoms are intermittent tonic spasms of voluntary muscles. Spasm of the jaw muscles accounts for the name lockjaw. Diagnosis is clinical. | Difficulty swallowing; restlessness; irritability; stiff neck, arms, or legs; headache; fever; sore throat; chills; and tonic spasms. Later, the patient has difficulty opening his/her jaw (triasmus). | Average 5–10 days Injection from infected soil particle; thorn, wood. | Treatment is immuno-globulin and intensive support. Immunisation. |
| Thalassaemia. Caused by problem with haemoglobin breaking down more quickly than usual in blood. | Anaemia. Breathlessness. Lack of energy. Headaches. Difficulty sleeping. | Inherited disease. | Regular blood transfusions. Injections. Management of symptoms as appropriate. |

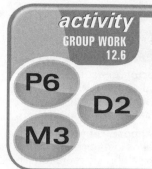

*activity*
GROUP WORK
12.6

P6

D2

M3

Split into two groups.

Group 1 chooses an infectious disease and Group 2 a non-infectious disease.

Both groups list and explain the appropriate methods of prevention and control for both diseases.

Write in detail about how effective these methods are for these diseases.

## Non-communicable diseases

Non-communicable diseases are diseases that cannot be transmitted from human to human. An example of this might be some cancers as in skin cancer.

### Skin cancer

There are two types of skin cancer, non-melanoma and melanoma (malignant) type skin cancer which is the one that can spread throughout the body if left undetected. In the UK the most common type reported is non-melanoma cancer which accounts for 60,000 cases each year.

The skin is made up of three layers:

■ the epidermis

■ the dermis

■ the supporting subcutaneous layer of loose tissue and fat.

Cancer can start from cells in any of these layers.

Figure 12.22 Section through the skin

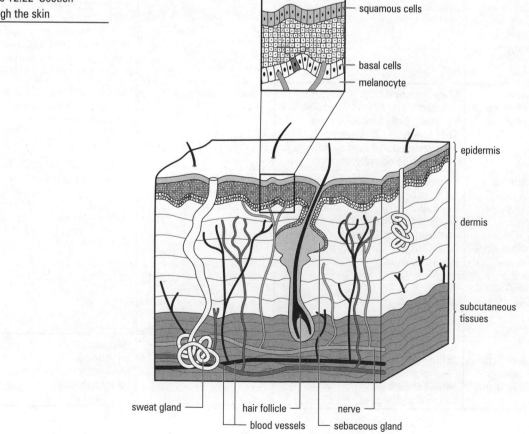

Different types of skin cancer can look different and grow at different rates. The malignant variety is usually fast growing and regular skin checks by yourself should be carried out. Similarly it is a good idea to carry out regular breast checks in females and testicular checks in males so that any out of the ordinary changes can be detected early and treated if problems are found.

Common symptoms include any spot or lesion on the skin that:

- changes in colour
- is irregular in shape and size
- oozes
- is inflamed
- feels different.

Figure 12.23 Detecting skin changes

| Normal mole | Melanoma | Sign | Characteristic |
|---|---|---|---|
| | | Asymmetry | when half of the mole does not match the other half |
| | | Border | when the border (edges) of the mole are ragged or irregular |
| | | Colour | when the colour of the mole varies throughout |
| | | Diameter | if the mole's diameter is larger than a pencil's eraser |

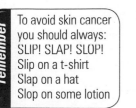

To avoid skin cancer you should always:
SLIP! SLAP! SLOP!
Slip on a t-shirt
Slap on a hat
Slop on some lotion

*remember*

Treatment is dependent on the type and severity of cancer. It may involve a range of treatments from chemotherapy, freezing with liquid nitrogen, surgical removal and or radio-therapy.

Some people are more susceptible to skin cancer than others, e.g. light coloured skin, freckles, previous sun exposure and burning, using a sunbed, family history of skin cancer, skin with abundant moles, exposure to UV rays, e.g. working outside.

**Professional Practice**

Recommendations for prevention and limiting the incidence of skin cancer are:

- Don't use sunbeds.
- Cover up skin – especially in peak sunlight hours 11 a.m. to 3 p.m.
- Wear appropriate sun screen applications and apply regularly.
- Check skin regularly.
- Visit the doctor if you notice any unusual changes.

Cancerbackup
0808 800 1234
www.cancerbackup.org.uk
British Association of Dermatologists
020 7383 0266
www.bad.org.uk

***Progress Check***

1. List the key aspects in protecting public health, e.g. monitoring

2. Discuss why is it important to identify the health needs of the population.

3. Identify where we might obtain statistics and information on diseases and illnesses in this country.

4. Describe and explain the main factors that affect public health.

5. Identify and explain how diseases and illnesses are spread giving two examples each from infectious, non-infectious and genetic diseases.

6. Evaluate the importance of public health strategies to reduce the incidence and spread of potential risks to health.

7. Explain how socio-economic factors affect the health of individuals and groups. Choose examples linked to social class, gender, employment status, environment, discrimination.

8. Critically evaluate the role of health promoters giving examples of how health is promoted.

9. What strategies would you employ to reduce the incidence of common transmissible diseases in teenagers? Choose a viral, fungal or bacterial infection to illustrate your points.

10. What have you learnt about public health since carrying out this unit?

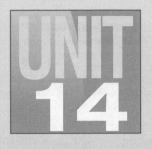

# Physiological Disorders

## This unit covers:

- The nature of physiological disorders
- The processes involved in diagnosis of disorders
- The care strategies used to support individuals through the course of a disorder
- How individuals adapt to the presence of a disorder

Health and social care workers need to have an insight into the ways in which different physiological disorders **present** themselves and how the caring services diagnose, treat and care for patients.

This unit aims to give you a basic understanding of a variety of physiological disorders. It describes their causes, the body systems involved and associated signs and symptoms. It looks at the investigations and measurements involved in reaching a diagnosis, patient care and the roles of the people involved in delivering care. Finally, it explores how individuals cope with the difficulties caused by their disorder and how its progression could affect them in the future.

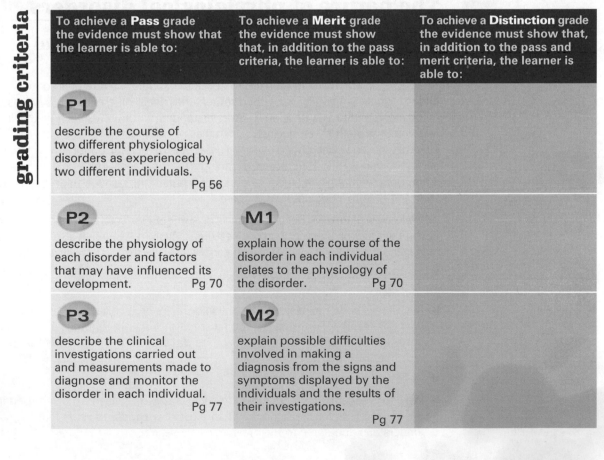

**grading criteria**

| To achieve a **Pass** grade the evidence must show that the learner is able to: | To achieve a **Merit** grade the evidence must show that, in addition to the pass criteria, the learner is able to: | To achieve a **Distinction** grade the evidence must show that, in addition to the pass and merit criteria, the learner is able to: |
|---|---|---|
| **P1** describe the course of two different physiological disorders as experienced by two different individuals. Pg 56 | | |
| **P2** describe the physiology of each disorder and factors that may have influenced its development. Pg 70 | **M1** explain how the course of the disorder in each individual relates to the physiology of the disorder. Pg 70 | |
| **P3** describe the clinical investigations carried out and measurements made to diagnose and monitor the disorder in each individual. Pg 77 | **M2** explain possible difficulties involved in making a diagnosis from the signs and symptoms displayed by the individuals and the results of their investigations. Pg 77 | |

## grading criteria

| To achieve a **Pass** grade the evidence must show that the learner is able to: | To achieve a **Merit** grade the evidence must show that, in addition to the pass criteria, the learner is able to: | To achieve a **Distinction** grade the evidence must show that, in addition to the pass and merit criteria, the learner is able to: |
|---|---|---|
| **P4** describe the care processes experienced by each individual case and the roles of different people in supporting the care strategy. Pg 86 | | **D1** evaluate the contributions made by different people in supporting the individuals with the disorders. Pg 86 |
| **P5** explain difficulties experienced by each individual in adjusting to the presence of the disorder and the care strategy. Pg 91 | **M3** explain how the care strategies experienced by each individual have influenced the course of the disorder. Pg 91 | **D2** evaluate alternative care strategies that might have been adopted for each individual. Pg 91 |
| **P6** compare the possible future development of the disorders in the individuals concerned. Pg 93 | | |

# The nature of physiological disorders

## Investigating individuals with physiological disorders

To achieve unit 14 you are required to develop and demonstrate an in-depth understanding of two physiological disorders that affect different body systems. It is recommended that you develop your understanding through research (see below) and demonstrate it by producing case studies of two individuals, each of whom has been diagnosed with a physiological disorder, has been referred for investigation and/or diagnosis, and is in receipt of care and/or treatment. This could include you, if appropriate, a family member, a friend, or a patient or **service user** if you have sufficient time to work closely with them.

Whoever you choose to use as individuals or **subjects** for your case studies, you must obtain their formal consent. If a **care setting** is involved, you must also obtain the manager's consent. An **ethical**, professional way to do this is to produce a document that:

- describes the purpose of your research and how you are going to use the information you collect
- reassures everyone involved that any information you collect will remain anonymous and confidential. For example, you must not include photographs or clinical reports in your case studies – by all means quote **data** but don't use details that could be attributed to specific individuals
- is easy to read and understand
- asks for your subjects' signatures, to show that they consent to being used in a case study; and asks for the signature of an **expert witness**, to verify that the subjects understand and agree to their role in your research.

Collecting information from an individual about their disorder is known as primary research. Primary research methods include interviews, observations, surveys and questionnaires. Primary research data is useful because it describes an individual's first hand experience of their disorder, for example, how they feel and how the disorder affects their life and their relationships. Descriptive information is known as qualitative data and is very important.

Secondary research is using information about physiological disorders that, for example, health and social care professionals and organisations such as charities have collected and published in books and specialist journals, on the internet, etc. Secondary research is useful because it gives quantitative (numerical) data, such as life expectancy and changes in blood pressure that are associated with a specific disorder. It is also useful in that it can describe and explain the physiology of different disorders and the factors that influence their development.

Figure 14.1  Primary and secondary research

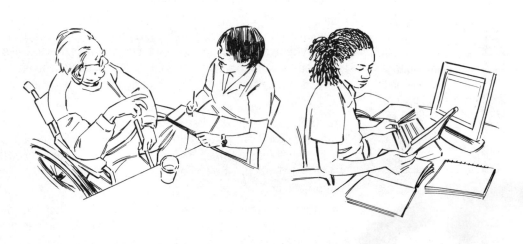

**Link** You will look more closely at primary and secondary research methods, quantitative and qualitative data and ethical codes in Unit 22.

## Appropriate disorders

To achieve unit 14, you are required to investigate two physiological disorders that are sufficiently different to allow you to gain an understanding of disorders relating to different body systems. You also need to choose disorders that you will be able to understand. The table below highlights a number of more common disorders and the principal body systems affected.

Table 14.1  Physiological disorders

| Physiological disorder | Principle body systems affected |
| --- | --- |
| Coronary heart disease (CHD) | Circulatory system |
| Stroke | Circulatory system |
| Diabetes (either IDD or NID) | Circulatory system |
| Asthma | Respiratory system |
| Emphysema | Respiratory system |
| Osteoporosis (fragile or brittle bone disease) | Skeletal system |

| Physiological disorder | Principle body systems affected |
|---|---|
| Rheumatoid arthritis (RA) | Skeletal system |
| Alzheimer's disease | Nervous system |
| Parkinson's disease | Nervous system |
| Multiple Sclerosis (MS) | Nervous system |
| Motor Neurone Disease (MND) | Nervous system |
| Inflammatory bowel diseases e.g. Crohn's disease and ulcerative colitis. | Digestive system |
| Cancer e.g. breast, lungs, bowel, skin, prostate | Dependent on the site of the cancer |

## Signs and symptoms

Changes in normal body functioning can indicate the presence of a physiological disorder and manifest themselves through signs and symptoms. To help ensure that patients and service users are diagnosed correctly and that they receive appropriate care and treatment, it is important that health and social care workers are able to recognise the signs and symptoms associated with physiological disorders.

Signs are things that are visible, can be smelled or heard, that are **palpable** and measurable. They include bad breath, bleeding, breathlessness, changes in appearance, behaviour, blood pressure and temperature, coughing, constipation, diarrhoea, discharges, frequent urination, loss of sight and hearing, loss of strength, rashes, redness and inflammation, sneezing, soreness, spots, swelling and lumps, vomiting, weight gain and loss, and wheezing.

Symptoms are feelings experienced by individuals. They include discomfort, aches and pains, feelings of bloatedness, buzzing or ringing in the ear, dislike of bright lights, feeling dizzy, irritation, itchiness, loss of appetite, smell and taste, nausea, numbness, tiredness, tenderness and tingling,

The signs and symptoms of physiological disorders vary between people and change from time to time. For example, people with Multiple Sclerosis (MS) don't necessarily have the same signs and symptoms as each other and those they do have vary in severity and duration.

Signs and symptoms change during the course of a physiological disorder, i.e. as it progresses, and it can be difficult to predict the future. In the example of MS, the younger a person is when diagnosed, the more gradually the disorder develops. There may be long periods of **remission** when damage to the body is repaired but after 10 to 15 years the number of remissions decreases and disability becomes more marked. If an individual is diagnosed at an older age, further signs and symptoms are likely and remissions unlikely.

The Multiple Sclerosis Society
www.mssociety.org.uk

> **remember**
>
> If you are involved in monitoring and recording signs and symptoms, make sure your skills and training are up-to-date; and if you have any doubts, always seek help or a second opinion.

Figure 14.2 The signs and symptoms of MS

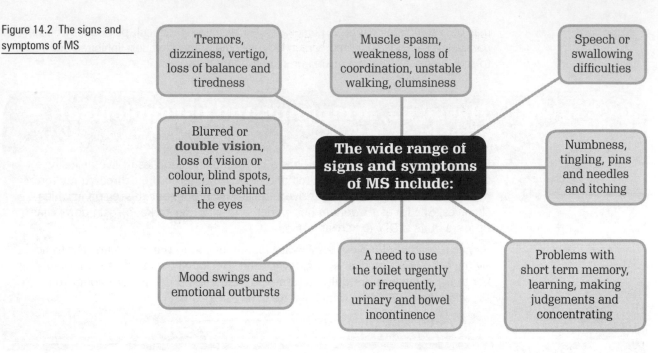

Tremors, dizziness, vertigo, loss of balance and tiredness

Muscle spasm, weakness, loss of coordination, unstable walking, clumsiness

Speech or swallowing difficulties

Blurred or **double vision**, loss of vision or colour, blind spots, pain in or behind the eyes

**The wide range of signs and symptoms of MS include:**

Numbness, tingling, pins and needles and itching

Mood swings and emotional outbursts

A need to use the toilet urgently or frequently, urinary and bowel incontinence

Problems with short term memory, learning, making judgements and concentrating

## Psychological effects

Being seriously ill or having to live with a disability can affect our psychological (emotional) health, altering the way we think and feel about things and the way we respond to people and situations. We may become anxious, depressed and apathetic, and we may experience personality changes. Effects like these are very common and, depending on the disorder, may fade with time or last for years.

### Depression and anxiety

Depression and anxiety are very common in people who are seriously ill or disabled. They usually set in once the person becomes aware of how their health or disability could affect their everyday life. For example, they may have to come to terms with chronic pain, the loss of their hopes and plans for the future, their changed role in the family and community, and the loss of a career. The signs and symptoms of depression and anxiety that health and social care workers should be on the alert for in the people they work with include:

- sadness, suicidal thoughts and feelings
- feelings of worthlessness, hopelessness or despair
- worry and changes in appetite
- loss of energy, an inability to concentrate and difficulty sleeping.

### Apathy

When people are seriously ill or disabled, they can become apathetic. This means they lose interest in everything going on around them, for example current affairs, their finances and hobbies, maintaining contact with family and friends and even emotional situations. In some cases they may lose the motivation to carry out simple everyday tasks or responsibilities.

Personality changes caused by illness and disability include exaggerated and rapid swings of emotion that can result in outbursts of laughter, tears and sometimes anger. This is called emotional lability. The emotional outburst of some people matches how they are feeling but is greatly exaggerated. In others, it is out of place and inappropriate to the situation they are in.

Some people who are ill or disabled become less sociable, more introverted, sometimes angry and aggressive. Usually, existing personality traits become exaggerated but there may be a complete change of personality. For example, a difficult person may become passive and a mild-mannered person may become aggressive, less inhibited and unable to stop themselves saying unkind or inappropriate things.

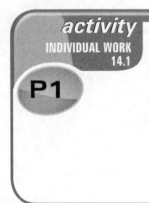

## case study 14.1

## The signs, symptoms and psychological effects of MS

Su is 35 years old. Although she has a boyfriend she chooses to live as a single mother with her two small children and elderly mother in their three-storey terrace house. Her job requires her to drive extensively throughout the region in which she lives. She loves to work in her garden and, in order to keep costs down, has become quite a DIY expert at home.

Su has recently been diagnosed with MS. She has read the literature sent to her by the MS Society and is feeling devastated. Her family, friends and colleagues tell her that her feelings are quite natural and that given time, she will adapt to her situation. None of their comments are of any help.

### activity
**GROUP WORK**

1. What signs and symptoms is Su likely to experience now and in the future?
2. How might having MS affect Su psychologically?
3. How might having MS affect Su's life?
4. How would you feel if you were in Su's shoes?

### activity
**INDIVIDUAL WORK 14.1**

**P1**

Think about two people you know who are experiencing and receiving treatment for a physiological disorder. The disorders must be different in that they each affect a different body system e.g. CHD (circulatory system) and asthma (respiratory system).

Use both primary research methods e.g. interviews, and secondary research methods e.g. a literature search, to find out:

■ the signs and symptoms that are manifested by each disorder over time

■ how the disorders have affected and continue to affect your subjects.

Use your findings to produce an information leaflet that could be given to people newly diagnosed with each condition.

## Physiology

The aim of this section is to give you a brief introduction to the body systems affected by some of the more common physiological disorders and to describe the changes caused by the disorder and its treatment.

### The circulatory system

The circulatory system is made up of blood, blood vessels and the heart.

Blood consists of about 55% plasma, which is mostly water, and 45% cells. There are three main types of blood cells:

1. red blood cells
2. white blood cells
3. platelets.

Red blood cells contain haemoglobin, a protein that contains iron which readily combines with oxygen. Haemoglobin in red blood cells enables them to transport oxygen from the lungs to all the body cells.

The main role of white blood cells is to respond to infection by producing antibodies and destroying anything that the body recognises as a 'foreign body'. This is called the immune response. The main types of white blood cell are neutrophils, lymphocytes, eosinophils, monocytes and basophils.

Platelets or thrombocytes are very important in the blood clotting process. They clump together to form a plug if bleeding occurs and then release other chemicals that help the blood to clot and the blood vessel to be repaired.

Blood circulates around the body carrying:

- oxygen, hormones, antibodies and nutrients such as glucose and amino acids to the body cells
- waste products such as carbon dioxide, urea, excess water and salt away from the cells to sites where they can be excreted from the body e.g. the lungs, kidneys and skin.

Without a permanent supply of blood, body cells die. Blood is pumped to all the body cells by the heart, a hollow muscular organ, through a system of blood vessels called arteries, veins and capillaries.

Arteries carry oxygen-rich blood from the heart to all parts of the body. As they get further away from the heart, they reduce in size and become arterioles and finally capillaries. The very small size of capillaries allows them to pass between cells so that oxygen, nutrients, etc. can diffuse from the blood into the cells and waste material such as carbon dioxide can diffuse from the cells into the blood. Capillaries become very small veins called venules that increase in size to become veins. Veins carry blood back to the heart, which pumps it to the lungs where it excretes the carbon dioxide it has collected from the cells and picks up more oxygen. Oxygen-rich blood then passes back to the heart from where it continues its circulation around the body.

Physiological disorders of the circulatory system include CHD, stroke and diabetes.

### Coronary Heart Disease (CHD)

In order to work properly, the muscle cells of the heart need a constant supply of oxygen. Blood containing oxygen is delivered to the heart muscle cells by the coronary arteries. CHD is caused by a build up of plaque (cholesterol) in the coronary arteries (arteriosclerosis). This build up narrows or blocks the arteries, thereby reducing or preventing a supply of oxygen to the heart.

### Angina

Angina is a symptom of CHD. It occurs when, due to a build up of plaque, there is a temporary reduction in blood flow to the heart. It causes pain but no damage; however, it does warn of an increased risk of a heart attack. A heart attack (myocardial infarction) happens when the blood flow to part of the heart is fully blocked, causing that part of the heart to die. This blockage can be caused by blood clots forming over plaques (coronary thrombosis) or when the coronary arteries go into spasm. Heart attacks can cause permanent damage to the heart and can be fatal.

Heart failure can also occur in people with CHD. This is when the heart gets too weak to pump blood around the body. As a result, fluid builds up in the lungs, making it difficult to breath.

Figure 14.3 The circulatory system

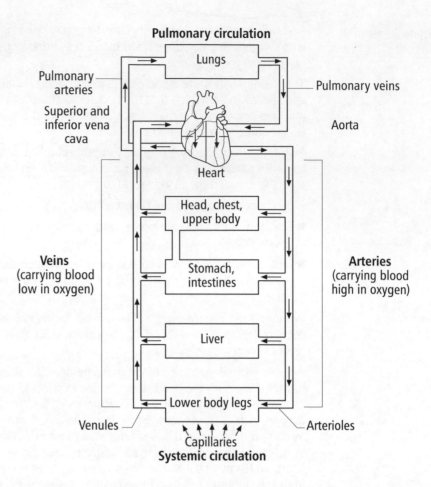

CHD can't be cured but it can often be prevented from getting worse by using medication and making lifestyle changes. You will read about the effect of lifestyle choices on health shortly. Medication that is prescribed for individuals with CHD includes:

■ aspirin, which helps prevent the blood from clotting

■ statins, which work by changing the inner lining of the coronary arteries so that plaques are less likely to form or get bigger

■ beta blockers, which improve blood flow by lowering blood pressure and slowing the heartbeat

■ ACE (Angiotensin Converting Enzyme) inhibitors, Angiotensin II receptor antagonists and nitrates, which reduce blood pressure by increasing the size of blood vessels

■ anticoagulants such as warfarin, which stop the blood clotting

■ cardiac glycosides e.g. digoxin, which strengthen the heart and slow the heartbeat. As a result, blood is pumped around the body with more force.

Surgery may be needed if the blood vessels are very narrow or if drugs don't help to open them up.

Figure 14.4 Treating CHD
with surgery

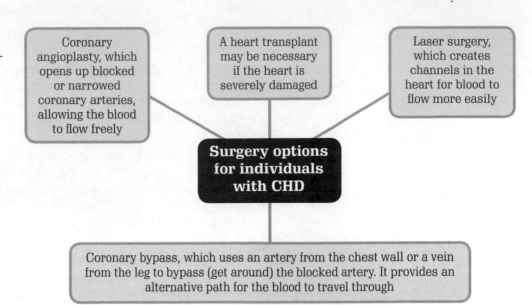

### Stroke

A stroke occurs when the blood and therefore oxygen supply to the brain is cut off. As a result, brain cells become damaged or die. The effects of a stroke can be mild but they can also be fatal.

There are two types of stroke:

1. Ischaemic stroke is when a blood clot blocks an artery that delivers blood to the brain. A blood clot can be triggered by plaque in the artery or it can form somewhere else in the body and be carried by the blood to an artery in the brain. Transient ischaemic attack (TIA) or mini-stroke happens when the blood supply to the brain is cut off for only a short time. Whilst recovery is usual, TIAs warn of an increased risk of a full stroke.

2. Haemorrhagic stroke occurs when a weakened artery bursts and blood leaks out, damaging nearby brain tissue. At the same time other parts of the brain that are fed by this artery become damaged because their oxygen supply is cut off.

Because a common effect of stroke is muscle weakness, treatment consists of exercise and physiotherapy for the parts of the body that have been affected. Exercise also helps maintain general good health and reduces the chances of having another stroke. In addition, medication is often prescribed to help prevent another stroke occurring, for example aspirin, which helps prevent blood clots forming, and drugs that reduce high blood pressure or blood cholesterol.

### Diabetes

Diabetes is a condition caused by having too much glucose in the blood. The blood glucose level is regulated by the hormone insulin, which is produced in the pancreas. Insulin is responsible for moving glucose out of the blood and into cells, where it is broken down to produce energy. If diabetes is not treated it can lead to many different health problems, because large amounts of glucose in the blood damage the blood vessels, nerves and organs.

There are two types of diabetes, IDD and NID:

1. Insulin-dependent diabetes (IDD) is a disorder in which the body produces little or no insulin. This is because the immune system attacks the insulin-producing cells in the pancreas, destroying them or damaging them sufficiently to reduce insulin

production. Sometimes IDD is caused because the body is not able to use insulin properly and, in some cases, it can be triggered by a viral infection.

Lack of insulin causes the blood glucose level to become too high and the person to have a hyperglycaemic attack. If left untreated, hyperglycaemia can lead to diabetic ketoacidosis, which is where the body starts to break down fats for energy. This leads to a build up of ketone acids in the blood, which can eventually cause unconsciousness and even death.

Treatment for IDD is to take insulin, by injection, pump or jet system. In addition, a healthy diet and regular exercise help to reduce blood glucose levels. But if blood glucose levels become too low, for example if too much insulin has been taken, the person can have a hypoglycaemic attack. Hypoglycaemic attacks can be brought under control by eating or drinking something containing fast-acting carbohydrates, such as a chocolate bar or sugary drink.

2. Non-insulin dependent diabetes (NID) is a disorder in which the body does not make enough insulin or cannot use insulin properly. This type of diabetes is often linked with obesity and occurs mostly in people over the age of 40. It is usually controlled by losing weight and dietary changes although some people may need to take tablets or insulin as well.

The British Heart Foundation

www.bhf.org.uk

The Stroke Association

www.stroke.org.uk

Diabetes UK

www.diabetes.org.uk

## The respiratory system

The respiratory system is made up of the nose, larynx (voice box), trachea (windpipe), bronchi, bronchioles and **alveoli**, blood vessels that circulate the alveoli, pleural membranes that surround the lungs, ribs and intercostal muscles (which run between the ribs), and the diaphragm.

There are two types of respiration:

1. external respiration or breathing, which involves taking oxygen from the air and excreting carbon dioxide from the lungs

2. internal or cellular respiration, which is when glucose is converted in the body cells to make energy. This requires oxygen and produces carbon dioxide.

The first stage of external respiration is when the muscular diaphragm and the intercostal muscles contract. This increases the size of the chest cavity, causing air to be sucked in. This is called inhalation and its function is to bring oxygen into the body. Air passes into the nose, down the respiratory tract i.e. the larynx, trachea, bronchi and bronchioles, and eventually into the alveoli. As air passes through the tract it is warmed and particles of dirt etc. are removed from it by sticky mucus produced by gland cells. Cilia (tiny hairs) move the mucus towards the nose and mouth from where it can be swallowed or expelled.

Inhaled air that fills the alveoli has a high concentration of oxygen and a low concentration of carbon dioxide. Blood in the capillaries that circulate the alveoli has a low concentration of oxygen and a high concentration of carbon dioxide. For this reason oxygen from the alveoli diffuses into the blood and carbon dioxide from the blood diffuses into the alveoli. This is called gaseous exchange.

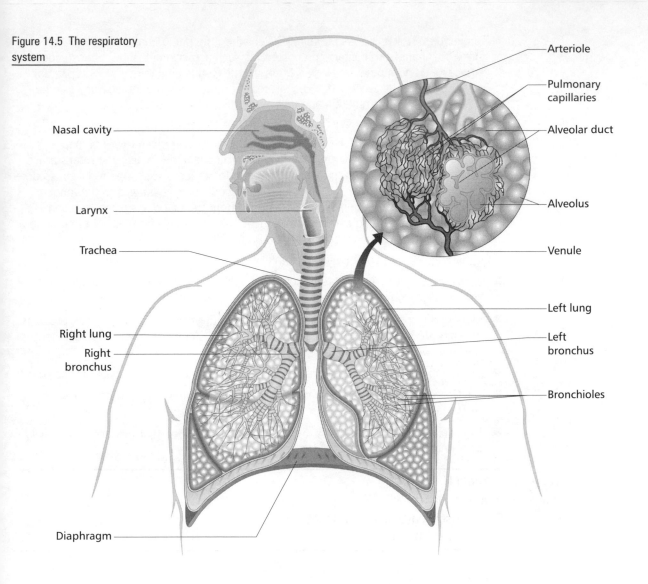

Figure 14.5  The respiratory system

Arteriole

Pulmonary capillaries

Nasal cavity

Alveolar duct

Alveolus

Larynx

Trachea

Venule

Left lung

Right lung

Left bronchus

Right bronchus

Bronchioles

Diaphragm

The second stage of breathing is when the diaphragm and intercostal muscles relax, decreasing the size of the chest cavity. This pushes air out of the lungs and into the atmosphere. This is called exhalation and its function is to excrete carbon dioxide from the body.

Internal or cellular respiration takes place in the body cells. Oxygen and glucose react together to form carbon dioxide, water and energy.

Physiological disorders of the respiratory system include asthma and emphysema.

### *Asthma*

The respiratory tract of people with asthma is very sensitive and when irritated, becomes swollen and narrow, its muscles tighten and there is usually an increase in the production of mucus. As a result, the chest feels tight, it becomes hard to get enough breath and the person coughs and wheezes.

The treatment for asthma includes:

■ relievers, which are inhaled during an asthma attack. Inhalers containing salbutamol and terbutaline (beta-2 agonists) deliver a small dose of drug directly to the lungs. This causes the muscles of the respiratory tract to relax and dilate (open up). Relievers don't reduce inflammation.

- preventers, which are used regularly, even when the person has no symptoms. They are also inhaled and contain corticosteroids such as beclometasone, budesonide, fluticasone and mometasone, which are used to reduce inflammation and prevent symptoms such as wheezing and shortness of breath. Steroid tablets may also be used to reduce inflammation and improve the way the lungs work.

### *Emphysema*

In emphysema, the walls of the alveoli break down, creating much larger air sacs in the lungs and reducing their elasticity. The larger the air sacs, the smaller the total surface area available for gaseous exchange. As the area for gaseous exchange reduces, so does the amount of oxygen that can diffuse into the blood from the lungs and the amount of carbon dioxide that can diffuse into the lungs from the blood. As a result, blood becomes oxygen-poor and carbon dioxide-rich. This results in shortness of breath and a reduced amount of oxygen reaching all the body cells.

Lung damage caused by emphysema can't be cured. Treatment includes:

- beta-2 agonists and bronchodiators, which are inhaled and dilate the respiratory tract, making breathing more easy

- alpha-antitrypsin replacement therapy. Alpha-antitrypsin is a protein which prevents an **enzyme** breaking down the walls of the alveoli. Alpha-antitrypsin replacement therapy may be used if the person has a deficiency of the protein.

- oxygen therapy, which can prevent death from hypoxia (a lack of oxygen in the blood)

- physiotherapy and exercise, which can help improve breathing and drain away any fluid that builds up in the lungs

- lung volume reduction surgery, which removes lung tissue that has lost its elasticity and so improves breathing.

Asthma UK

www.asthma.org.uk

**The British Heart Foundation**

www.bhf.org.uk

Figure 14.6 Relieving the symptoms of asthma

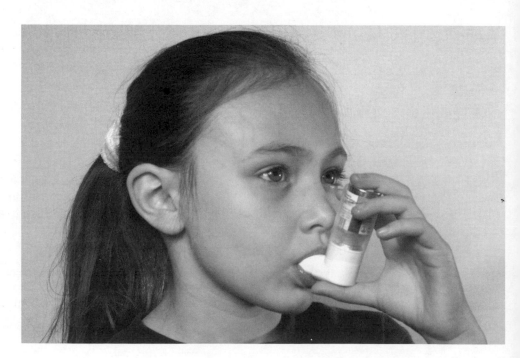

## The skeletal system

The human skeletal system is made up of about 206 bones. Its function is to protect and support the body's tissues and organs, provide a framework for muscles and enable locomotion (movement). In addition, bone marrow, which is a spongy material that fills some of the bones, produces **stem cells** which develop into the different types of blood cells you read about earlier.

Bone is made from bone cells (osteocytes), which multiply to replace old and damaged bone cells, and contains blood vessels and nerve cells. Bone cells are held together by a framework of non-living material comprised of tough, flexible protein fibres and hard deposits of minerals. Bone can either be compact or spongy. Compact bone is very dense and hard whilst spongy bone is lightweight due to the presence of spaces between the cells.

The strength and rigidity of bone is maintained by a supply of the minerals calcium and phosphorus, which are absorbed from the blood. The amount of calcium and phosphorus laid down in bones is controlled by growth and sex hormones. Changes in hormone levels can therefore affect the size and strength of bones.

Bones are covered at their ends by cartilage, which is a soft, smooth substance that allows smooth movement as well as acting as a shock absorber. Joints are formed when one bone articulates or connects with another. Bones of a joint are held together by bundles of tough fibres called ligaments, and between the bones of a synovial joint is a capsule that contains oily synovial fluid, which acts as a lubricant to reduce friction.

Physiological disorders of the skeletal system include osteoporosis and RA.

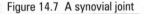

Figure 14.7 A synovial joint

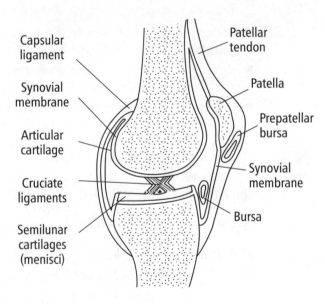

Capsular ligament

Synovial membrane

Articular cartilage

Cruciate ligaments

Semilunar cartilages (menisci)

Patellar tendon

Patella

Prepatellar bursa

Synovial membrane

Bursa

### *Osteoporosis*

From around the age of 35, more bone cells are lost than are replaced, which causes bone to become thinner and weaker. Osteoporosis is the name of the disorder associated with thin, weak, brittle bones. It happens more commonly in old age, as the body is less able to replace worn out bone, and in post-menopausal women.

There are a number of different treatments available for osteoporosis:

■ hormone replacement therapy (HRT). The female hormone oestrogen offers some protection against osteoporosis. After the menopause, oestrogen levels fall, often causing bones to thin quickly. HRT helps maintain bone density while the treatment lasts.

- Selective Estrogen Receptor Modulators (SERMs), which are drugs that work in a similar way to oestrogen.

- testosterone treatment. Osteoporosis can also occur because of insufficient male sex hormones. Testosterone treatment can be useful for men where this is the case.

- bisphosphonates, which also maintain bone density. They work by slowing down the rate at which bone cells break down and increasing the production of new bone.

- calcitonin, which is a hormone made by the thyroid gland and which inhibits the break down of bone

- calcium and vitamin D supplements. Calcium is necessary for strong, healthy bones, and vitamin D promotes the uptake of calcium by bones from the blood.

## RA

RA is an **auto-immune** disease. The normal function of the immune system is to produce antibodies that attack bacteria and viruses. In rheumatoid arthritis the immune system produces antibodies that attack the linings of the joints, making the joints become inflamed, swollen, stiff and painful. Over time, the inflammation can damage the joint, cartilage and bone near to the joint. In addition, tendons that attach bones to muscles can become inflamed.

Treatment of rheumatoid arthritis includes:

- Disease Modifying Antirheumatic Drugs (DMARDs), which slow down the disease and prevent joint damage

- Nonsteroidal Anti-Inflammatory Drugs (NSAIDs), which control pain and stiffness and reduce inflammation but don't slow the course of the disease

- corticosteroids, which are effective at reducing pain, stiffness and swelling but don't slow the progress of the disease or prevent joint damage

- cytokine inhibitors, which slow down the disease and prevent joint damage. They work by blocking the effects of cytokines, which are proteins that cause inflammation.

- surgery, which can be used to relieve severe pain and to correct joint problems. Joints in the body can also be partly or totally replaced e.g. knee and hip joints.

The National Osteoporosis Society
www.nos.org.uk
The National Rheumatoid Arthritis Society
www.rheumatoid.org.uk

## The nervous system

There are two parts to the nervous system:

1. The Central Nervous System (CNS), which consists of the brain and spinal cord. Different areas or centres of the CNS are concerned with different functions such as speech, hearing, smell, sight, movement, balance and maintenance of heart rate, blood pressure etc. Some of these centres are concerned with the information coming into the brain (sensory areas) and others are concerned with information leaving it for other parts of the body (motor centres).

2. The Peripheral Nervous System (PNS), the function of which is to relay information to and from different parts of the body via the brain and spinal cord.

The nervous system is made up of millions of neurones (nerve cells). Their role is to transfer information in the form of electrical signals from one part of the body to another. Neurones have:

- a cell body

- an axon sheathed in a fatty material called myelin. The myelin sheath acts as insulation, enabling nerve cells to conduct electrical signals without interfering with each another.

- tiny branches called dendrites on the cell body and at the end of the axon. The purpose of dendrites is to allow neurones to communicate with each other. However, the dendrites of one neurone don't actually touch the dendrites of another. For this reason there is no electrical connection between nerve cells. Instead, messages are passed across the gap between neurones i.e. the synapse by chemicals called neurotransmitters.

There are three types of neurone:

1. sensory neurons, which pass information about **stimuli** such as light, heat, touch and chemicals, from the internal (inside the body) and external (outside the body) environments to the central nervous system

2. motor neurons, which pass instructions from the central nervous system to parts of the body such as muscles or glands, causing them to respond to the stimuli

3. association or intermediate neurons, which connect sensory and motor neurons in the brain and spinal cord.

Figure 14.8 Neurones and synapses

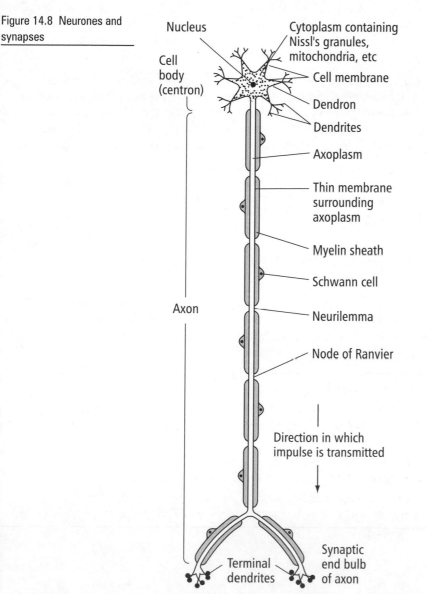

Nucleus

Cytoplasm containing Nissl's granules, mitochondria, etc

Cell body (centron)

Cell membrane

Dendron

Dendrites

Axoplasm

Thin membrane surrounding axoplasm

Myelin sheath

Schwann cell

Axon

Neurilemma

Node of Ranvier

Direction in which impulse is transmitted

Terminal dendrites

Synaptic end bulb of axon

Physiological disorders of the nervous system include Alzheimer's disease, Parkinson's disease, Multiple Sclerosis (MS) and Motor Neurone Disease (MND).

### Alzheimer's disease

Alzheimer's disease is a progressive disease and is the result of clumps and bundles ('plaques' and 'tangles') of certain proteins both inside and outside the brain cells. These clumps and bundles gradually destroy the connections between cells that are essential for normal mental activity.

There is no cure for Alzheimer's disease but treatments include:

- drugs such as donepezil, rivastigmine and galantamine, which slow down the progress of the condition in some people
- antioxidants, brain stem cell therapy and a vaccination, which are currently under investigation as they may help to stop the build up of plaques in the brain
- mood-controlling drugs (tranquillisers) and other forms of medication that can reduce the behavioural problems associated with Alzheimer's disease.

### Parkinson's disease

Parkinson's disease is caused by loss of dopamine, the neurotransmitter produced in the part of the brain that controls movement.

There is no cure for Parkinson's disease, but treatment includes drugs that increase the level of dopamine in the brain, stimulate the parts of the brain where dopamine works, or block the action of chemicals that affect, inhibit or break down dopamine.

### MS

MS occurs when there is a loss and/or scarring of the myelin sheath surrounding neurones. This is called demyelination. Where myelin is lost or damaged, electrical messages cannot travel normally from the brain to different parts of the body, which results in the signs and symptoms you read about earlier. There is also some evidence to suggest that MS is an autoimmune disorder, where antibodies attack and destroy the myelin sheath.

Treatments for MS include disease modifying drugs that can reduce the number and severity of MS **relapses** and scarring of the myelin sheath. MS disease modifying drugs are beta interferon 1a, beta interferon 1b and glatiramer acetate. In addition, corticosteroids can be taken to help reduce any inflammation; mitoxantrone and azathioprine to quieten down the immune system and reduce the number of relapses; and immunoglobin and plasma exchange, which can reduce disability.

### MND

MND is a highly debilitating disease that damages and kills the motor neurones in the brain and spinal cord. Evidence suggests that the neurones are killed or damaged by an overproduction of the neurotransmitter glutamate. There is no cure for MND. However, the drug Riluzole (Rilutek) can slow its progress, as can vitamin E.

The Alzheimer's Association

www.alzheimers.org.uk

The Parkinson's Disease Association

www.parkinsons.org.uk

The Multiple Sclerosis Society

www.mssociety.org.uk

The Motor Neurone Disease Association

www.mndassociation.org

## The digestive system

The function of the digestive system is to break food down into molecules of nutrients that are small enough to be absorbed into the blood. The digestive system consists of the intestine and a number of organs that produce digestive enzymes:

- the mouth, where chewing softens and moistens food and an enzyme in saliva commences the break down of carbohydrates

- the oesophagus, which receives chewed food from the mouth and propels it towards the stomach by muscular movements known as peristalsis

- the stomach, a muscular bag that further churns the food and secretes an enzyme that starts the digestion of proteins, and an acid that enables the enzyme to function and kills bacteria

- the small intestines, pancreas, liver and gall bladder, which produce enzymes that continue and complete the digestion of carbohydrates, proteins and fats. The nutrients produced – glucose, amino acids, fatty acids and glycerol are absorbed from the small intestine into the blood.

- the large intestine or colon, which is where undigested material from the small intestine passes and is stored. Absorption into the blood of any remaining nutrients and excess water also takes place in the colon

- the rectum, from which faeces are expelled from the body.

Physiological disorders of the digestive system include the inflammatory bowel diseases, Crohn's disease and ulcerative colitis.

Figure 14.9 The digestive system

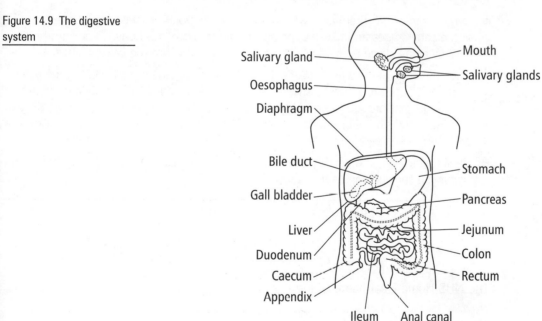

### Crohn's disease

Crohn's disease usually affects the lower part of the small intestine or the colon. Affected areas are red and swollen and sometimes ulcerated. As the ulcers heal, scar tissue forms that narrows the intestine, leading to obstructions.

### Ulcerative colitis

Ulcerative colitis is an ulcerated, inflammatory disease of the lining of the rectum and, sometimes, the colon.

Treatment for inflammatory bowel diseases includes:

■ corticosteroids, to reduce inflammation

■ antibiotics, in the event that there is an infection

■ aminosalicylates which can provide long-term relief from the symptoms of ulcers

■ laxatives and antidiarrhoeals, to help pass faeces or control diarrhoea

■ surgery, to remove damaged portions of the intestine and to treat obstructions, perforations and blood loss.

### Cancer

The body is made up of millions of cells, each of which is able to grow and multiply to replace old and damaged cells. A cancer develops when cells become 'abnormal' because they don't know when to stop multiplying. When a group of these rapidly multiplying cells clump together they form a 'tumour'. Benign tumours don't invade or spread to other parts of the body, whereas malignant tumours grow very quickly, invading and damaging nearby tissues and organs. They may even spread to other parts of the body and cause secondary tumours.

The circulatory system explains why some cancers nearly always spread to the same place. For example, cancers of the colon often spread to the liver, because blood circulates from the colon through the liver on its way back to the heart. If there is a cancer in the colon and some cancer cells escape into the circulation, they may stick in the liver as the blood passes through and begin to grow into a secondary cancer.

Treatment for cancer includes surgery, chemotherapy and radiation:

■ Surgical removal is the main treatment for most tumours, especially when they are in the early stages and haven't spread to other areas of the body. Some surrounding healthy areas of the body may also be removed to prevent the cancer returning.

■ Chemotherapy aims to kill cancer cells, stop them spreading or shrink the tumour to make it easier to remove. Chemotherapy works by attacking rapidly multiplying cells. Cells that produce hair and that line the mouth and intestines grow and divide rapidly, so the side affects of chemotherapy include hair loss, mouth sores, sickness and diarrhoea.

■ Radiotherapy aims to destroy cancerous cells with radiation from X-rays without damaging surrounding healthy tissue.

**National Association for Colitis & Crohn's Disease**
www.nacc.org.uk
**NHS Direct**
www.nhsdirect.nhs.uk
**The NHS Home Healthcare Guide**
www.surgerydoor.co.uk
**Net Doctor**
www.netdoctor.co.uk
**Patient UK**
www.patient.co.uk

## Influences on the development of disorders

There are a number of influences on the development of physiological disorders, as the following examples highlight.

### Lifestyle choices

Lifestyle choices can affect the development of physiological disorders in a variety of ways.

- We all know that smoking and passive smoking can harm our health. They contribute to arteriosclerosis, raised blood pressure (BP) and thrombosis, increasing the risk of disorders associated with the circulatory system. They also cause disorders of the respiratory system and are strongly linked with cancer of the mouth, tongue, throat and lungs.

- Excessive use of alcohol also raises blood pressure, causing disorders of the circulatory system. It damages the liver, causing problems in the digestive system, and is thought to be linked to conditions such as osteoarthritis.

- Physical activity. Regular exercise burns off excess calories, reduces blood pressure and cholesterol levels, strengthens the bones and improves the efficiency of the lungs. For these reasons, exercise reduces the risk of disorders associated with the circulatory, respiratory and skeletal systems.

- Mental activity. There is some evidence to suggest that staying mentally active can help reduce the risk of Alzheimer's disease.

- Where we live. According to research, the incidence of MS is greater in the temperate zones of the world than in the tropics, and asthma can be brought on by changes in the weather.

### Diet

Eating a diet that doesn't contain the recommended daily allowances of different food groups, or that contains excessive amounts of salt, cholesterol and sugar, can lead to nutritional deficiencies, obesity and raised blood pressure, which increase the risk of developing circulatory, respiratory and skeletal disorders. It can also reduce the effectiveness of the immune system and so increase the risk of acquiring viral infections thought to be associated with, for example, respiratory disorders, MS and Crohn's disease. In addition, some people find that certain foods increase their risk of developing inflammatory bowel disease and others, such as nuts and shellfish, cause allergies that trigger asthma.

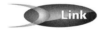 You will look more closely at diet in Unit 21.

> **remember**
>
> The role of a health or social care worker is to advise about, not dictate, healthy lifestyle choices.

Figure 14.10 Lifestyles

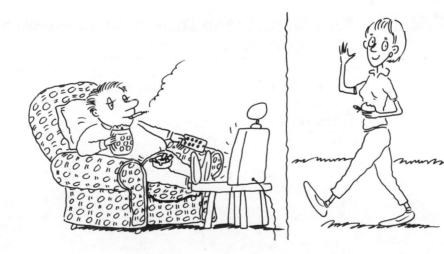

### Family

Some disorders are inherited and run in the family, for example NID diabetes, asthma, Alzheimer's disease, MND, breast cancer and inflammatory bowel disease. Yet others are linked with our gender, for example, RA and osteoporosis are more likely to occur in women than in men.

### Environment

The risk of developing respiratory disorders is increased by environmental factors such as bacteria and viruses, tobacco smoke and fumes from such things as cleaning products and vehicular exhausts. Asthma is often triggered by **allergens** found in the environment, for example, animal fur, pollen and house dust mite droppings; and exposure to ultra-violet (UV) radiation (sunlight) is known to cause skin cancer.

### Employment

Employment can expose people to industrial pollution and chemicals such as solvents and pesticides, which are associated with disorders of the respiratory and nervous systems such as emphysema and MND. Working with radiation – UV and X-rays – can cause cancers.

Patient UK

www.patient.co.uk

Government website promoting healthy living

www.healthyliving.gov.uk

Government website promoting healthy living

www.direct.gov.uk

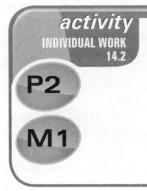

*activity*

**INDIVIDUAL WORK**
**14.2**

**P2**

**M1**

Look back at the two disorders you began to investigate for Activity 14.1. Develop your knowledge and understanding of each disorder by researching:

- its physiology.
- how its course or progression relates to its physiology.
- the factors that could have influenced its development in the individuals concerned.

Use both primary and secondary research methods and use your findings to produce a report for students studying a level 3 health and social care course.

# The processes involved in diagnosis of disorders

The processes involved in making a diagnosis of a physiological disorder include referrals, investigations, tests and measurements.

## Referrals

In order to provide appropriate care to someone who has developed a physiological disorder, their condition needs to be diagnosed. Referral is to do with the ways that people gain access to professionals within the health care services who are qualified to make a diagnosis.

There are three main types of referral:

1. Self-referral, which is where we choose to seek the opinion of a health care professional ourselves. We self-refer when, for example, we go to see our GP because we don't feel well.

2. Professional referral, which is where we are put in contact with a health care service by a professional health care worker. For example, a GP will refer us to a specialist doctor if they feel we need more specialised care or don't have the expertise to diagnose our condition.

3. Third-party referral, which is where we are put in contact with a health care service by someone who is not a health care professional, such as a friend, neighbour, relative, employer or teacher.

The following table describes health care services and examples of professionals that work within them who are able to diagnose physiological disorders.

Table 14.2 Health care services and examples of professionals working within them who are able to diagnose physiological disorders

| Health care services | Examples of professionals able to diagnose physiological disorders |
|---|---|
| Primary health care services, which are often the first point of contact that patients make with the health service. Patients usually self-refer or are referred by a third party. | The primary health care team i.e. General Practitioners (GPs), GP practice and community nurses, school nurses, midwives, health visitors, dentists, opticians, pharmacists, NHS walk-in centre staff and NHS Direct. |
| Secondary health care services, to which patients are usually referred by a professional within the primary health care team. They include hospitals, the ambulance service and services for people with a range of mental health needs. | **Triage** nurses, specialist hospital doctors and consultants, surgeons, dermatologists, chiropodists/podiatrists, complementary health therapists, speech therapists, occupational therapists, psychologists, mental health care specialists, pathologists, radiologists and special education and training staff. |
| Tertiary care, the third stage of investigation and treatment, which is usually provided in highly specialised centres and hospitals. Patients may be referred to tertiary care by primary or secondary health care specialists. | Highly specialised staff such as those working in hospices and those giving **critical care.** |

Department of Health
www.dh.gov.uk

# Investigations

A number of different investigations are used to diagnose physiological disorders. The type of investigation used depends on the individual concerned but can involve one or more of the following.

## Medical history

Taking a medical history involves a question-and-answer session between the health professional and the patient. A medical history is a very important diagnostic tool because it provides information that can help identify the cause and nature of the disorder. The information necessary for a medical history includes details about:

- the patient's age and sex. Many disorders are age- or sex-related.

- their signs and symptoms i.e. what is happening to their body that makes them think they may be ill, how they feel and how their signs and symptoms affect their day-to-day living

- whether they have experienced these signs and symptoms before

- whether anyone in their close family has a history of similar signs and symptoms. As you read earlier, some disorders are inherited and run in the family.

- their lifestyle, for example, whether they smoke, how much alcohol they drink, how much exercise they take, what they eat on a regular basis, their occupation and where they live. As you know, lifestyle, diet, employment and occupation can influence the development of a disorder.

Sometimes it can be difficult to establish a patient's medical history. For example, patients who have a limited vocabulary such as small children and those who have a learning difficulty or who don't use English as their first language may not understand questions or be able to express themselves adequately. In addition, patients who have difficulty talking, such as those who have a speech impediment, have had a stroke, are confused, have a hearing impairment, and patients who have difficulty remembering or who are anxious when visiting a health care professional may not be able to supply information that is asked of them. Health care professionals need to be alert to communication barriers and know how to overcome them.

Communication barriers are described in Unit 1 of Health and Social Care Book 1.

Figure 14.11 Establishing a medical history

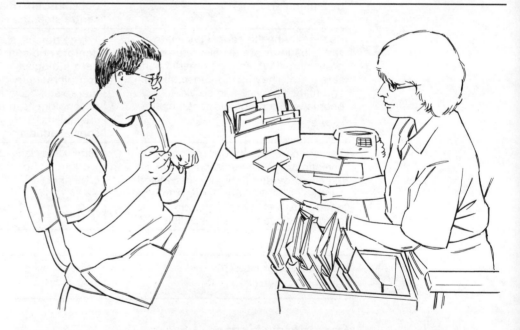

After taking a medical history, the health care professional may examine the patient to look for clues that will help them make their diagnosis. Examinations often include palpation.

## Palpation

If something is palpable, it can be touched or felt. **Palpation** is used to detect, for example:

- a raised body temperature, by feeling the forehead

- lumps in soft body tissues, for example in the breasts and testicles

- swellings in joints, for example in the spine and hands
- heart rate, by feeling the pulse.

Palpation can cause discomfort and pain, for example feeling for swellings in joints. And internal examinations such as vaginal and rectal, and feeling for lumps in sensitive, private areas such as the breasts and testicles, can cause anxiety and embarrassment. Patients can be helped by health care professionals who have a gentle hand and a sensitive attitude.

## Tests

### Blood tests

Blood is tested for a number of different reasons, for example to check for:

- blood group. Knowing a patient's blood group is essential if they need a blood transfusion or want to give blood

- antibodies. Antibodies are specific to the infection they fight, therefore the presence of antibodies identifies the presence of particular disorders, such as HIV. Checking for antibodies also identifies whether or not a patient has been vaccinated against a specific disorder, for example, rubella

- abnormal cells, for example sickle-shaped red cells indicate the presence of sickle cell anaemia

- numbers of cells and platelets. An abnormal count indicates the presence of a disorder, for example an increase in the number of white cells and a decrease in the number of red cells and platelets is associated with leukaemia

- cholesterol. As you know, high cholesterol levels cause arteriosclerosis, which leads to disorders of the circulatory system such as high blood pressure, angina and heart attacks

- sugar. Abnormal levels indicate a disorder, for example a raised blood sugar level suggests diabetes

- proteins. Again, abnormal levels indicate a disorder. For example, low protein levels can cause oedema, which is an accumulation of fluid in the body tissues. Oedema is a sign of a number of physiological disorders, including heart failure

- salts. The presence of high levels of salts such as potassium, sodium and urea in the blood can indicate that the kidneys aren't working properly

- DNA structure. By checking the DNA in blood, inherited diseases can be diagnosed. DNA can also be used for paternity testing i.e. to see if a man is the father of a particular child.

Some people are scared of needles and the sight of blood, and may feel faint when a sample of their blood is taken. They can be helped by being seated or lying down while the sample is taken. Others may be anxious that a blood test will confirm a diagnosis or predict the development of a disorder. As you will read shortly, counselling can be offered to help people come to terms with a diagnosis.

### Urine tests

Urine is produced in the kidneys and stored in the bladder. It is excreted to the outside of the body through the urinary tract. Urine testing is used to test for pregnancy, drugs and alcohol and to diagnose disorders such as:

- kidney disease and urinary tract infections. Blood in the urine can be a sign of disorders in the kidneys, bladder and urinary tract; protein can indicate kidney damage from diabetes; and bacteria can indicate infection such as cystitis.

- diabetes, which is signalled by the presence of glucose.

Although some urine samples need to be analysed in a laboratory, others can be tested very quickly using a strip of special paper that is dipped in the urine just after it has been passed. Some people need help to pass urine 'on demand', and may become embarrassed. A running tap, a drink of water and understanding staff can help. Counselling may also be offered to help patients who are anxious about their test results.

## Radiological investigations

Radiological investigations use electromagnetic radiation (EMR) or sound waves to scan and make images of tissues within the body, which can then be used to diagnose a range of physiological disorders. Radiological techniques include:

- X-rays. These are high energy particles that can penetrate most body tissues but are blocked by bone. They are used to create images that show up abnormalities in bone and certain other tissues, such as breast tissue. Some tissues such as the digestive tract and blood vessels don't show up on X-ray images. For this reason, substances like barium, through which X-rays can't pass and which make the area appear white, are swallowed or injected prior to an investigation.

- CAT (Computerised Axial Tomography) scans. CAT scans produce images similar to those produced using X-rays, but instead of using single X-rays, CAT scanners send several beams of rays from different angles so that pictures can be taken of an area of the body from different angles. CAT scans help diagnose many disorders, including cancers and disorders of the nervous system; and because CAT scanners can take pictures of moving parts of the body, they help diagnose disorders of organs such as the heart.

- PET (Positron Emission Tomography) scans. In PET scanning, a radiotracer attached to a chemical such as glucose is introduced into the body. The radiotracer goes to the part of the body where that chemical is used, where it breaks down, giving off particles called positrons and energy. This energy is used to make a 3-D image of activities going on inside the body where the chemical is used. PET scans are used to diagnose a range of conditions including cancer, Alzheimer's disease and Parkinson's disease.

- MRI (Magnetic Resonance Imaging) scans. When hydrogen atoms in water molecules in the body are exposed to strong magnets and radio waves from an MRI scanner, they give off a radio signal. This signal can be picked up by the radio-receiver in the scanner and converted into an image. Different types of body tissue contain different amounts of water, therefore the strength of the radio signal given off by different parts of the body varies. Because of this, during an MRI scan, detailed images from different parts of the body are created. MRI scans are commonly used to diagnose cancers and disorders of the nervous system such as MS and MND.

- Ultrasound. Ultrasound scanning uses sound waves that have very high frequencies. Different parts of the body have different densities and when ultrasound waves are directed at them, their different densities reflect the sound waves in different ways and the reflected waves are translated into an image. Ultrasound scanning is most commonly used to check on pregnant mothers and their unborn babies.

Scanning can cause patients great anxiety. In addition, although electromagnetic radiation is useful in diagnosing a number of disorders, it can be a health hazard. A risk assessment should always be carried out before exposing a patient to EMR.

Figure 14.12 Scanning as an aid to diagnosis

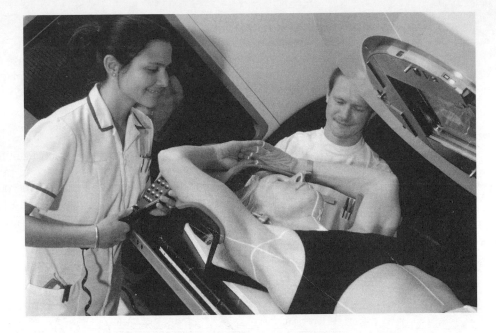

## Function tests

Body systems cease to function properly in the event of physiological disorders. Function tests assess how well different systems function and include:

- lung function tests. These assess lung volumes, the efficiency of the respiratory tract and gaseous exchange, and enable diagnoses to be made of different respiratory disorders.

- renal function tests. These require collection and assessment of urine over a 24-hour period and enable diagnoses to be made of different urinary disorders.

- cardiac function tests. These include chest X-rays, electrocardiograms (ECGs) and exercise tests, and enable diagnoses to be made of different circulatory disorders.

## Measurements

Some of the measurements used to diagnose physiological disorders are described below.

### Body mass index (BMI)

BMI is used as a guide to health and is calculated by dividing a person's weight in kilograms by the square of their height in metres. Obesity, which contributes to disorders of most of the body systems, is defined by a BMI of 30 or greater.

Table 14.3 BMI as a guide to health

| BMI | Comment |
| --- | --- |
| Less than 18.5 | Underweight |
| 18.5–24.9 | Ideal |
| 25–29.9 | Overweight |
| 30–40 | Obese |
| More than 40 | Very obese |

## Blood pressure (BP)

BP is a measure of the force that pumps blood from the heart, through the arteries, capillaries and veins and back to the heart. Although it increases with age and body weight, the expected range for an adult is between 90/60mmHg and 120/80mmHg. Anything either side of the expected range could indicate one or more physiological disorders.

## Peak flow

This is a measure of the efficiency of the respiratory tract. Peak flow readings vary according to age, sex, height, time of day and from person to person. However, anything above or below the published expected range can suggest the presence of a respiratory disorder, in particular asthma.

Figure 14.13 Measurements as an aid to diagnosis

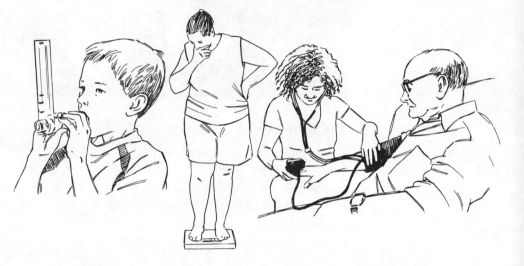

Some people become anxious when having to take part in function tests or have their weight, BP or peak flow measured. They need reassurance and encouragement. Risks associated with making measurements include faulty equipment and inaccurate recordings. When in doubt, even a competent worker should double check, by repeating the measurement or asking a colleague for a second opinion. And to avoid the risk of spread of infection where body fluids are concerned, health and safety procedures must be followed.

### Professional Practice

If you are involved in carrying out investigations and making measurements:

- be aware of communication barriers and try to overcome them
- be aware of how the patient feels and use your skills to support them and minimise their anxiety and discomfort
- make sure that any measurements you make are accurate
- always follow your organisation's health and safety procedures
- always follow your organisation's procedures for assessing risks.

Health and safety and risk assessment procedures are described in Unit 3 in Health and Social Care Book 1.

## Monitoring

As you read earlier, signs and symptoms change during the course of a physiological disorder. For this reason it is important to monitor a patient's condition on a regular basis. A change could mean recovery or remission, but it could also mean an increase in severity of the disorder. Unless changes are diagnosed, the patient will not receive appropriate care.

*i* NHS Direct
www.nhsdirect.nhs.uk

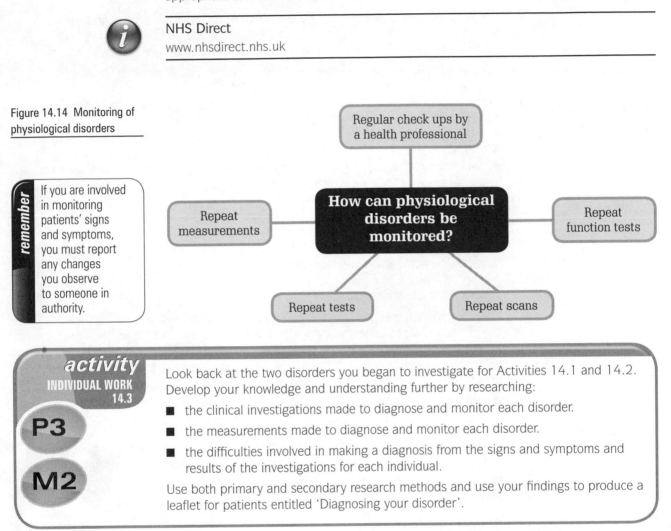

Figure 14.14 Monitoring of physiological disorders

**remember**
If you are involved in monitoring patients' signs and symptoms, you must report any changes you observe to someone in authority.

*Regular check ups by a health professional*

*Repeat measurements*

**How can physiological disorders be monitored?**

*Repeat function tests*

*Repeat tests*

*Repeat scans*

*activity*
**INDIVIDUAL WORK 14.3**

**P3**

**M2**

Look back at the two disorders you began to investigate for Activities 14.1 and 14.2. Develop your knowledge and understanding further by researching:

■ the clinical investigations made to diagnose and monitor each disorder.

■ the measurements made to diagnose and monitor each disorder.

■ the difficulties involved in making a diagnosis from the signs and symptoms and results of the investigations for each individual.

Use both primary and secondary research methods and use your findings to produce a leaflet for patients entitled 'Diagnosing your disorder'.

# The care strategies used to support individuals through the course of a disorder

The aim of this section is to introduce you to the strategies used to care for patients who have been diagnosed with a physiological disorder.

## Care settings accessed

Care setting is the term used to describe the location in which care is given.

### Own home

Most people who are experiencing or are disabled by a physiological disorder would choose to receive care in their own home, surrounded and comforted by familiar objects and where visiting is not restricted by busy hospital ward or care home schedules. Being at home supports a patient's rights and needs to be treated as an individual, to retain control of their life, to stay independent and care for themselves where possible, to make their own choices about how to be cared for by others, and to retain their privacy and dignity. With help from family and friends and from visiting health and social care professionals, many people can and do receive care at home, and with encouragement and support, learn to care for themselves.

## GP surgery or health centre

People who are ill or worried about their health or the health of anyone in their family should visit their National Health Service (NHS) GP surgery or health centre. GP surgeries and health centres are examples of primary health care service providers and every UK citizen has a right to be registered with a GP Surgery or Health Centre. They are usually the first point of contact that patients make with the health service.

Every surgery and health centre has a contractual agreement with its local Primary Care Trust (PCT). PCTs work with local health and social care organisations, outlining what services they must provide to ensure that the care needs of the community are met. GP surgeries and health centres look after and monitor the general health of people in the community, promoting health and wellbeing, disease prevention and self-help. When necessary, they refer patients to specialist health care professionals who work for secondary health care service providers.

## Hospital

NHS hospitals are examples of secondary health care service providers. They are run and managed by Acute Trusts, which make sure that they provide high quality health care and spend their money efficiently. They also decide on a strategy for how hospitals will develop, so that services can improve.

Hospitals provide specialised health care. Many people attend hospital with injuries that their GP is unable to treat, for example, as a result of a road traffic accident or in the event of an emergency such as a heart attack. Others are referred to hospital by their GP for specialised care, which is usually planned and **elective**, for example, cataract operations, hip replacements, kidney dialysis. Specialised care can be provided on an:

- outpatient basis, e.g. consultant appointments, clinics
- inpatient basis, where patients stay in hospital for e.g. investigations, surgery
- day case basis. Day case treatment includes procedures that are minimally invasive, such as keyhole surgery, and that allow patients to go home on the same day.

Foundation trusts are a new type of NHS hospital that are managed locally and meet the needs of the local population. They are an example of **decentralisation**.

## Social care settings

Social care settings include care homes and day centres. Care homes provide round-the-clock care for people for whom care in their own home is not possible, such as elderly people, people who are physically disabled, people who have mental health problems and people who are terminally ill. There are three main types of care homes:

1. homes with nursing. They used to be called nursing homes.
2. homes without nursing, which provide help with personal care such as bathing and dressing. They used to be called residential homes.
3. homes that offer both residential and nursing care.

Day care centres are located within the community and provide care for people who live at home but have been assessed by their Local Authority Social Services Departments as having special needs that affect their day-to-day living, for example physical disability, learning difficulty, and mental health problems such as memory loss. The services that day care centres provide include activities that are aimed at helping people maintain their independence, which in turn helps them to remain in their own homes for as long as possible.

Royal College of General Practitioners
www.rcgp.org.uk
Department of Health
www.dh.gov.uk

# People

There are over a million people working in the NHS, including over 30,000 GPs, 27,000 consultants and 370,000 nurses. They each have their own role to play in supporting patients with physiological disorders, which includes giving professional advice and supporting patients in managing their disorder.

## General Practitioners

General Practitioners (GPs) talk to and examine patients in their surgeries or in the patient's own home, with a view to diagnosing their disorders. When they have made a diagnosis, they may give professional advice to the patient, describe how the patient can contribute to managing their disorder, prescribe medication or treatment or carry out minor surgical operations. If they are unable to make a diagnosis or give treatment, they refer the patient to a specialist for further investigations. They also monitor the course of patients' disorders, through repeat visits and working with other professionals who are involved in the care team, such as nurses, health visitors, midwives, physiotherapists, dieticians, counsellors and administrative support staff.

## Clinical specialists

Clinical specialists have an in-depth knowledge and expertise of a particular area of physiology. Their role is to investigate, diagnose and prescribe treatment for patients who have been referred by their GPs, give professional advice to patients and their GPs, and ensure that the disorder is managed by monitoring its course, for example, through repeat consultations and investigations and adapting treatment regimes where necessary.

## Nurses

There are four branches of nursing: adult, child, learning disability and mental health. Nurses work in the community, for example in people's own homes, GP surgeries and health centres, care homes, NHS walk-in centres, schools, rehabilitation centres and prisons; and in hospitals.

In general, nurses assess, plan and implement health care; and they monitor the course of disorders through observation and evaluation of the patient's progress, adapting care regimes where necessary and in consultation with doctors. They may also counsel patients and their relatives. Examples of practical care that nurses give include:

■ health screening, e.g. taking measurements of weight, temperature, BP and peak flow, taking blood and urine samples

■ giving drugs, injections and immunisations and treating routine injuries e.g. cleaning and dressing wounds

■ assisting doctors with physical examinations and operations

■ administering blood transfusions and drips

■ promoting health and wellbeing through diabetes, asthma, sexual health, ante-natal and child health clinics, and helping patients to give up smoking or lose weight

■ giving professional advice to patients and support for managing their disorder as it progresses.

Figure 14.15 The main areas
of clinical specialism

Psychiatry. Psychiatrists work with patients who have mental health problems, prescribing drugs and treatment.

Medicine, i.e. the treatment of medical conditions and emergencies. Specialisms include cardiology, neurology, oncology, orthopaedics and radiology.

Surgery. Surgeons are responsible for patients before, during and after operations. Specialisms include cardiothoracic surgery, orthopaedics and neurosurgery.

**The main areas of clinical specialism**

Pathology. Pathologists diagnose disease by examining body tissues. For example, histopathologists diagnose disease from changes in the structure of tissues, chemical pathologists from biochemical changes in tissues, molecular geneticists from abnormalities in DNA and chromosomes, and medical microbiologists from micro-organisms present in tissues.

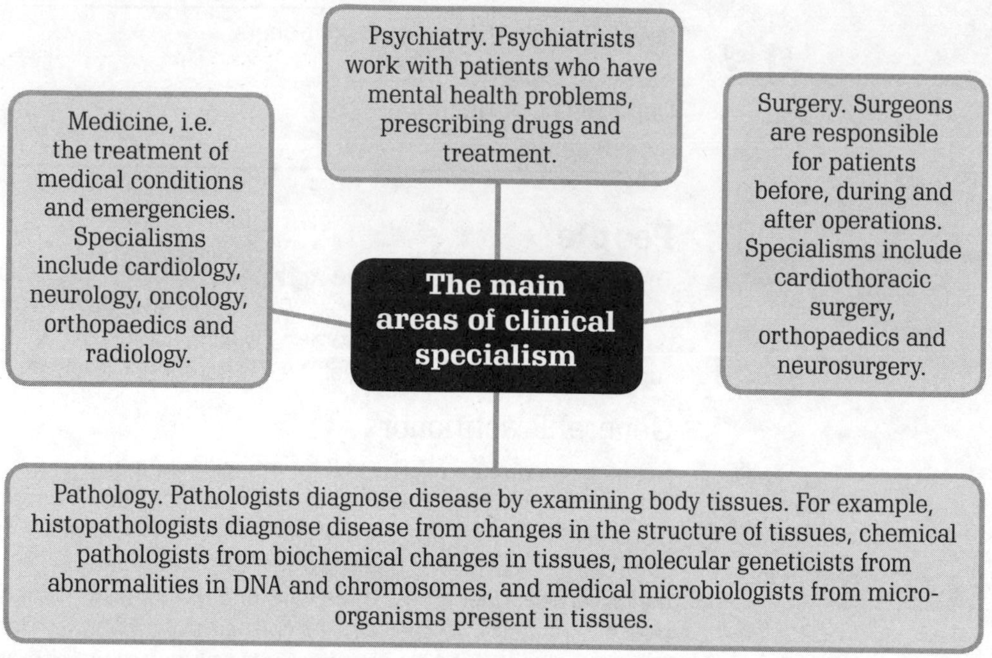

## Other professionals

Professionals allied to medicine include:

- physiotherapists, who assess and treat people with physical problems or disabilities caused by, for example, ageing and accidents
- occupational therapists, who use specific, purposeful activities to help people overcome the effects of disability, which promotes their independence in their day to day life
- chiropodists/podiatrists, who diagnose and treat disorders of the feet
- dieticians/nutritionists, who work with people to promote their nutritional wellbeing
- dance, drama, art and play therapists, who work with a range of people to help improve their physical, intellectual, emotional and social wellbeing
- speech and language therapists, who work with people with communication and/or swallowing problems
- prosthetists, who provide care, advice and artificial replacements for people who have lost or were born without a limb
- orthotists, who design and fit **orthoses**, for example braces and callipers
- orthoptists, who diagnose and treat disorders of the eyes
- psychologists, who help reduce the psychological distress caused by, for example, illness and depression.

## Pharmacists

Pharmacists specialise in the area of drugs (medicines). They work in industry, researching and developing new medicines; in the community, for example in shops, selling medicines over the counter; and in hospitals. Community pharmacists work with GPs, supporting patients through the course of their disorders by monitoring the effectiveness of their medication. And both community and hospital pharmacists prepare medication from prescriptions, give patients professional advice and information on how to use their medicines correctly, and work with other staff to keep them informed of new developments in the drug industry.

## Radiographers

As you read earlier, radiological techniques are used to diagnose a range of physiological disorders. Radiographers also use radiological techniques, for example X-rays, to treat disorders such as malignant tumours and tissue defects. Their work involves planning and delivering prescribed treatment, and assessing and monitoring patients before, during and after the course of treatment. Radiographers work as part of a multidisciplinary team alongside other health care professionals, for example radiologists, oncologists, physicists and radiologists.

## Medical laboratory assistants (MLAs)

Medical laboratory assistants, sometimes known as clinical support workers, work throughout the NHS in clinics, hospitals and laboratories, providing support to a range of different medical staff. They can specialise or work across a number of different areas, for example:

- biochemistry, which involves studying chemical reactions in the body and their link with physiological disorders

- cytology, which is the study of body cells and their link with physiological disorders

- histopathology, which is the study of diseased tissue

- haematology, which is the study of blood

- immunology, which is the study of the immune system and its link with physiological disorders such as allergies

- virology, which is the study of viruses and the diseases they cause

- transfusion science, which is to do with transferring blood and blood products from one person to another. You will read more about blood transfusions shortly.

MLAs can also work as phlebotomists, whose role is to take blood from patients and deliver it to a laboratory for analysis.

Figure 14.16 People who deliver care

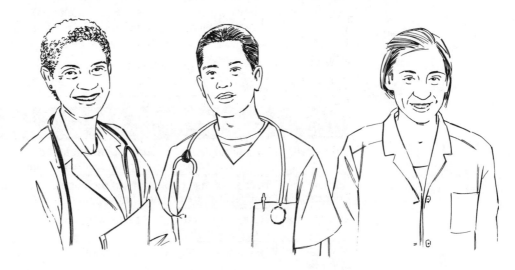

Being diagnosed with a chronic, possibly life threatening disorder can cause severe stress, distress, anxiety and depression. Many people go through a number of stages as they adjust to their diagnosis and new way of life.

Stage 1 is where they refuse to accept their illness or disability. This is called being in denial.

Stage 2 is where they are angry about their situation, often asking 'Why me?' and looking for something or someone to blame.

Stage 3 is where they become anxious, depressed, despairing.

Stage 4 is where they begin to come to terms with their disorder and its impact on their life.

## Counsellors

Counselling is offered by the NHS in GP surgeries, health centres and hospitals. Counsellors work with patients who have difficulty adjusting to a physiological disorder and/or disability and who are anxious or depressed. They help and support them in a safe and non-threatening environment by:

- exploring the problems caused by their situation

- helping them to understand their problems and see their situation from a different perspective

- helping them find their own solutions and develop a lifestyle in which they can cope.

Independent or voluntary organisations also offer counselling for relationship and family problems, anger management, smoking cessation, drug abuse, bereavement and so on.

## Health care assistants (HCAs)

Health care assistants, also known as nursing assistants and nursing auxiliaries, work in hospitals, care homes and patients' own homes, supporting patients and other health care professionals with their day-to-day care activities. For example, they talk to patients and help them wash, eat, dress and go to the toilet; they escort patients between different hospital departments; they make beds and help keep the ward or bedroom tidy; they collect and test urine samples; and they make routine measurements such as temperature, pulse and respiration rates.

## Care assistants

Care assistants, sometimes known as care workers, support people who are disabled, people who have learning difficulties, older people and so on with their day-to-day activities. They work in a variety of social care settings, such as people's own homes, care homes and day care centres. Personal Assistants (PAs) work on a one-to-one basis with people who are disabled, supporting them in their day-to-day life. The main role of a care assistant and PA is to get to know the people they work with so that they can help meet their basic needs.

Table 14.4  Basic needs

| Basic needs | Examples of basic needs |
|---|---|
| Physical needs | To be mobile (get about), move, eat and drink, rest and sleep, be warm, be comfortable, see and hear, be free of pain and take medication. |
| Social needs | To feel a sense of belonging, participate in group activities and maintain contact with friends and family. |
| Emotional needs | To be approved of, feel respected and loved, and to be able to give love and affection to others. |
| Intellectual needs | To communicate, be independent, be stimulated and be creative. |
| Cultural needs | To have one's values, expectations and dietary preferences respected, and to be free to observe religious requirements, practices and festivals. |

Care assistants and PAs also have to be willing to support patients with their personal care such as bathing, using the toilet, dressing and feeding; and to undertake general tasks such as housework, laundry and shopping.

## Informal carers or lay carers

Informal carers or lay carers are usually family members, friends and neighbours, who receive no payment for the care and support they give. Their place within the health care team is extremely important because their knowledge of the patient and how their disorder affects their day-to-day life is usually much greater than that of the health professionals. In addition, they have access to a wealth of information and support provided by numerous self-help groups that they can use to promote the patient's health and wellbeing.

Learndirect
www.learndirect.co.uk
Skills for Care
www.skillsforcare.org.uk

# Care

## Medication

People with physiological disorders receive care in a number of ways. You read previously about the different types of medication that are used to treat signs and symptoms. Note that disorders of different body systems may have similar signs and symptoms but because they have different causes are treated differently; and that different disorders of the same body system are not necessarily treated in the same way because they can present different signs and symptoms.

However, to recap, medication that is used to treat disorders of the:

■ circulatory system includes pain relievers, anti-inflammatories, drugs that strengthen the heart, and drugs that reduce the heart rate, blood pressure, blood glucose and cholesterol levels, and risk of plaques and blood clots.

■ respiratory system includes anti-inflammatories, oxygen and protein-replacement therapy, and drugs that relax and open up the respiratory tract.

■ skeletal system includes pain relievers, anti-inflammatories, hormone replacement therapy and drugs that slow down the course of the disorder and the breakdown of bone.

■ nervous system includes pain relievers, anti-inflammatories, disease modifying drugs, and drugs that control mood, increase the levels and functioning of dopamine, slow down the course of the disorder, prevent the build up of plaques in the brain and dampen down the effect of the immune system.

■ digestive system includes anti-inflammatories, antibiotics, laxatives, antidiarrhoeals and drugs that provide relief from the symptoms of ulcers.

Medication that is used to treat cancers includes chemo- and radiotherapy, both of which aim to kill tumour cells.

## Aids

Some physiological disorders cause patients to have sensory and mobility problems and difficulty with everyday living activities such as getting about, eating and drinking, personal grooming, taking medication and using the toilet. There are a number of different aids that can be used to help in such situations, for example:

■ aids for seeing, hearing, writing and reading include, in addition to glasses and hearing aids, magnifiers, tape recordings, orthoses for holding pens, pen grips and gadgets for holding books open.

■ mobility aids, which support movement from one place to another, such as ramps, grab rails, scooters, wheelchairs, stair lifts, bath lifts, walking frames, crutches, walking sticks, bed and chair elevators.

■ moving and handling aids, such as hoists, glide sheets, transfer boards and belts, which assist others in helping patients who have limited mobility.

- aids for restricted movement or flexibility, particularly in the hands, wrists and fingers, which can make preparing food, eating and drinking, personal grooming etc. more comfortable and manageable, for example, trays and trolleys, kettle tippers, jar and bottle openers, adapted cutlery, crockery, scissors, clippers and hair brushes, zipper pulls, and aids for doing up buttons and pulling on socks and tights. Patients who are unable to eat and drink normally because of their disorder may be fed using percutaneous endoscopically-guided gastrostomy (PEG). PEG feeding involves the surgical insertion of a tube through the abdomen wall into the stomach.

- medication aids, such as pill crushers and tablet organisers, which help patients who are unable to swallow tablets and who have problems remembering to take their medication.

- aids for using the toilet, which include commodes, toilet frames, toilet rails, bed pans and urinals. Continence pads are useful for patients whose disorder makes it difficult for them to use the toilet normally.

## Surgery

Some physiological disorders require surgery.

Figure 14.17 The use of surgery as a care strategy

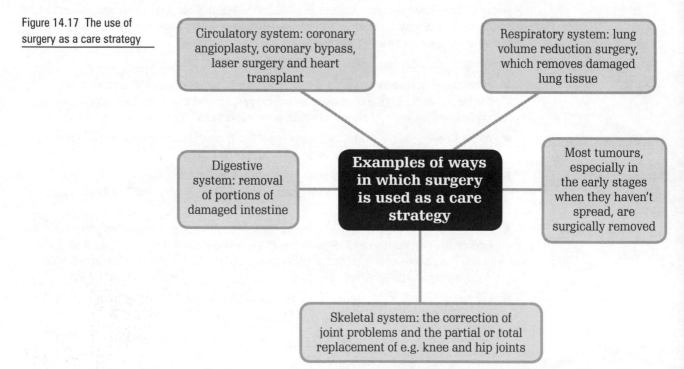

Circulatory system: coronary angioplasty, coronary bypass, laser surgery and heart transplant

Respiratory system: lung volume reduction surgery, which removes damaged lung tissue

Digestive system: removal of portions of damaged intestine

**Examples of ways in which surgery is used as a care strategy**

Most tumours, especially in the early stages when they haven't spread, are surgically removed

Skeletal system: the correction of joint problems and the partial or total replacement of e.g. knee and hip joints

## Blood transfusions

As you know, blood is essential to life: if our organs don't receive the oxygen and nutrients it carries, they fail to function properly, which can be fatal. Blood transfusion is the process of taking blood from one person and, in the event of massive blood loss, for example, as a result of an accident, giving it to another. More usually, however, it is the components of blood that are given to a patient. You will remember that the components of blood include red blood cells and platelets.

Red blood cells are used to:

- replace cells lost during surgery or in the event of haemorrhaging (heavy bleeding) within the body

- treat anaemia, a disorder in which where there is insufficient haemoglobin in the blood

- treat sickle cell disease
- replace broken down red cells in the blood of newborn babies.

Platelets are transfused to patients whose platelet count is low because, for example, they have been exposed to high doses of chemotherapy or they have had a bone marrow transplant.

Cells and platelets, along with dissolved nutrients, carbon dioxide, proteins and anti-bodies are transported around the body in a straw-coloured fluid called plasma. Plasma also contains chemicals that are important for blood clotting. It is therefore often transfused during surgery.

## Rehabilitation programmes

Rehabilitation programmes are used to improve symptoms and promote good health and are tailored to the needs of specific individuals. Teams of specialists are involved, such as GPs, nurses, physiotherapists, occupational therapists and speech therapists.

A rehabilitation programme prescribed for a patient with a disorder of the respiratory system would probably include exercises to increase their mobility and lung function, support for giving up smoking, which will help improve their breathing and reduce the risk of the disorder progressing, advice about diet, and information about the disorder to help them take control and improve their quality of life.

A rehabilitation programme prescribed for a patient who has had a stroke would include a variety of therapies to help them get back as much independence as possible. Physiotherapy in the form of exercise would play a major role, the type and amount depending on the seriousness of the stroke and the parts of the body that have been weakened. Occupational therapy would help the patient learn to use the parts of the body that have been weakened, and speech therapy would be used to help them make themselves understood. In addition, the programme might include advice about diet, support for giving up smoking, which would help reduce the risk of a further stroke, and counselling, to help them come to terms with any disabilities.

Figure 14.18 The role of rehabilitation programmes in care strategy

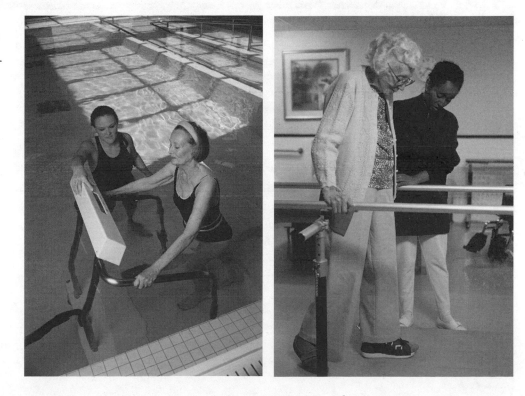

## Complementary therapies

Complementary therapies such as aromatherapy, acupuncture, hypnotherapy, chiropractic, herbal medicine, homeopathy, massage, osteopathy and different types of healing are increasingly being used alongside to complement conventional, scientific medicine. They are used to help in the treatment and prevention of a variety of disorders such as arthritis, asthma, digestive disorders, eczema, hay fever, the management of aches and pains, nausea and stress.

Unlike conventional medicine, which treats the part of the body that is affected by a physiological disorder, complementary medicine treats the whole person. Diagnosis takes into account a range of factors such as the patient's lifestyle, diet and environment, their relationships and their emotional (mental) health. Therapy is then tailored to the individual, with a view to relieving their signs and symptoms and promoting an improved feeling of health and wellbeing.

> **remember**
>
> Complementary therapies are designed to work alongside scientific medicine to help treat and prevent disorders, not cure them.

**NHS Direct**

www.nhsdirect.nhs.uk

**BBC website**

www.bbc.co.uk

---

**case study 14.2**

# Supporting individuals through the course of physiological disorders

Pippa, aged 16, has asthma; her mother, who is going through the menopause, has IDD diabetes; and her grandfather, who lives in a care home, has rheumatoid arthritis.

---

**activity**
**GROUP WORK**

1. What sort(s) of care might each individual receive and why?
2. Who could be supporting Pippa, her mother and her grandfather through the course of their disorders?

---

**activity**
**INDIVIDUAL WORK**
**14.4**

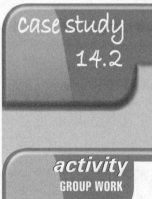

**P4**

Look back at the two disorders you investigated for Activities 14.1, 14.2 and 14.3. Develop your knowledge and understanding further by researching:

- the care processes or strategies experienced by the two individuals
- the roles of the different people involved in caring for them.

Use both primary and secondary research methods and use your findings to produce an information booklet for students studying a level 3 health and social care course who need to know about care strategies and the roles of people involved in supporting care strategies for them.

---

**activity**
**INDIVIDUAL WORK**
**14.5**

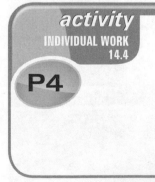

**D1**

Continue your studies by producing a PowerPoint presentation that evaluates the contributions made by the different people supporting the individuals with the disorders.

# How individuals adapt to the presence of a disorder

This section describes some of the difficulties patients face, how they can be helped to cope with their situation, and how their care may need to change as their disorder develops.

## Difficulties

Physiological disorders can make life very difficult. They can affect mobility and the ability to carry out everyday activities; they can disrupt the functioning of organs and body systems, which can be debilitating and cause relapses or long term ill health; they can have psychological effects, for example anxiety and depression; they can affect relationships between people; and they can impact on jobs and careers.

## Mobility

Mobility or movement is a fundamental human characteristic – it enables the body to act or react (behave). It is brought about by contraction and relaxation of muscles, which causes the bones to which they are attached to move, and which within the body causes, for example, facial expressions and movement of the contents of the intestines and of mucus in the respiratory tract. Movement is also brought about by bones articulating with each other in a joint.

Disorders that affect an individual's ability to move can have a profound disabling effect on their activities of daily living, for example:

- RA can make movement that involves joints, such as walking, bending, sitting, dressing, grooming, preparing food, doing housework, eating, driving etc. distressingly painful.

- MS, because it affects the neurones that deliver messages to muscles, makes balance and co-ordination difficult, movement clumsy and can cause problems with eating and drinking.

- CHD and respiratory disorders that prevent a sufficient supply of oxygen reaching the body tissues cause pain and breathlessness, which in turn impact on an individual's ability to carry out even the smallest of day-to-day activities.

Restricted movement can have a knock-on effect on an individual's relationships with others and their employment. For example, the breathlessness brought on by emphysema or the tremor and muscular rigidity or stiffness associated with Parkinson's disease can necessitate a change in job role; and it can mean a change in relationship, for example between a previously active grandfather and his young grandchildren with whom he is no longer able to play.

Individuals who suffer psychologically because of physiological disorders are also likely to experience changes in their relationships with other people. For example, sadness, suicidal thoughts and feelings, loss of energy, and personality changes such as low self-esteem, apathy, aggression, swings of emotion and isolation can make things difficult for family and friends, despite their caring natures. In addition, disorders such as Alzheimer's disease which include mood swings, confusion and changes in personality and behaviour can stretch relationships between individuals and their family and friends to their limits.

Figure 14.19 The difficulties caused by physiological disorders

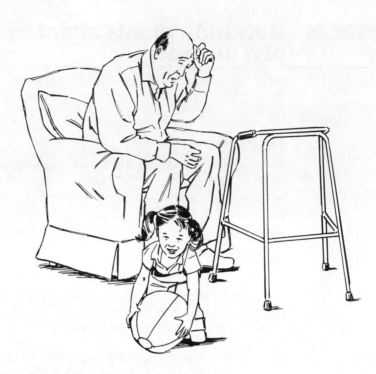

## Coping strategies

The issues that patients diagnosed with physiological disorders often have to cope with include:

■ their reactions to the diagnosis e.g. anger about what is happening now, fear about what the future may bring, worries about treatment and its side effects, loss of control and independence

■ anxieties about how the disorder will affect them personally, e.g. in their intimate relationships and in their careers

■ anxieties about how the disorder will impact on their family, e.g. how it will affect their children, partner and parents, and how it will affect their role within the family

■ anxieties about how they will deal with practical issues, for example their everyday living activities and mobility.

There are many ways of coping with reactions and feelings, but in general the most successful strategies are those that manage to change the way that the individuals concerned think about their situation and behave within it.

### Family and friends

Family and friends can be a useful source of help and advice about how to rethink and handle a situation. Seeking and accepting help from the people who know us best, who have our best interests at heart, who we respect, in whom we have confidence and with whom we can be open and honest can help us to deal with anxieties and adapt to new circumstances.

### Counselling

You read earlier that counselling is offered by the NHS and by independent and voluntary organisations. In health care, it is used to support patients undergoing investigations, patients who are traumatised because of a recent diagnosis, and patients who are living with disabilities, disfigurements and physiological disorders such as diabetes, MS, CHD and cancer.

Figure 14.20  Different types
of counselling

One-to-one counselling, which is where patients talk about their feelings and situation in private with a counsellor whose role is to help them cope by developing their own solutions.

Cognitive Behavioural Therapy (CBT), which is where a counsellor helps the patient to understand the thoughts that contribute to their feelings and behaviour. When these are understood, the counsellor can help the patient to change the way they think and behave, which helps them cope better.

**Different types of counselling**

Family counselling, which is where the family sees a counsellor together. The role of the counsellor is to provide an environment in which everyone feels safe to talk about how they feel and to understand each other and the situation. Family counselling is often used when a member of the family has e.g. cancer when the **prognosis** can be frightening and talking about it can be upsetting.

Group counselling or therapy, which is where a counsellor encourages a group of patients with similar problems to discuss their feelings and situations and share solutions. It can be very helpful for patients to realise that they are not alone with the problems and that other patients' solutions to problems may enable them to cope with theirs.

The British Association for Counselling and Psychotherapy
www.bacp.co.uk
Cancer Research UK
www.cancerhelp.org.uk

Stress can be good in small doses, for example it can energise us and help us deal with challenging situations. However, when we can't escape from something that causes us stress (a stressor), such as the diagnosis of a physiological disorder, it can be very damaging to our health.

Stress affects people physically, for example it can raise their BP and make them more prone to infections, asthma and ulcers. In other words, it plays a contributory role in a number of physiological disorders. Stress also has emotional effects, for example the stress caused by living with a physiological disorder can cause depression and reduce the patient's ability to cope. For these reasons, it is important that people know how to deal with stress.

## Lifestyle changes

Talking through a situation is useful in relieving stress. You read above about the roles of counsellors, family and friends in giving a patient an opportunity to tell someone how they feel. Making lifestyle changes can also help patients cope with stress:

- Stress produces energy, therefore it can be relieved by increasing levels of physical activity. This doesn't have to mean pumping iron at the local gym. Instead it could include taking short walks and participating in some form of gentle exercise.

- Rest and relaxation can also help reduce stress levels. Patients who regularly put time aside to unwind, perhaps with a good book, friend or TV programme, or to do muscular relaxing and deep breathing exercises, develop an increased ability to cope.

The ability to come to terms with having a physiological disorder is also very important in terms of coping. Patients can help themselves in this respect by making lifestyle changes such as:

- being prepared for a relapse e.g. starting medication as soon as fresh signs and symptoms appear
- eating more healthily or adapting their diets to avoid foods that trigger the disorder or make it worse
- avoiding environmental factors that trigger their disorder
- reducing their alcohol intake
- stopping smoking
- adapting their living accommodation and seeking out aids that will help them with their mobility and day-to-day activities.

EXTEND

www.extend.org.uk

Patient UK

www.patient.co.uk

## Complementary therapies

Some patients find complementary therapies beneficial in helping them cope with their disorder. Examples of complementary therapies include aromatherapy, reflexology and hypnotherapy.

### Aromatherapy

Aromatherapy involves the use of essential oils that are extracted from flowers, fruits and leaves, and which are either inhaled or massaged into the skin. Both inhaled oils and oils massaged into the skin stimulate the sense of smell, reduce stress and help the patient relax, sleep and deal with emotional problems.

### Reflexology

Reflexology involves applying pressure to parts of the foot and sometimes the hands or ears. The theory is that each part of the foot, hand or ear is related to a particular body part, for example, organ, muscle, bone, and that applying pressure can influence the function of that body part. A build-up of crystalline deposits under the skin causes tenderness and is said to reflect a malfunction in the corresponding body part. Reflexology breaks down the crystalline deposits, removing blockages in nerve and energy pathways, improving blood supply and aiding **detoxification**. Patients for whom reflexology works say it helps them with conditions such as stress, pain, digestive problems, headaches and sleeplessness.

### Acupuncture

Acupuncture is a branch of traditional Chinese medicine that involves inserting fine needles at selected acupoints on the skin. The theory is that life is based on the interaction between two forces (yin and yang). In the body, these forces are controlled by a flow of energy (chi) in channels called meridians that connect with particular organs. There are many acupoints along each meridian and inserting needles into them is said to promote the flow of energy and improve the function of the related organs. Acupressure uses fingertip pressure on the acupoints instead of needles.

Acupuncture is thought to cause the secretion of endorphins, which are chemicals that reduce pain and make us feel good. Patients for whom acupuncture works say it helps them with conditions such as asthma, digestive problems, high blood pressure and pain.

Figure 14.21 Acupuncture

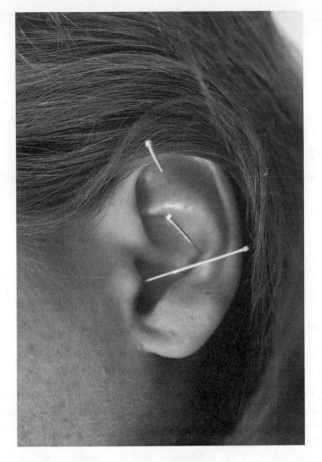

### Hypnotherapy

Hypnotherapy involves patients entering a very relaxed state known as a trance. They usually remain aware of everything that's going on but their state of mind means that they are open to suggestion. Suggestions are positive statements about changes in behaviour that allow the patients to deal with, for example, stress, anxieties such as phobias, addictions such as smoking, and weight problems and pain.

It is possible for patients to hypnotise themselves. First of all they self-induce into a state of deep relaxation, make positive suggestions to themselves, for example 'My pains are becoming less and less severe' and 'Stopping smoking is becoming easier and easier for me', after which they bring themselves back into consciousness.

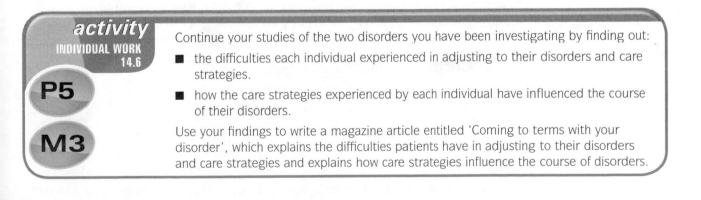

**activity**

**INDIVIDUAL WORK 14.6**

**P5**

**M3**

Continue your studies of the two disorders you have been investigating by finding out:

■ the difficulties each individual experienced in adjusting to their disorders and care strategies.

■ how the care strategies experienced by each individual have influenced the course of their disorders.

Use your findings to write a magazine article entitled 'Coming to terms with your disorder', which explains the difficulties patients have in adjusting to their disorders and care strategies and explains how care strategies influence the course of disorders.

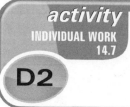

Explore alternative care strategies that could have been used to support the two individuals you have been studying and produce a PowerPoint presentation that describes and evaluates each one.

# Prognosis

To help you understand the likely progression of a disorder, its impact on an individual and how care strategies may have to change with time, you are going to look closely at Alzheimer's disease.

Alzheimer's is caused by a gradual loss of brain function which is why the risk of developing it increases with age. Below the age of 65, it is quite rare, but 1 in 20 of us is affected over the age of 65 and by the time we reach 85, nearly 1 in 2 of us will have the disease. Women have a slightly greater chance of developing Alzheimer's and at the time of writing about half a million people in the UK are affected.

The signs and symptoms of Alzheimer's disease vary but patients usually have progressive memory and language problems, confusion and unpredictable changes in behaviour.

## Memory problems

Short term memory i.e. memory of very recent events is affected first, but as the disorder progresses, problems with long term memory develop and patients start to confabulate and to invent conversations and events that never happened. Eventually their memory is so affected that they seem to live in the past or they completely lose both short and long term memory. Memory problems also contribute to a progressive difficulty performing everyday tasks and learning new ideas and skills.

## Language problems

At first, patients forget simple words and sometimes use the wrong words without noticing. As the disorder progresses, their conversation becomes simple, irrelevant and repetitive. Eventually, language problems can increase to the point where they develop dysphasia, which is the inability to find the right word.

## Confusion

Initially, patients are confused when meeting new people or going into new surroundings (disorientation). As the disorder progresses, they lose awareness of the time and date and recognition of familiar people and places. Eventually they become severely confused and disorientated, may take to wandering and may experience hallucinations, where they see, hear and smell non-existent sights, sounds and smells.

## Unpredictable behaviour changes

At first, patients are irritable and sometimes aggressive. As the condition progresses they may lose their inhibitions and begin to behave inappropriately, for example they may become demanding, rude and suspicious. Eventually they can become obsessive, repetitive, violent and paranoid, for example, they believe they are being persecuted. They also lose interest in the world around them, their family, friends and themselves, ignoring personal hygiene and household cleanliness, not eating properly, and so on.

Alzheimer's disease can cause other signs and symptoms, for example loss of appetite, difficulty in swallowing, changing position or moving, and because it weakens the body, an increased risk of infection.

## Impact

The impact of Alzheimer's disease on patients is far-reaching:

- loss of interest in their living environment increases risks of accidents
- loss of interest in their personal care and loss of appetite increases risk of infection, weight loss and general physical deterioration
- loss of memory causes frustration and anxiety, and confusion and disorientation cause agitation and alarm. Frustration, anxiety, agitation and alarm can, in turn, lead to unpredictable changes in behaviour.
- confusion, disorientation and behavioural changes can lead to social isolation, loneliness and depression
- hallucinations and paranoia cause disturbed sleep patterns.

## Care strategies

Care strategies for patients with Alzheimer's disease change as their disorder progresses. You read earlier about the use of mood-controlling drugs (tranquillisers). These are prescribed for patients when they develop, for example, sleeplessness, wandering, anxiety, agitation and depression. You also read about drugs that can reduce the behavioural problems associated with Alzheimer's disease. Specialist doctors decide which patients these drugs will benefit and when to prescribe them.

Patients in the early and intermediate stages of Alzheimer's disease are often able to cope well in their own homes, surrounded by familiar possessions. As the disorder progresses, they may need increasingly frequent home visits from family, friends and care workers, for example to stimulate their memory and interests, to support them in preparing meals and to encourage them to take their medication. Those who need nursing care but who have difficulty visiting their GP surgery may receive visits from district nurses.

As the disorder progresses, patients living in their own homes are usually assessed as needing day care services. You read earlier that day care centres provide activities aimed at helping people maintain their independence, which in turn helps them to stay in their own homes for as long as possible. An activity that has measurable success for patients with Alzheimer's disease is 'reality orientation'. This uses regular reminders of, for example, the time and date and where the patient is. Other useful activities include puzzles, memory games and board games, each of which can help patients who are losing their intellectual skills.

Patients with severe Alzheimer's disease can do little on their own and need full-time care, either in their own home or in a care home. Although the disease progresses at different rates in different people, most patients die about eight years after first experiencing the symptoms, usually from an infection such as pneumonia that develops as a complication.

*activity*
**INDIVIDUAL WORK 14.8**

**P6**

Complete your studies of the two disorders you have been investigating by finding out their possible future development in each individual.

Use both primary and secondary research methods and use your findings to produce a patient information leaflet entitled 'Living with your disorder – what the future holds', which compares the possible development of each disorder.

***Progress Check***

1. Describe the course of two physiological disorders, i.e. how the physical signs and symptoms, and emotional effects, change over time.

2. Describe the physiology of each disorder and the factors that may have influenced its development.

3. Explain how the course of each disorder relates to its physiology.

4. Describe the investigations and measurements that are made to diagnose and monitor each disorder.

5. Explain why it might be difficult to make a diagnosis from signs and symptoms and investigation results.

6. Describe the care strategies used for each disorder.

7. Compare and contrast the roles of the different people who provide care for individuals experiencing disorders.

8. Explain any difficulties that an individual might experience in adjusting to a disorder and the strategies used to care for them.

9. Explain how care strategies can influence the course of a disorder.

10. Suggest alternative strategies that could be used to care for individuals.

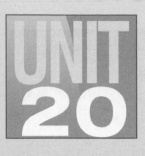

# Health Education

## This unit covers:

- The different approaches to health education
- The models of behaviour change
- How health education campaigns are implemented

Whatever role an individual has in health and social care, in some way or another, they will be involved with **health education**; either producing it, delivering or explaining it to clients. Hence, this unit introduces learners to the principles of health education, the approaches used and also to health education campaigns. Health education is a central component of **health promotion**, which in turn is a major component of public health and hence, this unit links with Unit 12, Public Health.

This unit aims to give both a theoretical understanding of health education and the opportunity for practical application. Learners will consider a range of different approaches to health education, including the role of the **mass media** and social marketing. Learners will also consider different models of behaviour change, relating these to the social and economic context. Learners will then have an opportunity to carry out their own small scale campaign; gaining skills in designing, planning, implementing and evaluating its success.

## grading criteria

| To achieve a **Pass** grade the evidence must show that the learner is able to: | To achieve a **Merit** grade the evidence must show that, in addition to the pass criteria, the learner is able to: | To achieve a **Distinction** grade the evidence must show that, in addition to the pass and merit criteria, the learner is able to: |
|---|---|---|
| **P1** explain three different approaches to health education. Pg 108 | **M1** compare three different approaches to health education. Pg 108 | |
| **P2** describe two different models of behaviour change, and the importance of the social and economic context. Pg 113 | | |
| **P3** describe the design and implementation of own small scale health education campaign. Pg 119 | **M2** explain the approaches and methods used in own health education campaign, relating them to models of behaviour change. Pg 119 | **D1** evaluate the approaches and methods used in own health education campaign relating them to models of behaviour change. Pg 119 |

**grading criteria**

| To achieve a **Pass** grade the evidence must show that the learner is able to: | To achieve a **Merit** grade the evidence must show that, in addition to the pass criteria, the learner is able to: | To achieve a **Distinction** grade the evidence must show that, in addition to the pass and merit criteria, the learner is able to: |
| --- | --- | --- |
| **P4** explain how own health education campaign met the aims and objectives, and explain the ethical issues involved. Pg 121 | **M3** analyse how own health education campaign met the aims and objectives and addressed any ethical issues. Pg 121 | |
| **P5** explain how own small scale health education campaign links to local/national/ international targets and strategies for health. Pg 121 | **M4** analyse the role of own small scale health education campaign in terms of local/ national/international targets and strategies for health. Pg 121 | **D2** evaluate own health education campaign. Pg 122 |

# The different approaches to health education

## Historical perspective

Health education is seen as a central component of health promotion and health promotion is seen as a central component of **public health**, and hence all three will be examined.

'Health education' as a term is one that we may recognise as a relatively recent phenomenon. However, people have been educating about health for many years. Consider Hippocrates stated claims that 'Those naturally very fat are more liable to sudden to death than the very thin.' and 'Walking is man's best medicine.' (Which, given societies' concern with obesity, should be taken heed of to today!) Consider the 'wise-woman' giving information about childbirth and how to breastfeed. Consider the time of the plague when people were told to stay indoors, away from others. This was 'educating' others on health. It may not have had the classification recognised now, but it was health education none the less.

Health education today is often defined as:

> 'working with people to give them the knowledge to improve their own health and working towards individual and behaviour change.'

(Ewles and Simnett, 2003, 24).

Figure 20.1 Components of public health

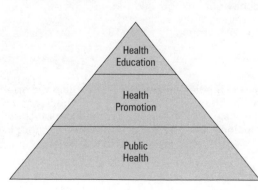

Hence health education is an activity that promotes health related learning and will bring about some relatively permanent change in the thinking or behaviour of an individual.

It is useful to consider at the outset why health education is needed. Unfortunately, it is necessary as individuals and groups do not always follow a lifestyle that is conducive to good health. This may be because of:

- unhealthy behaviour being seen as more 'pleasurable'
- peer pressure
- social conforming
- addictions
- marketing/advertisement of 'unhealthy' choices
- the real and perceived costs of healthy behaviour
- socialisation and culture
- lack of skills
- unavailability of healthy options
- lack of time to behave healthily
- lack of knowledge of the consequences of unhealthy behaviour
- disempowerment
- weak motivation.

Therefore throughout their lives, individuals and groups may need information and guidance that is available in the form of health education.

Health education is often seen as one element of health promotion, which is, according to the World Health Organization (WHO) defined as:

> 'the process of enabling people to increase control over, and to improve, their health.'

> (Ewles and Simnett:2003, 23)

Indeed, Tannahill (1985) uses a Venn diagram to explain how health education is just one element of health promotion:

Health protection is seen as measures for the population which will protect health. This could include legislative laws, e.g. laws on seatbelts, speed limits, the ban on smoking in public places, taxation on cigarettes, health and safety law, e.g. food hygiene.

Prevention is seen as measures to avoid the risks of ill health. These are mainly medical interventions, e.g. childhood immunisations, travel immunisations and preventions for those 'at risk', e.g. walking groups for those at risk of obesity.

As mentioned already, health education is seen as giving individuals or groups the information and advice needed to allow them to modify their behaviour and become 'healthier'.

Figure 20.2 Tannahill's model of health promotion (1985)

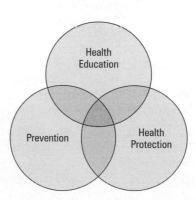

Health promotion is often seen as one element of public health, which is defined as: 'The science and art of preventing disease, prolonging life and promoting health through the organised efforts of society.'

(Ewles and Simnett: 2000, 26)

This therefore is much broader and incorporates more of the generic roles of those in authority. This ranges from keeping streets clean, ensuring neighbours are quiet, the weekly collection of refuse, cycle to school schemes, keeping green areas around towns, etc.

Public health tends to concentrate on large populations or communities. This is because public health acknowledges that people's health is often a result of their shared environment. Many challenges to public health have been a result of industrialisation, urbanisation, technological improvements and changing social attitudes. Hence, historically, important public health developments have been the development of sanitation, sewers, the clearance of slum housing, reducing smoke emissions, ending child labour and long working hours, developing public spaces, etc.

Dahlgren and Whitehead's model illustrates the need for public health as it outlines all the factors that can affect health. The main determinants of health were identified as: non-modifiable factors (age, sex, hereditary factors) and modifiable ones (individual lifestyle factors, social and community influences, living and working conditions and general socio-economic, cultural and environmental conditions).

Figure 20.3 Dahlgren and Whitehead's model of factors affecting health, 1991 (Dept of Health)

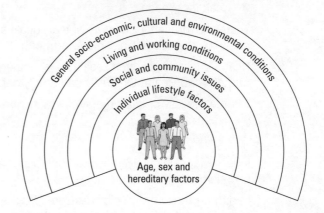

Over the years there has been development of the public health system. Internationally, one of the main milestones was the creation of the World Health Organisation (WHO). When diplomats met to form the United Nations in 1945, one of the items they discussed was setting up a global health organisation; hence WHO's Constitution came into force on 7 April 1948.

According to themselves, 'WHO is the directing and coordinating authority for health within the United Nations system. It is responsible for providing leadership on global health matters, shaping the health research agenda, setting norms and standards, articulating evidence-based policy options, providing technical support to countries and monitoring and assessing health trends.'

Source: www.who.int/en

Three major milestones of the WHO have been '**Health for All by the year 2000**' which aimed to meet basic health targets for all, the '**Alma-Ata declaration**' which aimed to develop primary health care and the '**Ottowa Charter for Health Promotion**' which aimed to develop health promotion.

Firstly, a major statement was made was in 1977 with 'Health for All by the Year 2000'. The Thirtieth World Health Assembly in 1977 identified the attainment, by all peoples of the world by the year 2000, of a level of health that would permit them to lead socially and economically productive lives as being a main social target of governments, international organisations and communities.

The indicators with target values are listed below:

*Health status:*

- life expectancy at birth of 70 years (male/female).
- infant mortality rate 30 per 1,000 live births.
- 10% or fewer newborns with a birth weight of less 2500 grams.
- 90% or more children with weight-for-age that corresponds to the reference values.
- reduction of maternal mortality by at least 50%.

*Essential Primary Health Care (PHC) programs:*

- 100% of pregnant women with access to prenatal care provided by trained personnel.
- 100% of deliveries attended by specialised personnel.
- 100% of puerperal women attended by trained personnel.
- 100% of women of childbearing age using family planning.
- 100% of children receiving growth and development monitoring.
- 100% of children fully immunized (DPT, polio, measles, TB) and 100% of pregnant women vaccinated with tetanus toxoid.
- 100% of the population with access to drinking water and excreta disposal services.
- 100% of the population with minimum nutritional needs satisfied.
- 100% of the population covered by primary health care services, including treatment of common diseases and injuries, provision of essential drugs and medications, and control of locally endemic diseases.

*(And two of the) Other indicators*

- Adult literacy rate for both men and women exceeds 70%.
- At least 5% of the gross national product is spent on health.

Source: www.who.int/en

This was significant as it highlighted inequalities in health across the world, given that many of these targets are commonplace for many people, yet for others completely unattainable. What is tragic though is that even after the year 2000, the world is still a long way from achieving all these targets.

## Alma-Ata declaration 1978

A further milestone was the 'Alma-Ata declaration 1978'. The International Conference on Primary Health Care in Alma-Ata 1978 expressed the need for urgent action by all governments, all health and development workers, and the world community to protect and promote the health of all the people of the world. The conference defined and granted international recognition to the concept of Primary Health Care as a strategy to reach the goal of 'Health for All in 2000'. A ten point declaration was then made to outline what could be done to improve the world's primary health care. (www.who.int/en)

According to the Declaration of Alma Ata, primary health care, is 'essential health care based on practical, scientifically sound and socially acceptable methods and technology made universally accessible to individuals and families in the community through their full participation and at a cost that the community and country can afford to maintain at every stage of their development in the spirit of self-reliance and self-determination.' (www.who.int/en). The Alma-Ata Declaration of 1978 emerged as a major milestone of the twentieth century in the field of public health, and it identified primary health care as the key to the attainment of the goal of Health for All. (www.who.int/en)

## Ottawa Charter for Health Promotion 1986

Building on this was the 'Ottawa Charter for Health Promotion 1986'. At the first International Conference on Health Promotion in Ottawa 1986, a charter to help achieve 'Health for All by the year 2000' was presented. The conference was primarily a response to growing expectations for a new public health movement around the world and it built on the progress made through the 'Declaration on Primary Health Care' at Alma-Ata and the World Health Organization's Targets for 'Health for All' document.

It claimed that health promotion is the process of 'enabling people to increase control over, and to improve, their health. To reach a state of complete physical, mental and social well-being, an individual or group must be able to identify and to realize aspirations, to satisfy needs, and to change or cope with the environment. Health was, therefore, seen as a resource for everyday life, not the objective of living. Health is a positive concept emphasizing social and personal resources, as well as physical capacities. Therefore, health promotion is not just the responsibility of the health sector, but goes beyond healthy life-styles to well-being.' (www.who.int/en)

According to the Charter, action on health promotion means:

- Building Healthy Public Policy.
- Creating Supportive Environments.
- Strengthening Community Actions.
- Developing Personal Skills.
- Reorienting Health Services.
- Moving into the Future.

The charter set out the pre-requisites for heath as being:

- peace
- shelter
- education
- food
- income
- a stable ecosystem
- sustainable resources
- social justice
- equity.

Source: www.who.int/en

It could be argued that not one country on the planet benefits from all of these; indeed some have very few at all.

The outcome of this international movement is that successive governments have had to try to implement and/or incorporate these nationally; although it does depends on the support of the government at the time. In 1990, the Conservative Government released 'The Health of the Nation' strategy which set targets for health improvement. In 1997, the Labour strategy was followed up by a revised strategy 'Saving Lives – Our Healthier Nation'. This linked to the Acheson Report and set out to tackle the **root causes of ill health**. In 2004, the Labour Government released 'Choosing Health' which recommended a new approach due to the increasing interest in health and the rapidly changing society.

International movements in health can affect national health policy.

Figure 20.4 The key
milestones in WHO's history

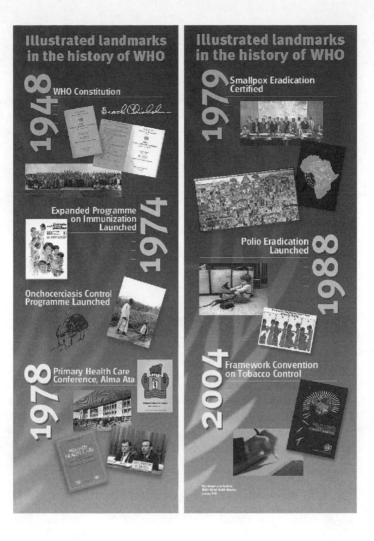

## Models

There are two main models within health education: the **'victim blaming' model** and the **empowerment model**. The 'victim blaming' model is one that is based on the concept that it is the individual's responsibility for his or her own health status and therein, it is the individual's own responsibility for his or her ill health. No one forces any individual to behave in any way, everybody has freewill. However, this has been criticised for being too black and white. Think of all the reasons people may be 'unhealthy'; were they always 'to blame'? Think of the individual born with an illness/condition, the individual living in poverty, the individual without a car, the individual with low education, the individual with a culture of 'unhealthy' behaviour, the individual with an addiction, etc. Can they exercise free will? Poverty, lack of opportunity, lack of choice and being disempowered can prevent people from adopting healthy lifestyles.

The empowerment model is based on a word within it, 'power'. This model is based on giving individuals or groups the 'power' to change their own health; empowering them. It is more a 'bottom-up' model that a 'top-down' model. It gives individuals the skills and the information to make informed decisions for themselves. Individuals can not be blamed for their health if they have not got the 'skills' to live healthily. One criticism of this is that people can use not having the skills or knowledge as an excuse for unhealthy behaviour; should they take more individual responsibility for their own health?

In terms of who sets the priorities, the 'victim blaming' model tends to work on priorities determined by those in authority. The empowerment model tends to work on the premise that individuals themselves should determine what is important to them and decide themselves what should be done about it.

In essence though, if we visualise the models on a spectrum most government initiatives would probably stay close to the centre; although there would be some movement depending on political stance. Where do you feel that action should be targeted?

Figure 20.5 A spectrum with 'victim blaming' at one end and 'empowerment' at the other.

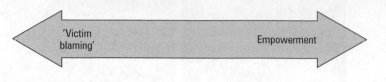

## Approaches

There are four main approaches to health education: **social marketing**, role of the mass media, **community development** and **two-way communication**; each of these shall be looked at in turn.

### Social marketing

Hubley (1993) describes social marketing as 'the application of commercial marketing and advertising approaches to health'. Commercial marketing has criteria it will utilise for the promotion of its goods; a logo, a brand, a slogan, a memorable advert. Take Coca Cola for example; most people will be able to visualise the red and white colours used, the way that 'Coca Cola' is written with the 'curly' font, the shape of the bottles and even memorable advertisements such as the Christmas themed ones, the polar bear ones, or the vending machine ones. It is evident therefore that marketing works; so why not use it for the benefit of health education?

According to the synopsis on the Institute of Social Marketing's website, the term social marketing was first coined by Kotler and Zaltman in 1971 to refer to the application of marketing to the solution of social and health problems. They follow with the explanation of social marketing as:

'the design, implementation and control of programs calculated to influence the acceptability of social ideas and involving considerations of product planning, pricing, communication, distribution and marketing research.'

They also state the difference to marketing *per se*, is that:

'while, for generic marketing the ultimate goal is to meet shareholder objectives, for the social marketer the bottom line is to meet society's desire to improve its citizens' quality of life.'

Hence social marketing is using the approach of marketing in health education materials.

If it is used however, then there needs to be a marketing mix; it has to be clear to the audience that it is useful information to take on board and not necessarily a specific 'brand' to be bought. Consider the marketing of the health education message about speed limits. The messages that are used are designed purposely to 'grab your attention' just like any other advertisement. They have a logo and a slogan. Therefore, they have a mix; they are noticeable enough to make you watch, but they are still essentially educating about health.

## case study 20.1 — Graeme

Graeme is a 34 year old man. He is married and has two children. Graeme works shifts for a local railway company. There is no canteen where he works, nor a kitchen. The only option for hot food is at a 24-hour garage along the road. At break time, Graeme will go and smoke with his work colleagues outside; he enjoys the social aspect of this and it relieves the boredom from work; he'd prefer not to sit with the non-smokers in the portakabin available at break time.

Because of his shift work, Graeme is usually too tired to exercise. Also, he is also not able to see his children, Ross and Jamie as much as he would like to. This upsets him greatly; he would love to be able to play rugby and football with them when they get home from school.

Graeme's sleep is often disturbed, sometimes due to his wife getting up and going to work herself; he feels he does not get enough quality time with her either.

What is also making Graeme feel down, is that despite all the sacrifices he feels he is making, once he takes out money for the mortgage, the money for the bills and the weekly shop, there is very little left. The only luxury he feels he has is a weekly night out with his friends at a local pub.

Graeme's parents are what his wife would describe as 'old-fashioned'. They smoke, eat lots of fried food and red meat, drink heavily, would never consider going to an exercise class or joining a gym. Graeme lost one grandmother recently to a heart attack and one grandfather to a stroke. His wife is worried that Graeme could be following a similar path and may have a premature death.

### activity
**INDIVIDUAL WORK**

1. Do you agree with Graeme's wife? Outline your reasons for agreeing or disagreeing.
2. If you were to follow the 'victim-blaming' model, what would you say about Graeme's health? Both in terms of causes and possible intervention.
3. If you were to follow the empowerment model, what would you say about Graeme's health? Both in terms of causes and possible intervention.
4. Do you think Graeme's current health and well-being is his own 'fault'?

It is important therefore to get the marketing right. The benefits need to be clear at the outset and the audience analysis and segmentation needs to be thorough. This means that it needs to be considered how the audience will respond to the message; it may be good to use humour, but what if the audience laugh at the joke, but do not act on the message? Audience analysis should mean that the approach is **needs-led**. An audience analysis on binge drinking would probably identify young people aged 16–25 as being most at risk, and their 'needs' would be specific to that age and culture. Knowing the audience means there can be a targeted approach; when is the best time and place to deliver that social marketing? Messages on alcohol that is presented during matinee films at the cinema will not be most effective as younger children will be the main audience.

However, one also needs to consider the limitations to the project in terms of the cost and the time involved. Once this has been done, one can analyse whether social marketing is the most effective way to educate on health.

Figure 20.6 An example of
earlier and current 'social
marketing'

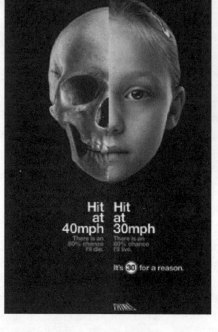

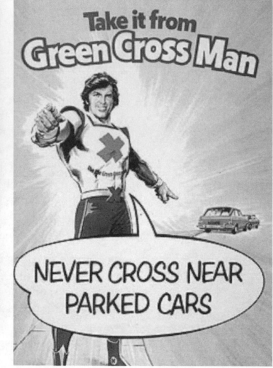

## Role of mass media

The media includes many different forms, e.g. television, radio, newspapers, magazines, posters, billboard displays, leaflets and all of these can be used to educate about health.

The benefit of using these formats is its effectiveness in:

- raising consciousness about health issues
- reaching large audiences
- conveying simple information
- placing health on the public agenda.

Clever usage of the mass media, which may involve a range of formats can ensure the message is clear in the minds of people. For example, consider the message about the dangers of smoking where information on this is found on the television, radio, newspapers, magazines, posters, billboard displays, leaflets, etc. then the campaign in many respects has been a success. Relating to the four benefits above, the smoking campaign has raised consciousness about the issue (people are aware – people may still smoke; but they are *aware* of the dangers); it has reached large audience (young, old, smokers, non-smokers); it is a simple message (smokers die younger); and the message is in the public agenda (people talk about wanting to quit, the risks, etc.).

### Limitation of mass media

However, it is also important to be aware of the limitations of using the mass media to educate about health. Firstly, there is its inability to convey complex information or teach skills. As the audience are getting only snippets of information, they might not always get the full picture or an in-depth account of the situation. As the information is usually only given verbally or audibly, it may not allow the audience to gain 'practical' skills. A

Figure 20.7 Information from the media

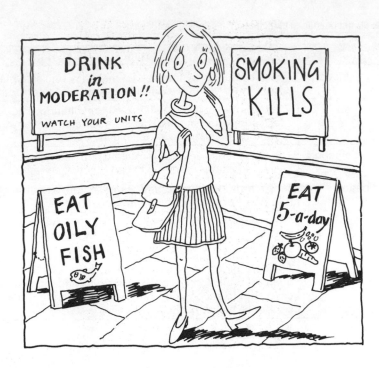

campaign may describe the benefits of having a fruit smoothie for breakfast; but what if an individual does not have the skills to buy fresh fruit or know how to cut fruit properly. Knowledge like that is usually best gained practically.

A second limitation is the situation that only less specific information can be presented. The mass media is not the place for detailed reports. Hence, the audience may feel like they are not being given all the facts.

Lastly, there is no opportunity for two-way communication. This means that if the audience has any questions or does not understand, they cannot ask for more information.

However, it may be the case that using the mass media can be the most appropriate approach to educate on health.

## Community development

This looks at health and well-being as a more **holistic** concept. Health and well-being are not just looked at in terms of how people will benefit physically from health education. By practicing community development, people's health can be developed intellectually, emotionally, socially, spiritually and mentally. This is because people will be involved at all levels.

Community development is described as 'much more than community participation. It means working with people to identify their own health concerns, and to support and facilitate them in their collective action.' (Ewles and Simnett: 2003, 299).

Therefore community participation is a foundation for community development.

Communities participation in health can vary as shown in Table 20.1.

As can be seen, there are many levels of community participation. Ideally, agencies should aim for the highest amount of participation and this will mean that community development is more likely to take place.

Table 20.1  Levels of community participation in planning health work

| No Participation | The community is told nothing, and is not involved in any way. |
|---|---|
| Very low participation | The community is informed. The agency makes a plan and announces it. The community is convened or notified of other ways to be informed; compliance is expected. |
| Low participation | The community is offered 'token' consultation. The agency tries to promote a plan and seeks support or at least sufficient sanction so that the plan can go ahead. It is unwilling to modify the plan unless absolutely necessary. |
| Moderate participation | The community advises through a consultation process. The agency presents a plan and invites questions, comments and recommendations. It is prepared to modify the plan. |
| High participation | The community plan jointly. Representatives of the agency and the community sit down together from the beginning to devise a plan. |
| Very high participation | The community has delegated authority. The agency identifies and presents an issue to the community, defines the limits and asks the community to make a series of decisions that can be embodied in a plan which it will accept. |
| Highest participation | The community has control. The agency asks the community to identify the issue and make all the key decisions about goals and plans. It is willing to help the community at each step to accomplish its goals, and even to the extent of delegating administrative control of the work. |

Source: Ewles and Simnet, 2003, 297

A community will only be able to develop their own communities, once that community is at a high level of participation. This will result in a great sense of empowerment for both individuals involved and the communities. This is a very 'bottom-up' scheme as opposed to 'top-down'. Communities develop the skills so that they themselves can decide what issues and risk factors apply to them. They will have the skills to investigate how these could be dealt with and what factors may hinder their efforts. They will develop the skills to implement their plans. Finally, they will develop the skills to evaluate the success of the initiatives. The alternative to this would be people in authority 'telling' people what their priorities should be.

Figure 20.8  What would your health priorities be?

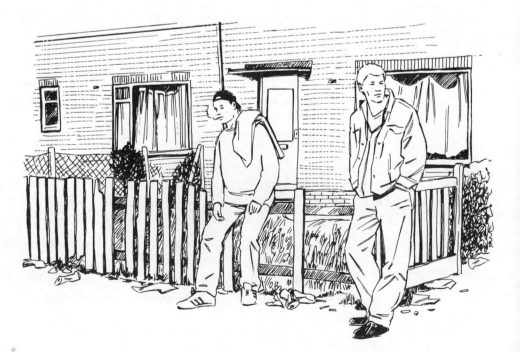

One benefit of community development at that it focuses on root causes of ill-health. It doesn't only focus on the outcomes; it doesn't just state what individuals should and shouldn't do. It looks at *why* people smoke, drink, use illegal substances, have sun exposure or eat a poor diet. It focuses on the individual's reasons.

Also, because communities that benefit most from community development are traditionally the less affluent and less skilled communities, a further benefit is that it helps to reduce inequalities.

Community development does have its limitations. Because development and participation is complex, it can be time consuming. This is possibly a reason why it doesn't always occur. The longer the process, the longer staff are needed and hence the greater the cost. Further, the process is difficult to quantify and evaluate. How can the benefits of local residents developing and implementing a traffic calming scheme be quantified. Self-esteem, empowerment, skill development, etc. are difficult to measure. Hence it will be difficult for health workers to justify the effort and funding to their superiors.

## Two-way communication

A final approach that may be used is two-way communication which is when dialogue between individuals or groups is used to educate on health. By *conversing* with individuals or groups, not only are health workers able to give information, but also the individuals are also able to:

- Ask questions.
- Clarify any misunderstandings.
- Challenge any myths.
- Find out more about support available.
- Find further contact details.

Figure 20.9 Health Education

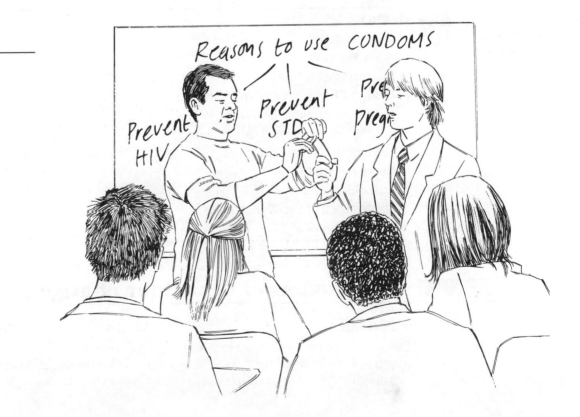

There is opportunity for two-way communication in health and social care settings. For example advice on pre-conceptual health could be given in GP surgeries and family planning clinics; advice on safe sex could be given in schools, youth clubs and family planning clinics; and advice on immunisations could be given in nurseries, schools, GP surgeries or child clinics. Also residential care, day centres and domiciliary care all provide opportunities for two-way communication with clients.

Two-way communication could be practiced using **peer educators** in schemes where people are 'trained' to inform their peers of the health issues. These can be a good approach as it is possible that individuals are more likely to engage and listen to their peers as opposed to a stranger, who may be seen as a 'do-gooder' or may be from a different culture and lifestyle.

When communicating, it is also possible to use resources to prompt discussion. The use of theatre and drama, interactive video and computer packages are all possible options. These will provide stimulus for discussion and questions.

*activity*
**INDIVIDUAL WORK 20.1**

**P1**

**M1**

You want to promote awareness of the childhood accidents.

1. Do a little background research into childhood accidents; numbers, types, preventions etc.
2. Choose three possible approaches and describe what you would do for each.
3. Justify your choices.

WHO
www.who.int/en
Alma Ata declaration
www.who.int/hpr/NPH/docs/declaration_almaata.pdf
Ottawa Charter for Health Promotion
www.who.int/hpr/NPH/docs/ottawa_charter_hp.pdf
Saving Lives: Our healthier nation
www.archive.official-documents.co.uk
Choosing Health
www.dh.gov.uk
The Institute of Social Marketing
www.ism.stir.ac.uk

# The models of behaviour change

## Models

As stated earlier, the aim of health education is to change behaviour. People act in certain ways for a variety of reasons, and hence action needed to change that behaviour can be complex. The models below all help to explain how behaviour change can occur.

## Health belief model

One model is the **Health belief model** developed by Rosenstock and Becker. This is where there is consideration of the possible psychological factors and the potential costs and benefits that could influence an individual's decision to engage with healthier behaviour. It is based on decisions made by people regarding health:

- belief on own susceptibility; can ill health be avoided?
- belief of the severity of the risk; how will life be affected?
- belief that the recommended health behaviour will reduce the risk of ill health
- belief of whether it is possible to do the recommended health behaviour.

Consider the consumption of alcohol. Someone may drink alcohol heavily one night; what could have influenced their behaviour?

Table 20.2 Applying the Health belief model

| Susceptibility? | Belief that ill health can be avoided; alcohol related illnesses will not affect them. |
| --- | --- |
| Severity? | Hangovers aren't really that severe. The other higher severity outcomes are unlikely anyway. |
| Benefits? | Staying sober will not guarantee longevity or indeed good health throughout life. |
| Barriers? | Do not believe it is possible to have the same quality of social life if alcohol wasn't consumed. |

Once the behaviour is broken down, it allows health agencies to plan health education. In the above scenario, it could be that health education is needed on:

- The prevalence of alcohol related illnesses and death. (Susceptibility)
- The possible severity of drinking in the short term (hospitalisation, stomach pumping, accidents, sexual attacks, violence, etc.) as well as the long term (liver failure, coronary problems, obesity, etc.) (Severity)
- The likelihood of 'years to life and life to years' from moderate alcohol consumption. (Benefits)
- Examples of how a social life is not negatively affected from moderate alcohol consumption. (Barriers)

## Theory of reasoned action

Another model is based on the **theory of reasoned action** developed by Ajzen and Fishbein.

This model focuses on a person's *intention* to behave in a particular way and assumes that most actions are under a person's individual control. Intention is the most important factor to behaviour change. A person may intend to exercise more, but may not actually do it, so it could be argued the intention wasn't strong enough. However, we are not always aware of individuals' intentions, as they are private and difficult to comprehend, so it is believed that one should look at two factors:

- The attitude towards the behaviour – whether positive or negative.
- The subjective norm – the individual's perception on how socially acceptable the behaviour is or isn't.

So to change an individual's behaviour on breastfeeding; an individual's intent to breastfeed is what is most important. To ensure they intended to breastfeed, the individual's attitude towards breastfeeding would have to be examined and challenged. How the individual sees society's perception of breastfeeding would also have to be understood, and perhaps challenged, too.

Figure 20.10 Individual perceptions

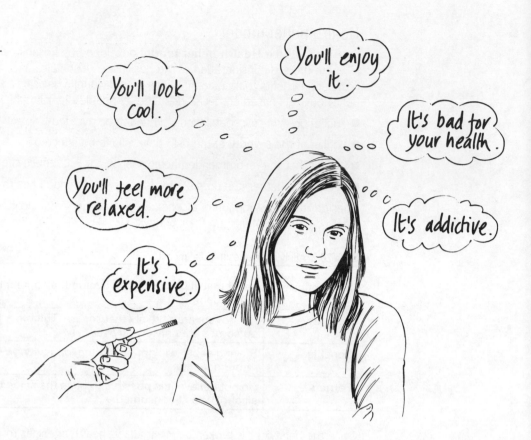

## Theory of planned behaviour

A further model to examine is the **theory of planned behaviour** developed by Ajzen and Maddens. This is an advance of the theory of reasoned action by Ajzen and Fishbein. It was developed to account for behaviours that are not fully under control of one's ability to choose; hence it incorporates a variable about the perceived ability to perform the behaviour. According to this theory, all behaviour is planned.

People consider all the outcomes of behaviour before they plan to do it. This may be an actual considered action, or it may happen instantaneously. However, an individual will consider:

- Behavioural beliefs – an individual's attitude about a behaviour and its consequences.
- Normative beliefs – an individual's perception of the social pressure to perform the behaviour and their motivation to comply with this.
- Control beliefs – an individual's perception of the control they have over the behaviour.

Because this method examines how an individual perceives the control they have over behaviour, it can be useful to utilise with addictions.

## Stages of change model

Another model is the **stages of change model** which was developed by Prochaska and DiClemente. It considers the stages an individual will go through before changing their behaviour.

Table 20.3 Stages of change model

| Pre-contemplation stage | An individual has no awareness of a need to change their behaviour. |
|---|---|
| Contemplation stage | The point of entry onto 'change'. Motivation/information has changed resulting in a desire to change behaviour. |
| Commitment stage | A commitment is taken to change behaviour. |
| Action stage | Commitment turns to action. Time/effort/resources are used to change behaviour. |
| Maintenance stage | An individual is coping with the change in behaviour. |
| Relapse stage | Occasionally, an individual may return to their former behaviour. |
| Exit stage | An individual is permanently behaving in the changed manner. |

Being aware of what stage a person is currently at will guide what the intervention and/or health education they are in need of. For example at pre-contemplation stage, an individual will need information about why their current behaviour needs to change whereas at the maintenance stage, individuals may need coping strategies.

 **Link**

See Unit 8 Psychological perspectives in Health and Social Care Book 1.

## Social learning theory

The last model utilises **social learning theory**. Using this theory, it is believed that individuals, especially children, learn from the world around them, and then imitate them. One advocate of this theory is the psychologist Albert Bandura. The most famous experiment demonstrating his belief had three groups of children who were each shown a film. The film involved adults physically abusing a Bobo doll (a doll that cannot be knocked down); however, all three films had different endings. One showed the adult being rewarded for the behaviour, one showed the adult being punished and the final one had no consequences for the adult. The three groups of children were then allowed to play with the doll themselves. The children who had seen the version where the adult was rewarded for their abusive behaviour, were more likely to hit the doll. Therefore, according to this theory, if children, or indeed anybody, see behaviour being rewarded or punished they will respond by imitating that behaviour or not. Hence, how people see others behaving and the consequences of their behaviour will affect their own behaviour.

If a teenager sees an adult being described as 'cool' and 'fun' for being drunk at parties, it may be that they will see that person as a role model and try to imitate them.

> **remember**
>
> Behaviour is complex and therefore so is an understanding of it.

## Importance of social and economic context

Whatever the model, health workers always need to consider the context. Individuals or groups may have to consider financial constraints, social constraints and/or peer pressure. All these aspects will affect whether behaviour can be changed or not.

Consider the ways that someone who has had a very bad day may choose to relax:

- sit in the back garden with a glass of wine
- go to the theatre
- meet up at a restaurant with friends
- go to the gym or for a swim
- go shopping
- have a long bath with candles and read a book.

**UNIT 20**

Figure 20.11 Observing what is 'right' in preparation to imitate.

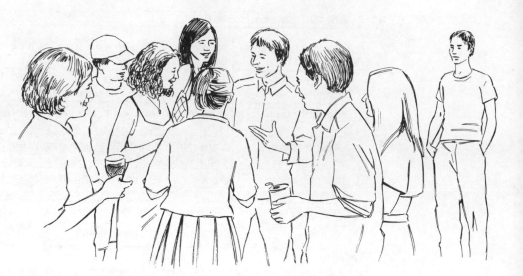

Figure 20.12 Is smoking her main concern?

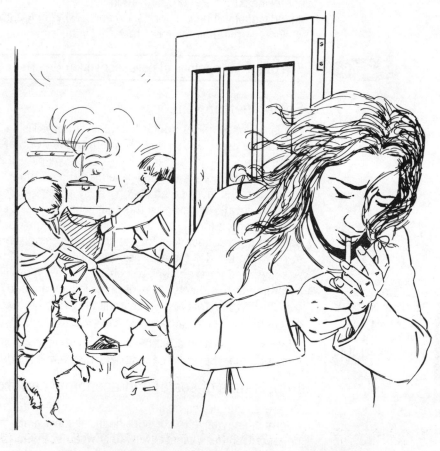

**remember**

Examining the 'real' cause of ill health by examining the cause of the 'unhealthy' behaviour can help to resolve the behaviour.

However, these methods are not accessible to all people. If someone had a low income, was a single parent, had not been socialised to see these as options, lived in poor housing, had noisy neighbours, did not have friends/family who shared an interest in the activities, worked shifts, etc., could they easily relax in the same way? Maybe the only way to reduce stress was to have a cigarette and 5 minutes to themselves to 'chill out'. It is not acceptable to preach to people on how to live their lives without due consideration to their circumstances.

The Acheson Report provides a good background to the importance of social and economic factors.

The Acheson Report
www.archive.official-documents.co.uk/document/doh/ih/ih.htm

## case study 20.2 — Adam

Adam is 8. He lives with his mum and dad and his older brother Peter who is 15. It has just been discovered that Peter has started smoking. His parents have said that Peter is old enough to know what is right from wrong, and if that is what he wants to do, then that is up to him; he'll be legally able to anyway soon when he is 16. Peter's mum is also concerned about fires in the house, so she has bought him an ashtray to use in his bedroom. Occasionally, Peter's father gives Peter one of his own cigarettes when he has one.

### activity — INDIVIDUAL WORK

1. Consider how the social learning theory could explain why Adam is now more likely to smoke in future.
2. Use the Health belief model to explain why Peter is smoking.
3. Use the theory of reasoned action to explain how Peter could be helped to stop smoking.
4. Use the theory of planned behaviour to explain how Peter could be helped to stop smoking.
5. Consider the stages of change model. Which stage do you think Peter is at?
6. Describe what social and economic issues could affect Adam in the future, making him choose to start smoking.

### activity — GROUP WORK 20.2

**P2**

In small groups, each takes a model of behaviour change.

1. Using the internet, research it and then produce one A4 sheet of information about it, focusing on the importance of the social and economic context.
2. Present this to your group with a verbal explanation.
3. When you have all presented, collect each sheet to collate and copy so that everyone has a 'book' of models of behaviour change.

## How health education campaigns are implemented

### Health educators

Many people and agencies are involved in educating about health. You will have already looked at one international agency involved in this earlier when you looked at the World Health Organization. Their role regarding public health is:

- providing leadership on matters critical to health and engaging in partnerships where joint action is needed

- shaping the research agenda and stimulating the generation, translation and dissemination of valuable knowledge

- setting norms and standards and promoting and monitoring their implementation

- articulating ethical and evidence-based policy options

- providing technical support, catalysing change, and building sustainable institutional capacity

- monitoring the health situation and assessing health trends.

Source: www.who.int/en

There are also national/local agencies involved in health education. The Department of Health is the government department that claims it is 'committed to improving the quality and convenience of care provided by the NHS and social services. Its work includes setting national standards, shaping the direction of health and social care services and promoting healthier living.'

## Department of Health

As well as directing and organising the NHS and social services, the Department of Health also has a public health role. There are nine Regional Public Health Groups (RPHGs) each linked with the nine regional offices. Their website claims 'They [the RPHGs] work alongside public health colleagues in NHS, local authorities and other agencies to improve and protect their local population. This involves addressing all determinants of health – such as diet, housing, the economy, transport and mental health – and factors that create health inequalities within their region.'

Source: www.doh.gov.uk

## Health Protection Agency

Established in 2003, the Health Protection Agency's role is 'to provide an integrated approach to protecting UK public health through the provision of support and advice to the NHS, local authorities, emergency services, other Arms Length Bodies, the Department of Health and the Devolved Administrations.' (www.hpa.org.uk). It exists to prevent and reduce the impact on human health of the consequences of infectious diseases, chemical and radiation hazards and major emergencies.

## Primary Care Trusts

Primary Care Trusts are, in their own words, 'at the centre of the modernisation of the NHS and are responsible for 80 percent of the total NHS budget. They are a free-standing NHS organisation with their own boards, staff and budgets. They work with other health and social care organisations and local authorities to make sure that the community's needs are met. PCTs provide some care directly and commission services from others, such as NHS acute trusts and private providers, with decisions on providers increasingly informed by the choices which patients make themselves.'

Hence Primary Care Trusts are almost the 'gate-keepers' to secondary care. Also, as they are responsible for their locality, they should be more likely to invest in health education.

# Health strategies

As mentioned earlier, over the years there have been numerous health strategies by the government. A strategy is an overall plan that will affect practice. Two key strategies affecting public health are 'Saving Lives: Our Healthier Nation' in 1999 and 'Choosing Health: Making Healthy Choices Easier' in 2004.

## 'Saving Lives: Our Healthier Nation'

The first strategy 'Saving Lives: Our Healthier Nation' was published in 1999 by the Labour Government who outlined a plan to tackle poor health. The aims were to:

- improve the health of everyone
- and the health of the worst off in particular.

This was because it claimed, although good health is fundamental to all our lives, too many people:

- are ill for much of their lives
- die too young from preventable illness.

It was believed that implementation of the plan could potentially save 300,000 unnecessary deaths. The plan set targets for the year 2010 in four key health concerns.

Table 20.4  Targets of Saving Lives: Our Healthier Nation 1999

| Cancer | To reduce the death rate in people under 75 by at least a fifth. |
|---|---|
| Coronary heart disease and Stroke | To reduce the death rate in people under 75 by at least two fifths. |
| Accidents | To reduce the death rate by at least a fifth and serious injury by at least a tenth. |
| Mental illness | To reduce the death rate from suicide and undetermined injury by at least a fifth. |

To achieve these targets many aspects were changed; more money was invested in health (£21 billion); they hoped to integrate health services with local government; they stressed health improvement as a key role for the NHS; primary care was prioritised and given more responsibility and Health Action Zones and Healthy Living Centres were established. A Healthy Citizens programme was introduced, establishing NHS Direct, Health Skills and Expert Patients.

The plan was significant as it boldly stated that 'the social, economic and environmental factors tending towards poor health are potent' (nhshistory), therefore recognising that many factors including poverty, low wages, unemployment, poor education, sub-standard housing, crime and disorder and a polluted environment can affect health. Herein it was accepting that the government has a responsibility to deal with health inequalities.

## 'Choosing Health: Making Healthy Choices Easier'

'Choosing Health: Making Healthy Choices Easier' was published in 2004 by the Labour Government. After consultation, the Government stated that they felt the public mood had changed and that people wanted to make their own choices about health, but that they wanted support and information. It was also felt that people did value the role that Government played in health and that they felt the Government should be trying to help people to be healthier.

There were three underpinning principals of 'Choosing Health', which were:

1. Informed Choice – giving people the facts to make their own decisions.
2. Personalisation – tailoring health promotion to the individual or groups.
3. Working together – all agencies involved in health working to the same goal.

Table 20.5  The key points in 'Choosing Health'

| |
|---|
| Make it easier for people to choose healthy lives |
| Help children and young people to be healthy |
| Help local communities to be healthier |
| Make health a way of life |
| Support the National Health Service to help people to be healthier |
| Help people to be healthier at work |

Table 20.6  What the Government wants to achieve through 'Choosing Health'

| |
|---|
| Fewer people to smoke |
| Fewer people to be overweight |
| More people to do exercise |
| Help people to drink alcohol sensibly |
| Help people to stay healthy sexually |
| Help people to be healthy mentally |

'Choosing Health' has already had significant effect. The ban on smoking in public places, the changes in food labeling and the changes to school dinners could be attributed to this.

The role of legislation is extremely important for three reasons.

1.  It affects thinking at national and local level. It can be easier for health agencies to promote a health message if the government is leading the way. When the Black Report in 1980 (a report into health inequalities, concluding that the national health strategy did not address the poorer health of the more disadvantaged in society) was submitted to the Secretary of State for the new Conservative Government, it is claimed only 260 copies were then made and there was neither a press release nor press conference. It was claimed the reception from the Government was 'frosty'. The dismissal of this report and hence the lack of any subsequent legislation clearly showed the thinking of the Government and hence affected the work national and local agencies did. (Townsend, Davison and Whitehead: 1998)

2.  It can result in funding becoming available to highlight the health message. The implications of 'Choosing Health' for example resulted in monies becoming available.

3.  It can make it easier for behaviour to be changed as individuals may have to. The compulsory wearing of seatbelts by drivers and passengers in cars has made it easier to deliver the message about the benefits of wearing seatbelts.

Health strategies can be relevant to all aspects of health, not just physical health. Intellectual, emotional, mental, social, spiritual and sexual health can all benefit from health strategies. For example, 'Choosing Health' looks at health in a very holistic way as it hopes to improve many facets of an individual's health and well-being.

## Aims and objectives

There are many reasons why health education campaigns are produced; some generic reasons are:

■  to improve the health of individuals in society, e.g. by providing health related learning

■  exploring values and attitudes

■  providing knowledge and skills for change

■  promoting self esteem and self empowerment

■  changing beliefs, attitudes, behaviour, lifestyle.

However, more specific aims and objectives will be needed for specific campaigns. An aim is what is hoped to be achieved overall. Objectives are the specific outcomes that are hoped to be achieved in order for the aim to be met. For example:

Aim: to reduce the amount of yearly deaths in road traffic incidents as a consequence of not using seatbelts.

Objectives:

■  to highlight the risks of not wearing seatbelts

■  to highlight the number of deaths per year that could have been prevented with the use of seatbelts

■  to outline responsibilities of drivers and adults

- to highlight legal consequences of not wearing seatbelts
- to increase understanding of who is most at risk, e.g. young males.

## Context

Health education can be done either on a one-to-one basis or on a group basis and each have their own benefits and limitations. Groups are rarely just random; they will usually have similarities that can be used when educating about health; for example intelligence, income, location, health status, age, etc. and hence this can be utilised when delivering health education.

## Design principles

When designing a health education campaign there are many considerations that need to be taken into account.

The importance of health policy is vital. Any education campaign should run parallel to current health policy otherwise the audience will be confused as to the message. Plus the audience is more likely to act on the message if it is reinforced by current health policy. For example, if you were to present a health education message about skin cancer, it would be inadvisable to outline the 'healthy ways to get a tan', as the current campaign is to avoid a tan altogether.

Figure 20.13   An antenatal class

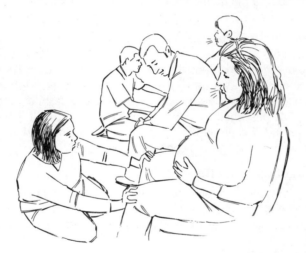

Before setting out on a campaign, it is important to spend time gathering and acquiring statistics. There is little point producing a health education campaign that is 1) incorrect or 2) not the message that the audience need. Find out about what your audience already know and what they'd like to know; then research that and use that.

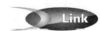 **See Unit 22, Research Methodology for Health and Social Care.**

Once background research has been done, it is then advisable to spend time target setting. This entails outlining what needs to be done and setting a date for it. A target will be needed for some or all of the following:

- research
- choosing the formats, e.g. presentation, video, display, leaflet, role play, posters, games, quizzes.
- designing the campaign materials
- producing the campaign materials
- producing any IT based information, e.g. PowerPoint presentations
- ordering of any resources
- photocopying.

Clear, realistic measurable objectives that acknowledge the starting point of the audience are needed. If presenting a campaign to a group of 16 year olds about the risks of unsafe sex, it may be unnecessary to spend time explaining about the reproductive system as they have probably had that education earlier. Maybe the needs of this audience are now more specific, e.g. risk of gay sex, prevalence of STIs, where to go if they feel they have put themselves at risk, etc. Common sense is a useful starting point, but maybe this needs some investigation as it should not be assumed that all the audience has a similar prior knowledge.

The choice of approach also needs to be considered. Approaches were covered earlier and include social marketing, the role of the mass media, community development and two-way communication. The appropriate approach for the message and the audience needs to be thought out.

When presenting your message, it is vital that you provide clear and accurate information which is conveyed appropriately. The message needs to be free of spelling and grammatical errors and be clearly set out ensuring the message is simple to take on board. Also the message must be presented appropriately for the audience, taking into account their intelligence, prior knowledge, age, ability, culture, etc. It is unlikely that a 14 year old will read an in-depth report into the potential negative socio-economic consequences of teenage parenthood; however, they may take more notice of a role play, a video or a magazine or cartoon-style booklet.

A further role of health education can be misinformation and prejudice challenged and corrected and hence this needs to be accounted for in the design. Misinformation is information that is incorrect and prejudice means a judgment is made on an individual or group based on prior, possibly stereotypical knowledge. For example, a health education message about drug use could challenge the myth that only people from 'certain backgrounds' take drugs; i.e. less affluent, from inner city areas, less educated, who could be described as 'more working class' youths. It is the case that any person of any age and background can and does become involved in illegal drug use, so it is responsible to challenge and correct this prejudice.

## Inter-agency working

Inter-agency working involves a variety of organisations working together with the motivation and working dynamics to achieve a common aim. Each agency may have its own individual aim; but when working together they may have a shared one. Take for example:

- high schools
- FE colleges
- sixth form colleges
- training providers
- local businesses.

All these agencies all have different aims; however, if they were to commit to a project to increase participation in education and training post-16, all would benefit; therefore in the case of the project, they would all have a similar aim.

When producing a health education campaign it may be the case that inter-agency working is beneficial. There is no point reinventing the wheel, so it is important to talk to other agencies and find out what they know. They may also have useful materials and resources. Also, they may want to partner in the project and this could be useful as it may bring extra staff, resources and funding.

Consider what links to national campaigns could be used. For example, if a message on childhood immunisations was being presented, a link to the NHS immunisations website would be useful to give out. If a message on breast cancer was being presented, a link to NHS Be Breast Aware campaign could be given. This allows the audience to gain more information and will allow the message to be reaffirmed.

When presenting any health education campaign, there are ethical considerations. Ethical considerations will be covered in more detail later. However, whatever your message or audience, health education must always be ethical and this must be taken into account when designing the campaign.

When designing a campaign, it is important to consider how evaluation will take place. How will it be assessed as to its success? Evaluation methods will be considered later, but it is important to consider this at the outset as; if any 'pre-campaign' information is needed it may be too late after the message has been delivered.

*activity*

**INDIVIDUAL WORK
20.3**

**P3**

**D1**

**M2**

1. Choose a health concern that is of interest to you.
2. Design a small scale health education campaign.
3. Explain and evaluate the approaches and methods used in your campaign, relating them to models of behavioural change.
4. Evaluate the approaches and methods used in your own health education campaign, relating them to models of behaviour change.

## Ethical considerations

**Link**    See Unit 2, Equality, Diversity and Rights in Health and Social Care Book 1

The Oxford Dictionary definition of ethics is 'the moral principles governing or influencing conduct; the branch of knowledge concerned with moral principles'. Hence, ethics are guidelines as to how society should behave – what is morally acceptable. All health educators should consider ethical issues; indeed it is so important that agencies such as the American based National Commission for Health Education Credentialing and the Society of Public Health Education both have a 'Code of Ethics for the Health Education Profession', which may be worth inspection.

National Occupational Standards for Professional Activity in Health Promotion and Care were launched in November 1997 and these were built on ten Principles of Good Practice. These will help to ensure that all working in health promotion and care are doing so ethically.

Table 20.7 Principles of good practice

| 1 | Balancing peoples' rights with their responsibilities to others and to wider society and challenging those that affect the rights of others. |
|---|---|
| 2 | Promoting values of equality and diversity, acknowledging the personal beliefs and preferences of others and promoting anti-discriminatory practice. |
| 3 | Maintaining the confidentiality of information, provided that this does not place others at risk. |
| 4 | Recognising the effect of the wider social, political and economic contexts on health and social wellbeing on people's development. |
| 5 | Enabling people to develop to their full potential, to be as autonomous and self-managing as possible, to have a voice and to be heard. |
| 6 | Recognising and promoting health and social well-being as a positive concept. |
| 7 | Balancing the needs of people who use services with resources available and exercising financial probity. |
| 8 | Developing and maintaining effective relationships with people and maintaining the integrity of these relationships through setting appropriate role boundaries. |
| 9 | Developing oneself and one's own practice to improve the quality of services offered. |
| 10 | Working within statuary and organisational frameworks. |

Source: Ewles and Simnett, 2003

One further way that ethics could be considered is in terms of the rights of individuals. No one has the right to tell someone else how to live their life. If an individual is not breaking the law then they are free to choose their own lifestyle; they can smoke, drink excessively, eat poorly, tan their skin, etc. However, the rights of others have to be balanced into this. What about the rights of children who may be exposed to second hand smoke? What about the rights of the neighbour woken up by drunken singing? What about the individual who takes care of their health who has been in an accident who has to wait longer for an operation because an overweight person has had a heart attack? What about the financial costs to society of treating people with skin cancer? Health education can produce lots of ethical issues which health educators have to consider.

## Professional Practice

When delivering any health education messages, it is important to behave and act professionally.

Your audience are more likely to listen to you and have faith in you if you are:

- well presented
- organised
- knowledgeable.

## Evaluation

See Unit 22, Research Methodology for Health and Social Care.

After delivering your health education message, it is vital that there is evaluation. It is important to evaluate as it allows for improvements in the future both for yourself and any other agencies who may be considering delivering a similar message.

The ways that the campaign could be evaluated are as follows:

- Has the campaign been a success with referral to the aims?
- Has the campaign been a success with referral to the objectives?
- Has behaviour been changed?
- Has the campaign been a success with referral to the strategies?
- Was the approach the best one to use?
- Were the materials the most appropriate ones to use?
- Has the campaign been a success with referral to the targets?
- Has the campaign been a success with referral to ethical issues?
- Were there any unexpected outcomes that were not intended?
- Was there successful engagement with the audience?
- What were the strengths of the campaign?
- What were the weaknesses of the campaign?

One way to do this would be to reflect, and any reflection will be improved by use of and inclusion of evidence. The best way to see if health education has been successful is to see if behaviour changes, but this can be difficult, as it may not be measurable in the short term. It may be useful to compare knowledge and attitudes before the campaign as well as to compare knowledge and attitudes after the campaign.

Consider Unit 22 on research methodology for health and social care, which provides a more in-depth description of methodologies that may be used to help answer the question 'Has the campaign been successful?' These methodologies could include questionnaires, observations, interviews or case studies.

A simple way which may be useful for a small scale campaign is a questionnaire that can be given to the target audience both before and after the message has been delivered. By comparing the two sets of answers, it should be possible to see if there has been any increase in knowledge or a change of attitudes. An example question after a campaign on using condoms could be 'Do you agree with the statement "People who carry condoms are more likely to be promiscuous."?' If the campaign has been a success, there should be more people answering no than before.

Evaluation could be formed on the basis of observations, which again could be performed before and after the message has been delivered. For example, after a campaign on the risks of second hand smoke, non-smoking individuals could be observed to see where they stand when with their friends who smoke.

Interviews with audience members could ask about the campaign, for example:

- Do you feel the campaign answered all your questions?
- Was there any information that you knew already?
- What information would you recommend is included?
- How would you make it more interesting/accessible?

This can be a useful way to get feedback. However, caution needs to be taken with content that may be sensitive or embarrassing as interviewees may not like to discuss this.

Case studies allow for a useful, more time-based analysis. Looking at how case studies behaviour changes over time can be a useful indicator as to the success of a campaign. For example, a case study who had been receiving health education on alcohol abuse could be monitored to see whether there was any change in behaviour. If any trends developed, it could be decided whether the material and approach were appropriate.

Once a thorough evaluation has taken place, the final stage is to consider the potential for improvement. What could be improved if a similar campaign was to be produced again?

This could be sectioned into four; the aim and objectives, the process, the content and the materials.

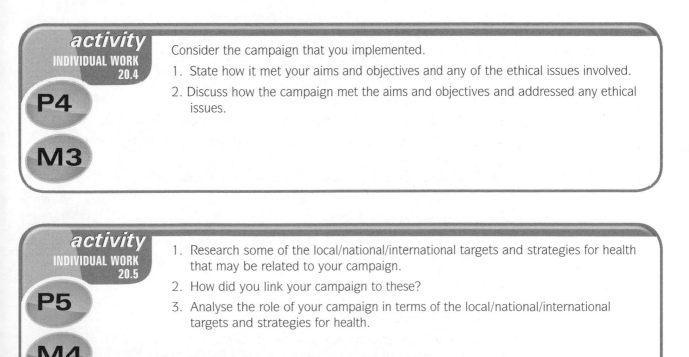

**activity**
**INDIVIDUAL WORK**
**20.4**

**P4**

**M3**

Consider the campaign that you implemented.

1. State how it met your aims and objectives and any of the ethical issues involved.
2. Discuss how the campaign met the aims and objectives and addressed any ethical issues.

**activity**
**INDIVIDUAL WORK**
**20.5**

**P5**

**M4**

1. Research some of the local/national/international targets and strategies for health that may be related to your campaign.
2. How did you link your campaign to these?
3. Analyse the role of your campaign in terms of the local/national/international targets and strategies for health.

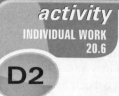

Using whatever evidence you have, evaluate your own campaign.

**D2**

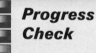

Regional Public Health Groups
www.gos.gov.uk/publichealth/?a=42496

Department of Health
www.dh.gov.uk

Health Protection Agency
www.hpa.org.uk

Saving Lives: Our Healthier Nation
www.nhshistory.net/savinglives.pdf
www.archive.official-documents.co.uk/document/cm43/4386/4386.htm

NHS Immunisations
www.immunisation.nhs.uk

Breast cancer screening
www.cancerscreening.nhs.uk/breastscreen/

National Commission for Health Education Credentialing
www.nchec.org/index.htm

Society of Public Health Education
www.sophe.org/index.asp

**Progress Check**

1. Outline why health education is needed.
2. Outline three important documents produced by the WHO.
3. Describe two models of health education.
4. Choose one approach used in health education and briefly outline it.
5. Briefly describe the 5 models of behaviour change.
6. Explain why it is important when educating on health to always consider the social and economic context.
7. Name some of the agencies involved in health education.
8. Outline one important health strategy the UK has had in recent years.
9. What is meant by ethics?
10. Produce a checklist of issues that would need consideration when designing a health education campaign.

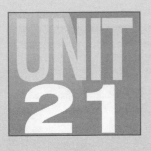

# Nutrition for Health and Social Care

## This unit covers:

- The concepts of nutritional health
- The characteristics of nutrients
- The influences on food intake and nutritional health
- How to use dietary information from an individual to make recommendations to improve nutritional health

Because improvements in nutrition have such a huge influence on the improvement of people's health, health and social care workers need to have a good understanding of what makes for good nutrition.

This unit aims to give you both a scientific and a **socio-economic** understanding of nutrition. It explores the language of nutrition and describes nutrients, the components of food, in terms of their chemical composition and digestion. It looks at nutritional requirements for different individuals and the influences on, and of, their food intake. Finally, it gives you an opportunity to reflect on your learning and analyse dietary information with a view to planning for improved health.

## grading criteria

| To achieve a **Pass** grade the evidence must show that the learner is able to: | To achieve a **Merit** grade the evidence must show that, in addition to the pass criteria, the learner is able to: | To achieve a **Distinction** grade the evidence must show that, in addition to the pass and merit criteria, the learner is able to: |
|---|---|---|
| **P1** explain concepts of nutritional health. Pg 130 | | |
| **P2** describe the characteristics of nutrients and their benefits to the body. Pg 138 | **M1** explain the potential risks to health of inappropriate nutrition. Pg 138 | |
| **P3** identify the different factors that influence dietary intake for different population groups. Pg 145 | **M2** explain the factors affecting the nutritional health and wellbeing of different groups of individuals. Pg 145 | **D1** evaluate the relative importance of different factors affecting the nutritional health and wellbeing of two different groups of individuals. Pg 146 |

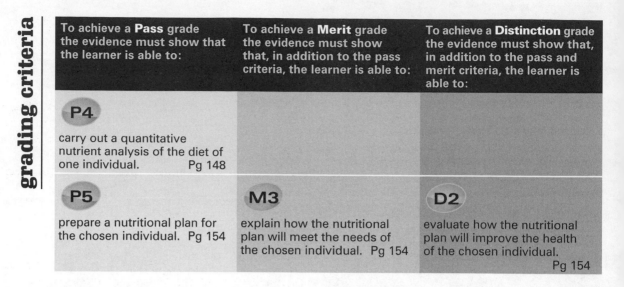

grading criteria

# The concepts of nutritional health

## Nutrition

The study of nutrition is the study of food and of the body processes that depend on its digestion i.e. the breakdown of food into molecules that are small enough to be absorbed from the digestive tract into the blood. You will read about digestion and the digestive tract shortly.

Food is anything we eat or drink that the body can convert into:

- energy, which is produced in the body cells by a process called internal (cell) respiration

- material that enables body cells to grow, repair and reproduce

- material that enables the body to function, for example **enzymes** that regulate the physiological processes taking place in the body.

You can read about cells, internal (cell) respiration and physiological processes in Unit 5 of Health and Social Care Book 1. You will read more about enzymes shortly.

Food is composed of the nutrients proteins, vitamins and minerals, carbohydrates and lipids. It may also contain fibre and water, which, although not nutrients, are used by the body to promote and maintain good health.

Proteins and minerals are used by the body for growth and repair of cells, and vitamins and minerals to help regulate physiological processes. Carbohydrates and lipids are known as energy foods because the body uses them to produce the energy needed for physiological processes and for muscular movement. The body can also convert carbohydrates and lipids into fat, which gives it shape and provides insulation, thereby helping to maintain body temperature.

A healthy diet is one in which the amount of energy consumed is balanced by the amount the body needs to expend. This energy balance is tipped if:

- the diet contains more energy than the body needs, in which case more body fat is made. Individuals who consume large amounts of carbohydrates and lipids and who don't use up or 'burn off' energy that is superfluous to their bodily needs become overweight and, eventually, obese. Obesity and being overweight contribute to a range of physiological disorders, including diabetes, Coronary Heart Disease (CHD), high blood pressure (BP) and some cancers.

remember

Eating too much energy food and not using up energy the body doesn't need causes weight gain and obesity!

■ the diet contains insufficient energy for the body's needs, for example because of ill health or a psychological eating disorder. In this case, body weight decreases, which further threatens health.

## Body mass index (BMI)

Body mass index (BMI) is used as a guide to health and is calculated by dividing a person's weight in kilograms by the square of their height in metres. Overweight is defined by a BMI of 25 and over, obesity by a BMI of 30 or greater, and underweight by a BMI of less than 18.5.

**Link**

You can read about BMI in Unit 14.

## Diet

Diet is the term used to describe the food we eat on a day-to-day basis. It is often used in the context of slimming, in which case it is more correctly called a 'weight reduction diet'. Other types of diet include weight increasing, vegetarian, vegan and lactose-free diets.

A healthy diet for an individual is one that contains nutrients from a wide variety of foods and energy in sufficient amounts to meet their nutritional or dietary needs. Nutritional needs vary between individuals and depend on their:

■ basal metabolic rate (BMR) i.e. the rate at which basic life processes such as heartbeat, breathing and the maintenance of body temperature need to proceed when we are at complete rest. BMR varies and some people have a higher BMR than others. As a result they have greater energy needs.

■ body size and composition, for example, short, slight people generally need fewer nutrients and less energy food than men or women who are taller and more muscular

■ sex, for example women who are menstruating, pregnant or breastfeeding require additional nutrients to replace the iron lost in menstrual blood, to support the growth and development of the foetus and to sustain their energy levels when pregnant and when caring for the baby

Figure 21.1 The energy balance

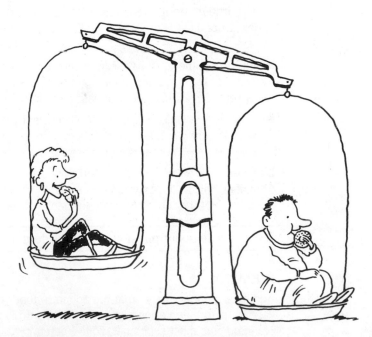

- age, for example growing children have a greater need for energy foods and nutrients that promote growth than adults and older people who are less active and not growing

- state of health, for example people with diabetes, coeliac disease or food allergies need to eat a diet that avoids particular nutrients

- level of physical activity, for example an adult who has a sedentary office job has different dietary needs from a physically active social care worker.

**Dietary Reference Values** (DRVs) spell out the amounts of nutrients needed by different individuals. There are three categories of DRV:

1. Estimated Average Requirement (EAR), which is an estimate of the daily amount of energy needed by people at different ages, for example a male aged 15 to 18 years needs 2755 **kilocalories (kcal)** of energy every day and a female of the same age 2110 kilocalories. EARs are very general and most people need more or less than the estimate for their age.

2. **Reference Nutrient Intake** (RNI), which is the amount of each nutrient that is enough for people at different ages, for example a male aged 15 to 18 years needs 11.3**mg** of iron each day and a female of the same age 14.8mg. RNIs are higher than most people need and for this reason people who consume their RNI are unlikely to suffer deficiency diseases (see below).

3. Lower Reference Nutrient Intake (LRNI), which is the amount of each nutrient needed by people with low nutritional needs. Most people need more than the LRNI and people who consume less are likely to develop deficiency diseases.

### Malnutrition, overnutrition and undernutrition

Malnutrition is caused by taking in too few or too many nutrients. Overnutrition results from taking in too many nutrients. You read earlier how overconsumption of carbohydrates and lipids affects the energy balance and leads to overweight and obesity. Overconsumption of other nutrients can also affect health, for example a very high intake of protein affects kidney function, high intakes of sodium (salt) are linked with high blood pressure, and high levels of vitamin A taken during pregnancy can adversely affect the unborn child.

Undernutrition results from taking in too few nutrients over a period of time; continued undernutrition leads to starvation. Examples of disorders caused by undernutrition include:

- mirasmus, more usually seen in children in less developed countries and which is caused by a sustained inadequate diet. It is a 'wasting' disease, causing stunted growth, emaciation, poor appetite and slow intellectual development.

- kwashiorkor, which is caused by insufficient protein in the diet. It too is more usually seen in children in less developed countries, and signs and symptoms include stunted growth, lethargy, diarrhoea and a swollen abdomen.

**Deficiency** diseases are caused either because the diet lacks particular vitamins or minerals or because the body is not able to absorb them from the diet. A brief description of the more common deficiency diseases is given in the table below.

You can read about physiological disorders associated with diet in Unit 14.

## Additives

Additives are ingredients that are added to food, either to preserve it or to improve its flavour, texture and appearance. The law controls the use of additives in food and lists of ingredients must show the additive category name and its serial number, for example, E500.

Table 21.1 Examples of deficiency diseases

| Examples of deficiency diseases | Vitamin/mineral concerned | Examples of effects on the body |
|---|---|---|
| Night blindness | Vitamin A (retinol) | Vitamin A helps us see in the dark. A deficiency makes night vision difficult and sometimes causes eye lesions (xerophthalmia) and complete blindness. |
| Scurvy | Vitamin C (ascorbic acid) | Vitamin C is needed for maintaining healthy skin and gums and helping wounds to heal. Signs and symptoms of a deficiency include swollen and bleeding gums, loose teeth and slow healing of wounds. |
| Anaemia | Iron | Iron is needed to make haemoglobin in red blood cells, which transports oxygen to other body cells where it is used to make energy. Signs and symptoms of a deficiency include tiredness and weakness because of a lack of energy, breathlessness as the body fights to maintain its oxygen supply, dizziness and palpitations (rapid heartbeat). |
| Goitre | Iodine | Iodine is an important constituent of the hormones produced in the thyroid gland. A deficiency causes the thyroid to enlarge and if it presses on the trachea or oesophagus, it can cause difficulty in breathing and swallowing respectively. |
| Rickets and osteomalacia | Calcium and vitamin D | Vitamin D is necessary for the absorption of calcium from food in the digestive tract and calcium is needed to give strength to bones. A deficiency of both causes rickets (stunted growth and deformed legs) in children, and osteomalacia (thin, weak bones) in adults. |

Food can be spoiled by mould, which makes it inedible; by bacteria, some of which cause life threatening food poisoning; and chemical action such as oxidation, which causes food to go rancid. Preservatives added to food include sulphur dioxide and sodium nitrite, which prevent the growth of mould and bacteria, and anti-oxidants, which prevent food going rancid.

Additives that are used to improve flavour, texture and appearance include emulsifiers such as those used in margarine and mayonnaise, stabilisers that help food to set and prevent it separating out, and colourings and flavourings.

## Nutritional supplements

Nutritional supplements are useful for people who don't or can't eat properly, for example because they're ill, have problems swallowing or have lost weight as a result of being ill or having treatment. Nutritional supplements are taken to provide energy or particular nutrients, such as proteins, **oils**, vitamins and minerals. They can be consumed in a variety of ways, for example in drinks, soups, puddings and tablets, and include lactase enzyme, folic acid, glutamine, glucosamine, chondroitin and fish oil.

Foods such as margarine, bread and yoghurt may be fortified with various vitamins and minerals to replace those lost during manufacture or to bring their nutritional content up to the minimum required by law. Texturised vegetable proteins, for example soya beans, may be fortified with vitamins and minerals to meet the dietary needs of **vegetarians**.

General Practice Notebook
www.gpnotebook.co.uk
Netdoctor
www.netdoctor.co.uk
NHS Direct
www.nhsdirect.nhs.uk
The Vegetarian Society
www.vegsoc.org

Figure 21.2 Nutritional
supplements

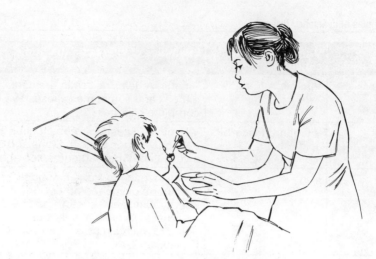

## Dietary intake

To stay healthy, we need to eat the right amount to retain a healthy BMI, drink plenty of fluid and enjoy a healthy, balanced diet.

Food is divided into five different food groups. Although we all have individual nutritional and energy needs, we can achieve a balance of good health by eating a variety of foods from each food group in the following proportions:

1. plenty of bread, potatoes, cereals and grains e.g. rice and wheat

2. plenty of vegetables and plenty of fruit

3. moderate amounts of milk and dairy foods

4. moderate amounts of meat, fish and alternatives such as pulses, nuts and seeds

5. very small amounts of foods containing lipids and sugar.

The balance of good health is often represented pictorially as a:

- pie chart. This is composed of five segments, one for each food group, with the size of each segment representing the proportion of food from each group that we should consume.

- food pyramid. There are a number of different designs of food pyramid but generally the pyramid is divided horizontally into five bands, each band representing one of the five food groups with a key that describes the proportion from each group that we should consume.

Key 'food pyramids' into internet search engines, for example Google and Yahoo! to see examples of foods within the different food groups and the proportions of them that we should be eating.

Bread, potatoes, cereals and grains are starchy carbohydrate foods. They are a good source of energy, low in lipids and contain a range of vitamins and minerals, including the B vitamins and calcium and iron. They are also a good source of fibre.

Fruit and vegetables are also low in lipids, an excellent source of fibre, vitamins and minerals, and they protect us from diseases such as CHD and some cancers. We should eat at least five portions a day. A portion of fruit and vegetables weighs about 80g.

Figure 21.3 What is a portion of fruit and vegetables?

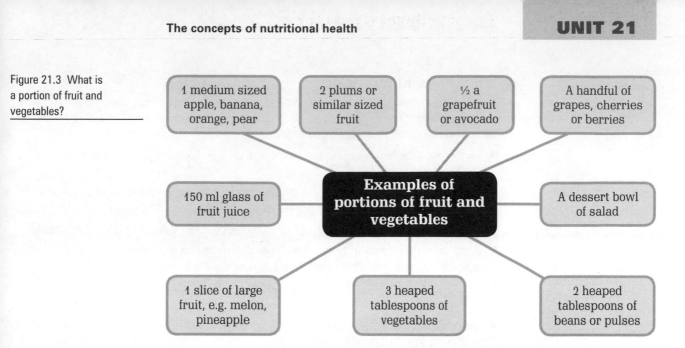

Meat is a good source of protein, minerals such as iron, selenium, zinc, and the B vitamins, for example vitamin B12, which is only found in meat and animal products such as milk. Some types of meat are high in saturated **fat**, which can raise cholesterol levels and increase the chance of developing CHD.

Fish is also a good source of protein, of vitamins such as A and D, and minerals such as calcium, phosphorus and iodine. White fish, for example cod and haddock, are low in lipids; and oily fish, for example sardines and salmon, are rich in healthy fatty acids.

Nuts, seeds such as sesame, poppy and sunflower, and pulses (seeds that grow in pods) such as beans, peas and lentils are useful protein-rich alternatives to meat and fish. They are also starchy, a good source of fibre, vitamins and minerals such as iron, and some are high in unsaturated fats that help reduce the blood cholesterol level.

Milk and dairy foods such as cheese and yoghurt are also good sources of protein, and of calcium and the vitamins A, B12 and D. However, some dairy products contain salt and large amounts of saturated fats, which is why we are recommended to eat them in moderate amounts only.

It is important to have some lipids, particularly unsaturated fats, in the diet because they're a good source of energy and help maintain body temperature. Some are a good source of **essential fatty acids** and some help the body absorb vitamins. But as you read earlier, overconsumption of lipids tips the energy balance and causes weight gain. This is why we are recommended to eat them in small amounts only.

You will read about fatty acids and saturated and unsaturated fats shortly.

Like starch, sugar is a form of carbohydrate. It is not a nutrient but a rich source of energy. It occurs naturally in foods such as fruit (fructose) and milk (lactose) and is added to very many processed foods (usually as sucrose). Because it has no nutritional value, decays teeth and overconsumption leads to weight gain, we are recommended to include it in our diets in small quantities only.

The Food Standards Agency
www.eatwell.gov.uk

## Preparing and processing

Preparing and processing raw food makes it more appetizing, more easily digested and prolongs the amount of time it can be kept before eating. However, food preparation and **processing** methods can affect nutritional content, for example:

- skimming milk removes fat, and pasteurising, sterilising and evaporating milk can destroy vitamins
- cooking meat and fish destroys vitamins; and minerals can be lost in the juices produced when meat and fish are defrosted and cooked
- cooking eggs destroys vitamins; and when fried, their lipid content rises markedly
- removing the germ and bran from wheat grains during milling means that white flour has less protein, vitamin, mineral and fibre than wholemeal flour
- heat treating, puffing and flaking grains to produce breakfast cereals destroys vitamins
- peeling potatoes loses vitamins and minerals, mashing them loses more vitamins than keeping them whole, and frying them greatly increases their lipid content
- storing, preparing and cooking fruit and vegetables reduces their vitamin and mineral content.

## Hidden ingredients

The hidden ingredients or 'unwanted extras' in food can also affect its nutritional content and our health, for example:

- some food labels don't list additives or preservatives or make their presence clear. This makes it hard for people who suffer with allergies to identify problem ingredients
- some food labels make it difficult to work out how much lipid, sugar or salt is present, which makes it difficult to monitor their consumption
- some food labels seduce customers into buying food by describing it as, for example, 'low fat', even though it may contain huge amounts of unwanted extras such as sugar and salt
- some foods, for example alcoholic drinks, restaurant meals, take-away meals and unwrapped bread and confectionery have no ingredient list at all. It is therefore impossible to know what additives or how much lipid, sugar or salt is present.

*activity*
INDIVIDUAL WORK
21.1

P1

Produce an information leaflet for students studying a level 3 health and social care course that explains the concepts used in the field of nutritional health.

# The characteristics of nutrients

This section introduces you to the science of nutrition.

## Characteristics

Table 21.2  The characteristics of nutrients

| Nutrient | Main sources in the diet | Main function in the body | RNI for different groups |
|---|---|---|---|
| Carbohydrates: sugars and starches | The main sources of sugar in the diet are table sugar (sucrose), milk (lactose), fruit and fruit juice (fructose), sweets, chocolate and foods made using sugar. The main sources of starch in the diet are bread, potatoes, cakes, biscuits and other cereal products. | To provide energy. 1g of carbohydrate provides 3.75kcal of energy. | The EAR for energy increases markedly from birth, peaking at between 15 and 18 years for both sexes, remaining relatively stable until early old age when it gradually begins to decrease. |
| Lipids: fats (animal, solid at room temperature) and oils (vegetable, liquid at room temperature) | The main sources of animal fats in the diet are meat and meat products, butter and whole milk. The main sources of vegetable oil in the diet are margarine, cooking oils, cakes and biscuits. | To provide energy. 1g of lipid provides 9kcal of energy. | See above. |
| Proteins | Meat, fish, milk and dairy products, bread and other cereals. | Growth and repair of the body. Excess protein can be used to provide energy. 1g of protein provides 4kcal of energy. | The RNI for protein increases at the same rate for both sexes from birth until about age 15, when it becomes greater for males. Pregnant and breastfeeding women need additional amounts. |
| Vitamins: fat-soluble (A, D, E and K) and water-soluble (B group, C). | Bread, breakfast cereal, eggs, fruit, fruit juices, margarine, meat, milk, vegetables and oily fish such as sardines and herring. Vitamin D is also manufactured by the body due to the action of sunlight on the skin. | To help regulate physiological processes. | We need different amounts of different vitamins but in general, the RNI for vitamins increases at the same rate for both sexes from birth to young adulthood when it plateaus. Men need some vitamins in greater quantities then women; and pregnant and breastfeeding women need additional amounts of e.g. folic acid and vitamin C. |
| Minerals, for example iron, calcium, magnesium, sodium, potassium, selenium and zinc. | Bread, breakfast cereals, cheese, meat, milk, vegetables. | For growth and repair and to help regulate physiological processes. | We need different amounts of different minerals but in general, the RNI for minerals increases at the same rate for both sexes from birth to about 11 years, when males and females start to need differing amounts. For example adolescent males need more calcium than adolescent females and menstruating females need more iron. Pregnant and breastfeeding women need additional amounts of calcium and zinc. |

You read above that food processing can affect the nutritional content of different foods. This is because heat causes physical and chemical changes to nutrients, making them less usable by the body, and also because water-soluble vitamins and minerals are lost as they dissolve into cooking water or steam.

Freezing has little effect on nutrients, especially if food is frozen directly after harvesting. It is therefore a good method of storage. However, drying food and preserving it through the addition of preservatives can destroy vitamins.

All food should be stored appropriately, to maintain its storage- or shelf-life. The shelf-life of a food is the period of time during which it can be stored under specified conditions of temperature, light and humidity, so that it remains in the best possible condition and suitable for consumption.

- 'Use by' dates on labels tell us the date after which we should no longer consume the food. Using food after its 'Use by' date increases the risk of food poisoning.

- 'Best before' dates tell us when food is no longer at its best, for example it might have lost its flavour or texture.

'Use by' and 'Best before' dates are usually given in conjunction with conditions of storage, for example in 'store in a cool, dark place'. If food isn't stored as instructed, 'Use by' and 'Best before' dates cease to be valid.

## Availability to the body

Nutrients become available for the body to use through digesting and the action of sunlight on the skin. You read at the beginning of this unit that digestion is the breakdown of food into molecules that are small enough to be absorbed from the digestive tract into the blood. Molecules of starch, protein and lipid, and some of the sugars, are too big and too complex to be absorbed – they are broken down by action of enzymes. The resultant smaller, more simple molecules are used by the body to manufacture the complex molecules that are necessary for the maintenance of life. You will read about the fate of absorbed nutrients shortly.

Digestion of sugars, starch, protein and lipid into simple molecules is also known as catabolism; and the manufacture of complex molecules from simple molecules is known as anabolism. The processes of catabolism and anabolism constitute metabolism, and the speed at which metabolism takes place is known as the metabolic rate.

 **Link**   See the diagram of the digestive system in Unit 14.

Digestion of sugars and starch:

- Salivary amylase in the mouth and amylase secreted from the pancreas into the small intestine break starch down into maltose. Maltose is a disaccharide sugar.

- Maltase, sucrase and lactase in the small intestine break the sugars maltose, sucrose and lactose down into glucose, fructose and galactose, which are monosaccharides (simple sugars). Monosaccharides are the basic building blocks of carbohydrates and small enough to be absorbed across the intestinal wall into the blood.

You will read more about mono- and disaccharides shortly.

When absorption has taken place, glucose is transported by the blood to cells where it is converted into energy. Excess monosaccharides are transported to the liver, muscle cells and fat cells where they are converted to glycogen and fat, both of which readily release energy when needed.

Digestion of proteins (polypeptides):

- Pepsin in the stomach breaks proteins down into peptides. Peptides are short chains of amino acids.

- Trypsin and chymotrypsin secreted from the pancreas into the small intestine break proteins down into peptides and amino acids. Amino acids are the basic building block of proteins and small enough to be absorbed across the intestinal wall into the blood.

- Proteases in the small intestine complete the digestion of proteins into amino acids.

You will read more about polypeptides, peptides and amino acids shortly.

When absorption has taken place, amino acids are transported by the blood to cells where they are used to build the proteins that the body needs, for example antibodies, hormones, enzymes, keratin (in skin and hair), collagen (in bones, cartilage and tendons), and actin and myosin (in the muscles). They can also be used as a source of energy.

Digestion of lipids:

- Bile, which contains bile salts, is produced in the liver and stored in the gall bladder. It is secreted into the small intestine where the bile salts emulsify fats, assisting their digestion.

- Lipase from the pancreas and small intestine break emulsified fat down into fatty acids and glycerol, molecules of which are small enough to be absorbed across the intestinal wall into the blood.

As fatty acids are absorbed they are built into triglycerides and carried in the lymph to the blood. The blood transports triglycerides to body cells, where they are used as a source of energy or are converted into body fat.

You will read more about fatty acids, glycerol and triglycerides shortly.

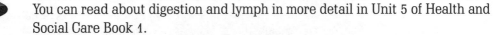

**Link** You can read about digestion and lymph in more detail in Unit 5 of Health and Social Care Book 1.

Fat soluble vitamins are absorbed along with fatty acids whilst minerals and water soluble vitamins are absorbed directly into the blood. Vitamin D is obtained from the diet, for example in margarine, oily fish, dairy products, fortified breakfast cereals and eggs, but as you read earlier, it is also manufactured when the skin is exposed to sunlight. Some groups of people need to take dietary supplements to increase their vitamin D levels, for example people who are housebound, people who for personal or cultural reasons choose to keep their skin covered, children, and pregnant and breastfeeding women whose needs for vitamin D are especially high.

## Carbohydrates

Carbohydrates exist in three forms: sugars and starches, which you have already been introduced to, and fibre. They are all **compounds** of a basic common unit made from the elements carbon, hydrogen and oxygen. This basic common unit is usually the glucose molecule.

Sugars are either single basic common units called monosaccharides (glucose, fructose, galactose) or disaccharides (sucrose, maltose, lactose), which are two monosaccharides chemically linked.

Starches are polysaccharides i.e. they are made from large numbers of glucose molecules linked together. The linked molecules can form straight chains, such as amylose, or branched chains, such as amylopectin. Branched chain starches cause cooked food to be sticky, for example, sticky, waxy rice, whereas straight chained starches cause cooked food to fluff and separate, for example, long grained rice.

Glycogen, which you read about above, is a starch that is only made by animals.

Non-starch polysaccharides (NSP) are made from many thousands of linked glucose molecules and form the structure of the cell walls of fruit, vegetables, pulses and cereal grains. Some NSPs, for example pectin, are digestible; their function is to help reduce the amount of cholesterol in the blood. Others, for example cellulose, provide us with fibre and cannot be digested; their function is to provide bulk to the contents of the digestive tract, keeping it moving and preventing constipation.

Figure 21.4 The chemical structure of carbohydrates

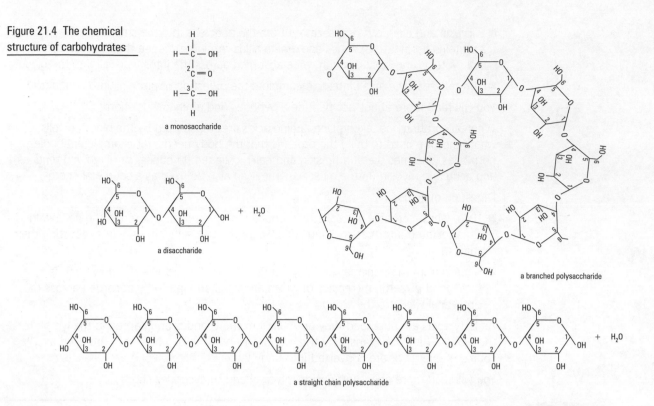

a monosaccharide

a disaccharide

a branched polysaccharide

a straight chain polysaccharide

Sugar substitutes, for example sorbitol and mannitol, occur naturally as sugars in some fruits or are manufactured. They are a source of energy but because they are broken down very slowly, they are used in, for example, diabetic foods. Artificial sweeteners, such as saccharin and aspartame, are known as food additives because they have no nutritional value and don't provide energy. They are used by people who have to restrict their sugar intake.

## Proteins

Like carbohydrates, proteins are compounds of a basic common unit made from carbon, hydrogen and oxygen. This common unit is called an amino acid. But unlike the carbohydrate common unit, all amino acids contain nitrogen, most contain sulphur and some contain phosphorus.

There are two types of amino acids:

■ indispensable amino acids, which cannot be made in the body and so must be present in the diet. They include isoleucine, phenylalanine and tryptophan.

■ dispensible amino acids, which the body can make from other amino acids in the diet. They include alanine, glutamine and tyrosine.

Figure 21.5 The chemical structure of proteins

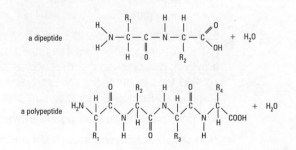

a dipeptide

a polypeptide

When amino acids join together, they become peptides. Dipeptides are molecules made from two amino acids and polypeptides are molecules made from chains of more than 50. Proteins are made from a single polypeptide molecule or from several linked together.

Whilst there are only about 20 amino acids, there is a huge variety of proteins because of the infinite number of ways that amino acids can be ordered or sequenced in a chain.

As you know, sources of protein include both animals and plants. Animal protein has a high biological value, i.e. it supplies many indispensable amino acids in the amounts we need. Plant protein has a low biological value. For this reason, people who may not or who choose not to eat meat need to have a diet that contains a wide variety of different fruits and vegetables. Texturised vegetable protein, for example soya mince, mycoprotein, for example Quorn, bean curd (tofu) and miso (fermented bean paste) are all useful protein-rich meat alternatives.

## Lipids

Figure 21.6  The chemical structure of lipids

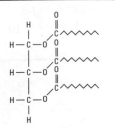

Like carbohydrates and proteins, lipids are compounds of carbon, hydrogen and oxygen. They consist of mixtures of triglycerides, which are made from three fatty acids joined to a unit of glycerol. Fats and oils are different because they contain different fatty acids.

Fatty acids are different because of the numbers of carbon atoms they contain and the number of hydrogen atoms they can hold. Saturated fatty acids have as many hydrogen atoms as they can hold. This makes them chemically stable so that food containing them, for example hard fats such as butter, lard and cocoa butter keep quite well. However, saturated fatty acids are linked with increased blood cholesterol levels.

Unsaturated fatty acids have missing hydrogen atoms. This makes them chemically less stable than saturated fatty acids so that when exposed to oxygen in the air, food containing them becomes rancid. Most unsaturated fatty acids occur in vegetable, seed and fish oils although others occur in very small amounts in some animal fats. Unsaturated fatty acids, particularly omega-3s and omega-6s, are thought to be very good for health.

Unsaturated fatty acid molecules can exist in two different forms, cis and trans. They exist naturally in the cis form but during **hydrogenation**, for example when oils are hardened during the manufacture of margarine, some of the unsaturated fatty acids become saturated and are changed into the trans form. Trans fatty acids have been linked with rises in blood cholesterol and heart disease.

Cholesterol is made by the body and not needed in the diet. It is used for the production of bile salts, vitamin D, hormones, cell membranes and so on, and is carried in the blood within molecules of lipoprotein:

■ low density lipoprotein (LDL), is often known as 'bad cholesterol' because if it increases to a high level, it can be deposited on the blood vessel walls. This helps to form the plaques that cause arteriosclerosis and CHD.

■ high density lipoprotein (HDL), is often known as 'good cholesterol' because it transports cholesterol away from where it has accumulated to the liver, where it is broken down, thereby protecting against the risk of heart disease.

## Vitamins and minerals

Like the nutrients you have read about so far, vitamins are organic i.e. they contain the element carbon. Minerals, on the other hand, are inorganic i.e. they don't contain carbon.

Vitamins are found in plants and animals. You read earlier that there are two groups of vitamins:

1. fat-soluble (A, D, E and K) vitamins, which are absorbed into the body along with fat and transported by fat through the body. They may be stored in fat and liver cells for short periods of time, until needed.

2. water-soluble (B group, C) vitamins, which are absorbed into and transported through the body in water. They need to be eaten every day as they can't be stored for any length of time. The B vitamins are B1 (thiamin), B2 (riboflavin), B3 (niacin), B5 (pantothenic acid), B6 (pyridoxine), B9 (folate), B12 (cobalamin) and biotin.

Apart from vitamin D and niacin, vitamins can't be made by the body so they must be present in the diet. You read earlier about some of the diseases caused by a deficiency of vitamins.

Minerals originate in the soil and are absorbed by plants (fruits and vegetables) as they grow. Like vitamins, they can be divided into two groups:

1. major minerals, which the body needs in large amounts. These include iron, calcium, magnesium, sodium, potassium, selenium and zinc.

2. trace elements, which the body needs in smaller amounts. These include fluoride and iodine. Most of the trace elements are poisonous when eaten in excess.

About 15 minerals are essential to life and must be included in the diet. You read earlier about some of the diseases caused by a deficiency of minerals.

Key "vitamins and minerals" into internet search engines, for example *Google* and *Yahoo!* to find out more about their functions, main sources and benefits to the body.

# Other diet-related consumption

## Water

Our bodies are approximately two-thirds water and whilst we can do without food for some time, without water the body's survival time is limited to a matter of hours or days. Water is needed for almost all body processes but is continually lost through urine, sweat and expired air. Although it is made as a by-product of chemical reactions within the body, we need to take in about two and a half litres of water every day. It is recommended that we drink six to seven glasses of water per day, more during periods of hot weather or during and after periods of physical activity; the rest should come from solid foods, in particular fruit and vegetables.

## Dietary fibre

Dietary fibre is provided by indigestible NSPs that form the structure of the cell walls of wholegrain cereals, pulses, fruits and vegetables. As you read earlier, the function of fibre is to add bulk to the faeces, helping it move along the digestive tract and prevent constipation. It is recommended that we eat about 18g of NSP per day.

Figure 21.7 Other diet-related consumption

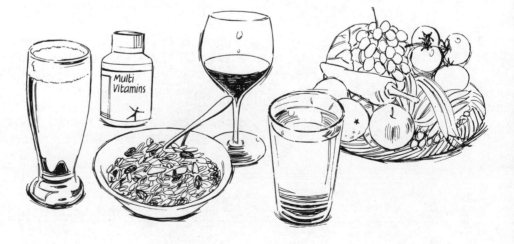

## Alcohol

Alcohol is produced when the sugar in fruit, for example grapes, and in cereals, for example barley, is fermented by yeast. It is a high source of energy but has little nutritional value: although some alcoholic drinks contain traces of vitamins and minerals, they aren't in amounts that make a useful contribution to the diet. And whilst drinking alcohol in moderation is thought to help reduce the risk of CHD, in excess it is linked with a wide range of physiological disorders, for example high blood pressure, gastritis, ulcers, liver disease and cancer, as well as mental health and behavioural problems.

Recommended daily amounts of alcohol are:

- women – two to three units
- men – three to four units.

In general, one unit is equivalent to a small glass of wine, half a pint of beer (284ml) or a pub measure of spirits. A large (175ml) glass of wine is equivalent to two units and some stronger beers and lagers contain as many as 2.5 units of alcohol per half pint. To calculate the number of units, multiply the amount of drink in millilitres by its strength (%ABV), and then divide by 1,000.

## Nutritional supplements and substitutes

Nutritional supplements and substitutes include slimming foods and nutrient pills. Slimming foods fall into two groups:

1. formula or 'dietetic' foods. These are products that have been fortified with low calorie nutrients, thereby enabling people to lose or control their weight without reducing their nutritional intake. They are regulated by legislation and labels are not allowed to refer to the speed or amount of weight loss, reduced appetite or feeling of having eaten enough that users can expect.

2. low or reduced calorie foods or portion controlled ready meals. Products like these are not dietetic foods but 'normal' foods that have been modified, usually through a change in ingredients, to contain fewer calories.

Because of their eating patterns and the amount of junk- and fast-food available, many people don't eat a balanced diet. The body's need for nutrients can be met by taking nutrient pills, for example those that contain:

- vitamins and minerals, e.g. calcium, iron, zinc, vitamin C, vitamin E and the B-complex vitamins, i.e. the vitamins and minerals most commonly missing from the diet
- omega 3, an unsaturated fatty acid which must be present in the diet for good health
- folic acid (folate, vitamin B9), which is recommended for women a month before conception and during the first 3 months of their pregnancy, to reduce the risk of birth defects such as spina bifida (abnormal spinal cord).

**case study 21.1**

## You are what you eat

Jon, aged 13, refuses to eat fruit and vegetables. His younger sister Amy, aged 9, refuses to eat anything other than food from the local fast food outlet and his older sister Caroline, aged 16, will only eat low calorie ready meals, which she has been told will enable her to lose weight quickly. His mother and father drink a couple of bottles of wine every night. None of the family makes an effort to drink water.

**activity**
**GROUP WORK**

1. How will each individual's diet affect their health?
2. How could they change what they eat to ensure that each has a balanced diet?

# Physiological principles

Figure 21.8 Physiological systems associated with nutrition

Digestive system, which breaks food down into molecules that are small enough to be absorbed across the intestinal wall into the circulating

Circulatory system, which transports the products of digestion around the body to cells that use them to make the complex molecules needed by blood in the body

**Physiological systems associated with nutrition and the metabolism of carbohydrates, fats and protein**

Endocrine system, which produces hormones such as insulin that regulates the level of glucose in the blood, and thyroxine that regulates the rate of all physiological processes

Renal system, which plays a role in maintaining the concentration of the blood and the excretion of the products of digestion

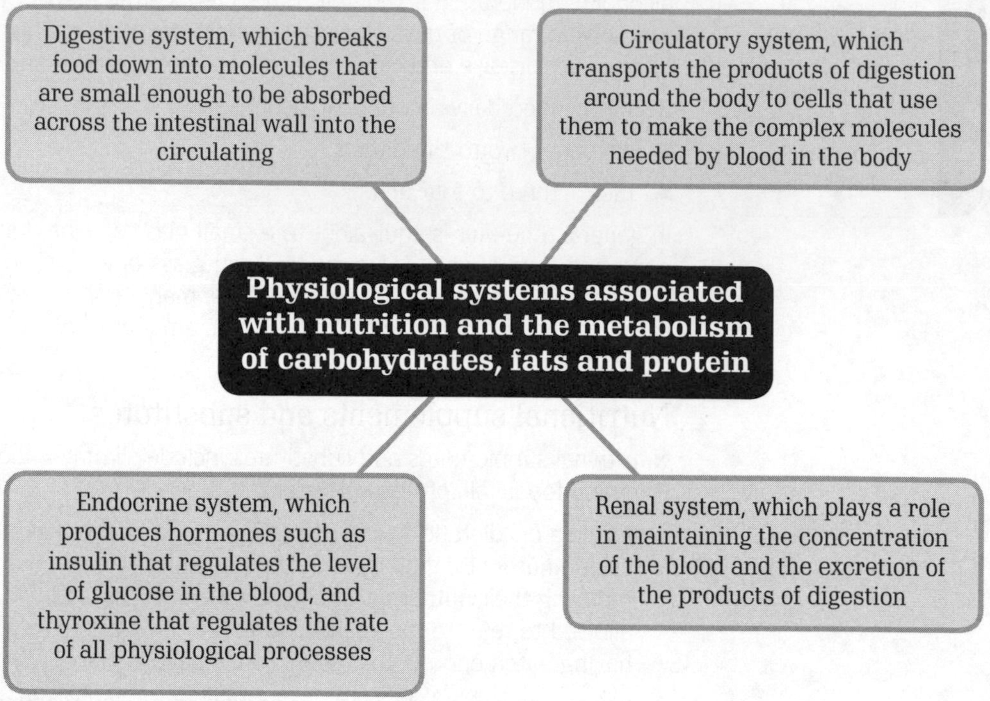

**Link**

You can read about the role these different systems play in the process of nutrition in more detail in Unit 5 of Health and Social Care Book 1.

The British Nutrition Foundation
www.nutrition.org.uk
The Vegetarian Society
www.vegsoc.org
NHS Direct
www.nhsdirect.nhs.uk
The BBC website
www.bbc.co.uk
Infant and Dietetic Foods Association
www.idfa.org.uk

*activity*
GROUP WORK
21.2

P2

M1

Produce a display that:

■ describes the characteristics of nutrients and their benefits to the body.

■ explains the potential risks to health of inappropriate nutrition.

# The influences on food intake and nutritional health

The food intake and nutritional health of different population groups is influenced by a wealth of different factors. This section aims to develop your understanding of the impact, including the risks to health, of some of these factors.

## The developed world

The food intake of people who live in the **developed world** is different from what it was two or three generations ago, for example:

- there are many more food outlets and a much greater choice of food available, which allows people to satisfy their personal taste for a wide variety of different foods

- dietary habits have changed. There has been an increase in snacking and the eating patterns of families have changed, for example many no longer eat together at the table.

- much of what is eaten, such as high energy snacks and high fat ready meals, contains too little fibre and too much sugar, salt and saturated fat, i.e. it doesn't reflect a balance of good health

- portion sizes continue to increase. According to the Economic and Social Research Council (ESRC), the average size of a hamburger has doubled since 1980.

In sum, the diets of many people in the developed world are not nutritionally healthy – they don't meet their specific nutrient needs and the amount of energy they consume is more than their body needs.

You learned about specific nutrient needs earlier in this unit (page 126) when you read about RNI.

### Lifestyles

Lifestyles have also changed in the developed world over the last fifty years:

- levels of physical activity have greatly declined, for example many of us choose to take the car or catch a bus rather than walk, and ride in lifts or on escalators rather than use the stairs

- occupations are much more sedentary, for example there has been a huge growth in numbers of people whose work requires them to sit at a computer station

- leisure pursuits require less exercise – for many people, leisure time is synonymous with sitting and watching the television or playing computer games

- there has been an increase in social eating and drinking, and as you read earlier, alcoholic drinks have little or no nutritional value and there are no labels on the food served in restaurants to tell us what we are eating.

The influence of changing lifestyles and of a diet that is not nutritionally healthy has resulted in a dramatic rise in levels of overweight and obesity (as measured by BMI) in the developed world. For example, the proportion of obese English men increased from 13.2 per cent and of obese English women from 16.4 per cent to 23.6 and 23.8 per cent respectively between 1993 and 2004. As you know, obesity increases the risk to health of a range of physiological disorders including non-insulin dependent diabetes, high blood pressure (BP), coronary heart disease (CHD) and some cancers; and an excess of alcohol increases accident risk and the risk of alcohol-related diseases.

Levels of obesity in the developed world are higher among women and people who:

- are unemployed and have insufficient income to invest in a well balanced diet or to keep fit, for example by paying to enter or join a sports centre or sports club
- do routine work and for whom snacking and alcohol can be an escape from boredom
- are seduced into buying unhealthy food because of the way it is marketed
- are seduced into heavy, binge drinking by, for example, peer pressure and cheap 'happy hour' prices
- are unable to understand food labelling because they are less well educated or have a learning difficulty
- remain unexposed to health education and healthy eating campaigns.

They are also high among some cultural and ethnic minority groups within developed world societies because, for example, their dietary beliefs include eating high fat diets, food plays an important role in their family, community and social life, they have a lower socio-economic status or there is a genetic tendency to being overweight.

## The less developed world

The 'obesity epidemic' is not restricted to the developed world. In the less developed world, economic development is introducing developed world dietary habits, lifestyles and employment practices, and over 115 million people suffer from obesity-related ill health. The World Health Organisation expects that the global total of people overweight will rise to 1.5 billion by 2015.

According to the ESRC, the global total of obese people in the year 2000 was roughly equal to the total of those suffering from malnutrition. As you read earlier, malnutrition is a nutritional health disorder and includes both overnutrition and undernutrition. Undernutrition is to do with taking in too few nutrients. It is a characteristic within some groups of people in the developed world but is more significant in the less developed world.

Undernutrition manifests itself as health conditions such as mirasmus and kwashiorkor and as the vitamin and mineral deficiency diseases that you read about earlier. It is also brought about as a result of mental health conditions such as the eating disorders anorexia and bulimia nervosa. Whilst eating disorders affect all social groups and almost all cultural groups, they predominate in young women between the ages of 15 and 25.

People with anorexia nervosa have an intense fear of gaining weight and a distorted perception of their body shape. In order to control their weight, they make themselves vomit; and some over-exercise and take appetite suppressants, laxatives and **diuretics**. As a result, they progressively lose weight (adults with anorexia have a BMI of less than 17.5) and develop physiological disorders caused by nutritional deficiencies, such as osteoporosis which is due to low calcium levels. Anorexia can also be fatal due to dangerously low levels of essential minerals in the blood, dehydration and starvation.

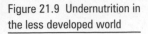

Figure 21.9 Undernutrition in the less developed world

| Poverty, which prevents people meeting the cost of good quality, nutritious food |
| Deficient and contaminated water supplies |
| Lack of transport, which makes travelling to buy food difficult |

**Influences on the food intake and nutritional health of people living in the less developed world**

| Extreme weather conditions such as tsunamis, drought and flooding, that destroy harvests and cause famine |
| Natural and man-made disasters, such as earthquakes and war, which kill people, destroying the workforce; and deforestation, which denudes the soil of nutrients, reducing levels of food production |
| Government food policies that affect food availability, for example sanctions that withhold food imports |

## Bulimia nervosa

People with bulimia nervosa crave and binge eat large quantities of food, often in secret, then purge themselves by making themselves vomit. They may also purge by fasting for periods of time or by taking laxatives and diuretics; and some exercise excessively. As a result, their weight fluctuates. Like anorexia, bulimia nervosa can cause dangerously low levels of essential minerals in the blood and dehydration.

# Children and young people

Children and young people grow quickly and are very active. Their nutritional health needs change as they grow and develop but are initially influenced by the quality of milk they are fed as babies. Breast milk is ideal as it contains all the nutrients a baby needs in the right proportions; antibodies to protect against disease; and because it is a natural product, it doesn't cause allergies. In addition, breastfeeding helps develop a close bond between mother and baby.

## Socialisation

Socialisation plays an important role in the nutritional health of children and young people. Close family and carers are the first role models to whom children are exposed, and their:

- religious and personal beliefs about what may and may not be eaten
- dietary habits, for example their personal tastes for food and drink, their snacking and meal patterns
- values, for example coming together as a family to eat.

Are markedly influenced by these people.

Figure 21.10 Dietary habits
and eating patterns

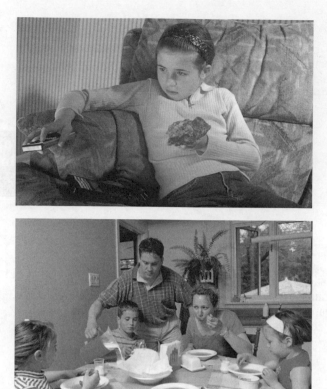

Children and young people are also influenced by food manufacturers and retailers, who aim to persuade them through advertisements, food packaging, shop displays and so on into eating their products. Unfortunately some of the food targeted at this age group is not nutritionally balanced, encourages snacking and exploits a taste for highly flavoured (sweet, salty) and fatty foods. As you read earlier, the EAR for energy and the RNI for different nutrients increases from infancy through to young adulthood. Unless children and young people develop sensible dietary habits that meet their specific needs but avoid excess sugar, salt and fat, their health is at risk.

## Childhood obesity

There has been a marked growth in childhood obesity over recent years. Worldwide there are about 155 million obese children, 22 million of whom are under the age of 5. Whilst parents and carers have a responsibility to ensure that children eat a healthy diet, UK legislation, regulations and policies, such as the Children Act 2004, Every Child Matters and the Nutrition Standards for School Lunches and Other School Food 2006 are in place to ensure that their nutritional health rights are met. To this end, health professionals such as public health nutritionists and dieticians are employed to support everyone involved in the care of children and young people to understand what makes for a nutritious, balanced diet; and public health policies and procedures, including health education and healthy eating campaigns, target different groups of people with the aim of educating them about sensible eating.

**Every Child Matters**
www.everychildmatters.gov.uk
**Food in Schools**
www.foodinschools.org
**Healthy School Lunches**
www.healthyschoollunches.org

# Adults, pregnant and breastfeeding mothers, and older people

The nutritional health needs of adults are influenced by their body size and composition, sex, age, state of health, BMR, level of activity and, to a certain extent, where they live in the world. Pregnant and breastfeeding mothers have additional nutrient and energy needs in order to provide for:

- the developing foetus i.e. their diet must contain energy foods, proteins and the range of vitamins and minerals necessary for building foetal bones, teeth, muscles and so on
- physiological changes within their own bodies, such as growth of the uterus and production of milk, and their increased need for energy whilst carrying the foetus or caring for the baby.

Most adults have roughly the same nutritional needs. However, as people get older, their BMR reduces and they become less active, which influences their appetite, reducing it such that many don't take in sufficient nutrients. In addition, some older people are unable to get to the shops, don't have the resources to buy good quality food, have lost the motivation or skills to prepare nutritious meals, and so on. Resultant undernutrition leads to general weight loss as well as disorders such as osteoporosis and night blindness, which increase the risk of falls.

To avoid risks to nutritional health, older people are advised to eat food that contains:

- enough energy to meet their decreasing level of activity, in the form of starchy foods rather than fats and sugars. Older people who take in more energy than they need quickly become overweight, which further increases the risks to health associated with old age, makes movement difficult and generally reduces quality of life.
- high concentrations of protein, vitamins and minerals.

They are also advised to take in plenty of fluid.

Health professionals such as doctors and nurses are able to identify when elderly people are not eating a balanced diet and others, such as dieticians, to make recommendations that will improve their nutritional health.

Some people have specific nutritional requirements because they have a metabolic disorder, a sensitivity or allergy to or intolerance of a certain food, restricted movement

Figure 21.11 Undernutrition in older people

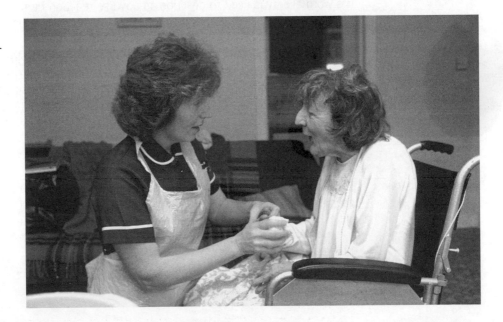

for feeding or a diet-related disease such as obesity, diabetes, CHD, cancer and osteoporosis.

You can read about diet-related diseases in Unit 14.

## Diet-related diseases

Metabolic processes are processes that go on within the body and are necessary for life. Metabolic disorders occur as a result of these processes being defective. For example, phenylketonuria (PKU) is a metabolic disease in which the enzyme that converts phenylalanine to tyrosine is defective. As a result, there is an accumulation of phenylalanine in the body tissues, which causes infantile spasm, developmental delay, disturbed behaviour and hyperactivity. PKU is diagnosed at birth through the Guthrie test (heel prick test) and people who are tested positive must restrict their intake of foods that contain phenylalanine.

## Coeliac disease

Coeliac disease is a disorder caused by a sensitivity to gluten, a protein found in wheat, rye and barley. When gluten reaches the small intestine, it activates the immune system to attack the intestine lining, destroying the finger-like projections called villi which are involved in the absorption of nutrients. Loss of villi means there is a reduced area for absorption and as a result, deficiency diseases can occur due to insufficient vitamins and minerals being processed by the body. People with coeliac disease must eat a strict gluten-free diet.

## Lactose intolerance

Lactose intolerance is caused by a lack of lactase. As you read earlier, lactase is the enzyme produced in the small intestine that is needed to digest lactose into glucose and galactose. Milk and milk products such as cheese are the only source of lactose in the diet. When people who are lactose intolerant take in milk and milk products they can experience indigestion, stomach cramps, wind and diarrhoea. They must therefore adjust their intake to levels they can tolerate. Alternatively, they may take lactase enzyme before eating, either added to milk or taken as drops or capsules, to help digestion.

## Allergies

The word allergy is used to describe an adverse reaction by the body to a protein within an allergen. Allergens include pollen, dust mites, antibiotics and some foods, for example milk, egg, wheat, soya, seafood, fruit and nuts.

An allergic reaction to food usually happens quickly and symptoms include itching and swelling of the mouth, lips, throat and skin, vomiting and diarrhoea, dizziness, coughing, wheezing and streaming of the eyes and nose. Anaphylaxis, or anaphylactic shock, is a whole-body allergic reaction and can be fatal. People who have food allergies must avoid any food to which they are allergic and replace it with alternatives that make sure they don't miss out on essential nutrients.

## Restricted movements

Some people have restricted movements for feeding, for example they have a physical disability such as tremor or spasticity, a weak grip, joint pain that makes it difficult for them to eat and drink independently, or they are unable to sit up. There is a wealth of eating and drinking equipment to help people with restricted movement, including adapted cutlery and crockery and feeding systems.

Figure 21.12 Adapted
cutlery and crockery

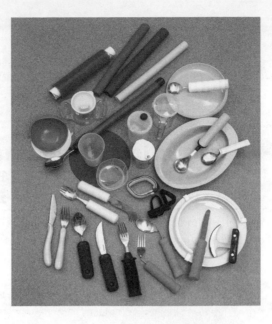

Nutritional support is used to help people who aren't able to eat or drink normally, for example because they have difficulty chewing and swallowing, cancer of the throat or they are losing weight and dietary supplements don't help. Liquidised food can be useful but some people require:

1. nasogastric feeding, which is where nutritional fluid is fed into the stomach through a tube down the nose

2. percutaneous endoscopically-guided gastrostomy (PEG) feeding, which is where nutritional fluid is fed into the stomach through a tube in the stomach wall

3. parenteral nutrition (PN), which is where nutritional fluid is fed directly into a vein.

### Economic and Social Research Council
www.esrcsocietytoday.ac.uk
### Disabled Living Foundation
www.dlf.org.uk
### NHS Direct
www.nhsdirect.nhs.uk
### Cancerbackup
www.cancerbackup.org.uk

---

**activity**
**INDIVIDUAL WORK
21.3**

**P3**

**M2**

Write case studies featuring a child, young person, adult, older person and pregnant/breastfeeding mother in which you:

■ identify the different factors that affect their dietary intake.

■ explain how each factor affects their nutritional health and wellbeing.

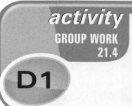

**activity**
GROUP WORK
21.4

**D1**

Working with a partner, choose two different groups of individuals, research the factors that affect their nutritional health and wellbeing and give a presentation that evaluates the relative importance of the different factors.

# Using dietary information from an individual to make recommendations to improve nutritional health

The aim of this section is to enable you to apply your developing knowledge and understanding of nutrition to yourself or someone you know with a view to making recommendations for your or their improved nutritional health.

**Professional Practice**

When making suggestions to someone you know about how they can improve their nutritional health, you must:

■ obtain their consent first

■ be positive i.e. focus on how they might improve their diet. Negative, critical feedback won't help.

■ maintain their confidentiality at all times.

In order to make recommendations to an individual for their improved nutritional health, we need to assess whether their typical consumption reflects a balance of good health. In other words, we need to know what and how much food and drink they consume, how much energy their intake contains and to measure these amounts against their personal nutritional and energy needs.

## Record of food intake

There are a number of ways to assess and record an individual's dietary intake. One method is to use recall. This involves them recalling or remembering all the food and drink that they consume during a period of time (usually about three days) in which intake is typical. It's the least complex way of identifying and measuring dietary intake but it's also the least accurate, because it's easy to forget exactly what and how much was consumed. Completing a diary or diet sheet helps with recall of what and how much has been taken in, as does taking photographs and keeping an oral record e.g. on audio tape, but recall only ever gives an approximation.

A second method is for the individual to complete a questionnaire that asks how often and in what quantities foods from a given list are eaten over a given time period. This is a quick and easy method of assessing the intake of particular food types or nutrients but can be inaccurate, particularly when assessing amounts.

A third method is to record what and how much food and drink was bought by or for the individual over a period of time and to subtract what and how much they did not consume, for example what was stored and not eaten, thrown away during preparation, wasted on the plate and so on. This is quite a cumbersome method of assessment and generally inaccurate.

A fourth method is to weigh all the different foods and drinks that the individual actually consumes over a period of time in which intake is typical. This is probably the most accurate way of assessing consumption but it can be time-consuming. In addition, care is needed when reading labels if pre-packaged food and drink, including mixer drinks, are consumed; and in assessing consumption such as when a meal is shared and the individual

**remember**
When recording dietary intake, only include what is actually consumed. Don't include food thrown away during preparation or food wasted on the plate etc.

Figure 21.13 Other factors to bear in mind when assessing dietary intake

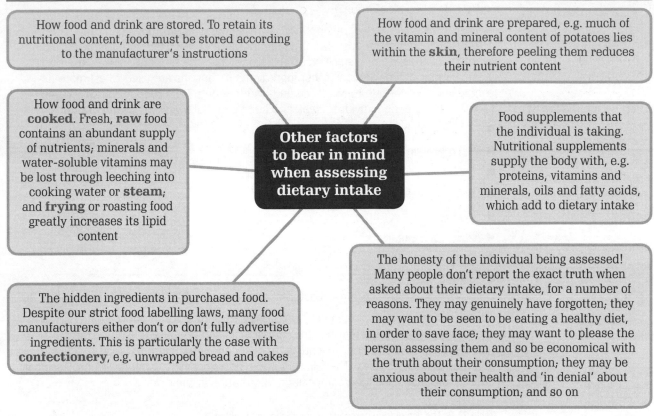

How food and drink are stored. To retain its nutritional content, food must be stored according to the manufacturer's instructions

How food and drink are prepared, e.g. much of the vitamin and mineral content of potatoes lies within the **skin**, therefore peeling them reduces their nutrient content

How food and drink are **cooked**. Fresh, **raw** food contains an abundant supply of nutrients; minerals and water-soluble vitamins may be lost through leeching into cooking water or **steam**; and **frying** or roasting food greatly increases its lipid content

**Other factors to bear in mind when assessing dietary intake**

Food supplements that the individual is taking. Nutritional supplements supply the body with, e.g. proteins, vitamins and minerals, oils and fatty acids, which add to dietary intake

The hidden ingredients in purchased food. Despite our strict food labelling laws, many food manufacturers either don't or don't fully advertise ingredients. This is particularly the case with **confectionery**, e.g. unwrapped bread and cakes

The honesty of the individual being assessed! Many people don't report the exact truth when asked about their dietary intake, for a number of reasons. They may genuinely have forgotten; they may want to be seen to be eating a healthy diet, in order to save face; they may want to please the person assessing them and so be economical with the truth about their consumption; they may be anxious about their health and 'in denial' about their consumption; and so on

consumes a portion only. It doesn't work for food and drink, including alcoholic drink that is consumed at a restaurant or from a take-away food outlet when the exact content and amount cannot be determined. In such situations, a sensible estimate is necessary.

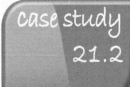

## case study 21.2

## Recording food intake

Maggie is 83 years old. She is very obese and has difficulty moving around, which makes it hard for her to look after herself. She has been referred to a dietician to plan for improved nutritional health in order that she may have an improved quality of life. Maggie lives alone and has short term memory problems. She is anxious about seeing the dietician as she has heard that obesity is linked with heart disease, from which her mother and father both died.

### activity
**GROUP WORK**

1. Describe, with reasons, how you would assess Maggie's food intake over three days.
2. What factors would you need to bear in mind when assessing her food intake?

## Sources of nutritional information and quantitative analysis

Having assessed what and how much an individual eats and drinks, it is possible to carry out a quantitative analysis of their diet i.e. calculate the amounts of energy and various nutrients that they have consumed. Food composition or analysis databases and tables provide detailed information about the amounts of energy, protein, fat, carbohydrates, vitamins and minerals that an item of food or drink contains, as well as information about the amounts of fibre and water. Nutrient amounts or values are usually quoted 'per 100g of edible portion'.

Nutrient values are based on laboratory analyses of different foods or, in the case of composite (combined foods), from the composition of the different ingredients. For example, in the case of a small steak and kidney pie, the nutrient value of the pastry, steak, kidney, onions and any other ingredients it contains are used to estimate its composition. According to McCance and Widdowson's *The Composition of Foods* (*1991*), 100g of an individual steak and kidney pie (allowing for waste) contains:

- 323 kcal energy
- 9.1g protein
- 21.2g fat
- 8.4g saturated fat
- 25.6g carbohydrate
- 2.3g total sugars
- 0.9g fibre NSP
- 42.6% water.

Source: Food Standards Agency Manual of Nutrition HMSO 2005

There are very many food composition databases and tables in publication. They are used by a variety of different health professionals and organisations, for example dieticians, nutritionists, food scientists, home economists, caterers, food manufacturers and food advisory bodies. The following table describes how some health professionals and organisations use food composition information in their work.

Table 21.3  The use of food composition databases and tables

| Examples of professionals and organisations who use food composition information | Reasons for the use of food composition information |
|---|---|
| Health and social care researchers | To find out the nutritional intake among different population groups in order to look for links between diet and disease. |
| Health professionals | To develop meal and menu plans for patients to ensure that their specific nutritional needs are met. |
| People who are concerned with food sustainability and security | To ensure that foods developed locally provide sufficient nutrients for survival or to develop food products that can be used for famine relief. |
| Health educators and policy developers | To produce health promotion campaigns and other messages aimed at educating the public about healthy eating. |
| Food manufacturers and producers | To calculate the nutrient values for food labelling purposes. They may also use the information to develop new products e.g. supplements with particular nutritional qualities. |

**activity**

INDIVIDUAL WORK 21.5

P4

Use food composition databases or tables to carry out a quantitative analysis of the energy and nutritional content of the diet of yourself or someone you know over a three day period, quoting the values per 100g of:

- energy, including the proportion of energy obtained from fat alone
- nutrients, including fat, protein, sugar, iron, vitamin C and fibre.

## case study 21.3
## Determining the nutritional content of foods

A dietician has successfully assessed Maggie's typical daily intake and recorded it in the following table.

| Breakfast | Midday meal | Evening meal | Drinks & snacks |
|---|---|---|---|
| 50g cornflakes<br>200g whole milk<br>20g sugar<br>70g white bread<br>20g butter<br>30g marmalade | 200g pork chop (lean, grilled)<br>200g chips<br>100g peas<br>500g rice pudding | 140g white bread<br>40g butter<br>100g tuna (canned in oil)<br>80g tomatoes<br>500g cheesecake | 100g salted roasted peanuts<br>50g digestive biscuits<br>100g whole milk<br>250g beer<br>1 litre of water |

## activity
### GROUP WORK

Use food composition databases or tables to carry out a quantitative analysis of the water, energy and nutritional content of Maggie's typical daily consumption, quoting the nutrient value per 100g of food for the following nutrients:

- protein
- fat
- saturated fatty acids
- carbohydrate
- fibre
- calcium
- iron
- vitamin A
- vitamin C.

## Lifestyle needs

In order to recommend how to improve their nutritional health, it is necessary to compare an individual's nutritional and energy intake with their nutritional and energy needs.

Our nutritional and energy needs are dictated by our lifestyles or ways of living, which include:

- our eating patterns – what we eat and when
- the way we prepare our food
- our BMI
- our levels of activity.

You are already familiar with RNIs, which spell out the amounts of nutrients needed by individuals at different life stages. You are also aware that different individuals have specific nutrient needs according to factors such as their state of health, allergies, sensitivities and tolerances; and that the way food is prepared, for example frying and cooking with water, affects its nutritional content. It follows that when making recommendations for improved nutritional health it is important to take these factors into account.

## Eating patterns

Individual eating patterns should also be considered when planning for improved nutritional health. For many people, a pattern of three balanced meals a day ensures that they remain satiated and healthy. But people who have a high BMR may soon feel hungry after a meal and be tempted to eat too much. Similarly, people who have a low BMR may find it difficult to eat three meals a day. Individual needs for meals should be taken into account, with recommendations to eat three nutritionally-balanced meals a day; to eat little and often, for example five or six smaller but nutritionally-balanced meals; or simply to consume sufficient food and drink to maintain good health and a healthy BMI.

People snack i.e. eat little and often for many reasons, for example they may:

- be too busy to prepare or sit down to eat a 'proper' meal
- crave the energy boost (raised blood glucose level) delivered by high energy (sugary, fatty) foods
- be addicted to the feelings of pleasure caused by the release of **endorphins** when eating food such as chocolate.

When making recommendations for improved nutritional health, people's need for snacking must be taken into account. Drinking plenty of water (we often mistake thirst for hunger) and planning snacks as mini-meals that include a variety of nutritious foods, for example fruit, unsalted nuts, raw vegetables (raw food aids digestion and promotes weight loss) and low fat dips, fruit scones, rice cakes with low fat cheese, wholemeal toast and low fat spread, can help maintain blood sugar levels, ward off cravings, and prevent overweight and associated health risks.

Many people, for religious reasons or as a method of personal choice for removing toxins from the body, desist from eating and drinking for periods of time. This is known as fasting. Fasting properly can improve health, for example studies have shown that blood glucose and cholesterol levels become lower during Ramadan fasting, reducing the risk of NID diabetes, high BP, CHD etc. Proper fasting, as opposed to crash dieting and binge eating during periods of relief from fasting, requires careful planning. Individuals should be recommended to plan to consume normal quantities of food, when appropriate, from the five food groups you read about previously.

## Body Mass Index (BMI)

Body Mass Index, which you read how to calculate earlier, is used as a guide to health. The following table describes the significance of BMI for health.

Table 21.4  BMI as a guide to health

| BMI | Comment |
|-----|---------|
| Less than 18.5 | Underweight |
| 18.5–24.9 | **Ideal** |
| 25–29.9 | Overweight |
| 30–40 | Obese |
| More than 40 | Very obese |

In general, if an individual's BMI is:

- over 25, they need to think about losing weight
- over 30, they need to change their lifestyle in order to get their weight down, for example by eating a weight-reducing diet and increasing their activity levels
- below 18.5, they need to think about putting weight on.

When making recommendations for improved nutritional health that are based on an individual's BMI, the following factors should be taken into account:

- their build – BMI's aren't necessarily accurate for lean, muscular individuals such as athletes and people who weight-train
- their state of health – calculation of BMI doesn't take into consideration pregnancy or physiological disorders
- their age – people lose weight as they get older and BMI doesn't allow for age.

## Activity levels

EAR values are the estimated amounts of energy needed by individuals for expenditure on basic life processes and physical activity. They are very general and most people need more or less than the estimated amount. Therefore when planning for improved nutritional health it is important to take into account the individual's particular energy needs.

Energy derived from food is used to maintain the BMR i.e. the rate at which basic life processes such as heartbeat, circulation, breathing and maintenance of body temperature need to proceed when we are sleeping or at complete rest. It is measured in kcals and is the minimum amount of energy the body needs to expend on a daily basis.

BMR varies according to:

- body size – in general, the larger the person, the greater their BMR
- sex – because women have a smaller muscle bulk than men and are usually lighter, they have a lower BMR
- age – it is relatively higher in infants and actively growing children than in adults, and lower in older people.

Table 21.5 Energy expenditure of various activities

| Activity | Intensity of the activity | kcal of energy used over a 30 minute period (approx) |
|---|---|---|
| Sitting (driving, doing sedentary work) | Light | 60 |
| Ironing | Light | 60 |
| Cleaning and dusting | Light | 70 |
| Walking (slowly, 2mph) | Light | 75 |
| Walking (briskly, 4mph) | Moderate | 150 |
| Tennis (doubles) | Moderate | 150 |
| Aerobic dancing | Vigorous | 195 |
| Football | Vigorous | 210 |
| Tennis (singles) | Vigorous | 240 |
| Cycling (12–14 mph) | Vigorous | 240 |
| Running (6mph) | Vigorous | 300 |

Energy derived from food is also used to expend on activities such as thinking, reading, eating, sitting, standing, walking and exercising. For this reason, an individual's energy needs are also dictated by their levels of activity and when making recommendations for improved nutritional health, reference should be made to how active they are.

The Physical Task Force, 2003, recommended that adults do at least 30 minutes of moderate activity on most days of the week, to help them maintain their weight and prevent them from gaining more. People who need to lose weight should think of 30 minutes as a starting point and gradually increase the intensity of the activity or spend more time being active.

# Other needs

Other factors that need to be considered when making recommendations for improved nutritional health include the individual's personal preferences, for example for food and drink; their personal financial resources; their social and cultural background; and the time they have available, for example to buy, prepare and eat food, and to participate in physical activities.

## Personal preferences

We all have a preference for one type of food over another and develop our likes and dislikes throughout life. Personal preferences are important when planning for good health. There is no point recommending that someone drink orange juice or eat liver to boost their vitamin C or iron level respectively if they don't like orange juice or can't stomach liver! Similarly, there's little point asking someone to give up certain foods or drinks unless they are motivated and supported to do so, for example through the realisation of the benefits of changing their diet and by being offered acceptable alternatives.

## Economic situation

An individual's economic situation can have a huge impact on their dietary intake. According to the National Consumer Council, low cost and economy range foods in Britain's leading supermarkets are much less healthy than more expensive products, for example they contain significantly more salt and slightly more fat and sugar than the supermarkets' own-brand products. In other words, buying cheap food is false economy (*The Guardian*, Friday December 1, 2006) and better quality food remains more expensive.

Transport from rural areas into town or from town to out-of-town supermarkets to buy food is another problem for poorer people, because of its cost. For these and other reasons, recommendations for improved nutritional health have to be sensitive to people's spending power.

## Social and cultural needs

Social and cultural needs also impact on dietary intake and nutritional health, for example:

- different people have different beliefs about what they need to eat to stay healthy. Many of our beliefs about nutrition originate from our parents and what we were taught at school. However, knowledge of nutrition is constantly evolving and what was 'good' to eat just a few years ago may not be considered a healthy option today! For example, margarine has for years been sold as a healthy substitute for butter but we now know that some brands contain trans fatty acids.

- different religions, for example Islam and Judaism, and social groups, for example vegetarians and vegans, also have beliefs about what they need to consume.

- attitudes and ideas about what is 'normal' to eat and drink. People from different parts of the world need to consume different things, because of food availability, traditions, customs and so on.

- peer pressure and the media can be very successful in persuading people what they need to eat in order that they can conform to a certain body image, for example muscle bound or very thin.

- living conditions. People who lack access to adequate food storage, preparation and cooking areas, and people who live alone may need to eat ready-prepared meals or eat out as opposed to cook at home or for themselves.

Figure 21.14 The bargain
basement

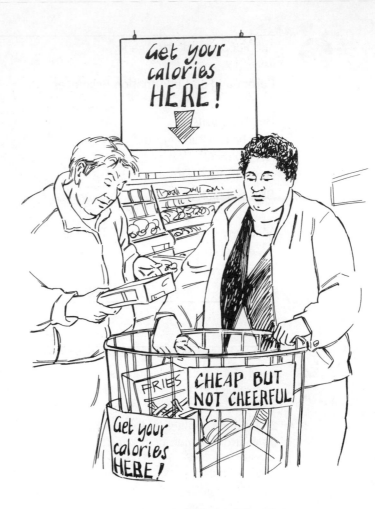

- language differences mean that some people need help in understanding food labels
  and health promotion messages and campaigns.

For these and other reasons, recommendations for improved nutritional health have to
be sensitive to people's social and cultural backgrounds.

## Time

Time also plays a role in people's nutritional health. Changes in the way they live
and work mean that many people are continually on the move. As a result they have
insufficient time to think about and plan what they are going to eat and drink, and to
shop for and prepare their own meals. Recommendations for improved nutritional health
must take account of the way people need to spend their time.

By comparing an individual's intake with their needs, it is possible to plan for their
improved nutritional health.

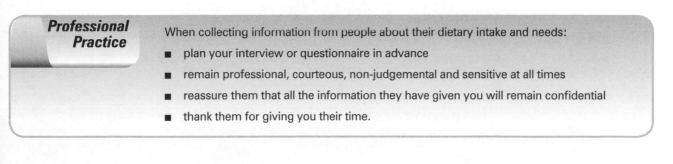

**Professional Practice**

When collecting information from people about their dietary intake and needs:

- plan your interview or questionnaire in advance
- remain professional, courteous, non-judgemental and sensitive at all times
- reassure them that all the information they have given you will remain confidential
- thank them for giving you their time.

The Food Standards Agency
www.food.gov.uk
European Food Information Resources
www.nutrition.org.uk
Healthy Living
www.healthyliving.gov.uk
NHS Direct
www.nhsdirect.nhs.uk
BBC website
www.bbc.co.uk
Matthew Robinson Personal Training
www.mrpt.co.uk
Fitness First
www.fitnessfirst.co.uk

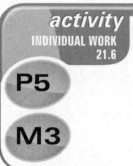

*activity*
**INDIVIDUAL WORK**
**21.6**

**P5**

**M3**

- Prepare a plan for improved nutritional health, for yourself or the individual you used for Activity 21.5, which meets their lifestyle, personal preferences, financial, social and economic needs, and which takes account of the way they use their time.
- Produce a leaflet to accompany your plan that explains how your suggestions meet your or the individual's needs.

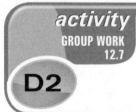

*activity*
**GROUP WORK**
**12.7**

**D2**

Write a report that evaluates how the plan you devised for Activity 21.6 will improve your or your chosen individual's health

*Progress Check*

1. Describe what is meant by the following terms: food, diet, nutrients, additives, nutritional supplements, fortification of food, malnutrition, undernutrition, deficiency, overnutrition, overweight, obesity, energy balance, body mass index, Dietary Reference Values, Reference Nutrient Intakes.

2. Describe the following terms as they relate to dietary intake: balance of good health, food groups, food pyramid, five a day, the effect of food preparation/processing methods, hidden ingredients.

3. Identify sources of the following nutrients and describe why we need to include them in our diet: carbohydrates, proteins, fats, vitamins, minerals.

4. List the nutritional requirements of different groups of people.

5. Describe the effects of food processing on nutrients.

6. Describe the chemical structure of carbohydrates, proteins and fats, and the processes involved in making them available to the body.

7. Explain the function within the body of water, dietary fibre, alcohol, and nutritional supplements and substitutes.

8. Compare and contrast factors that influence the dietary intake of: people living in the developed world and people living in the less developed world, children and adults, young people and older people.

9. Explain the impact of the factors you identified above on the health and wellbeing of the individuals concerned.

10. Why is it necessary to carry out a quantitative analysis of the diet when planning for improvements in nutritional health?

11. What factors need to be born in mind when planning for improvements in nutritional health?

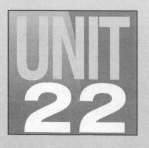

# Research Methodology for Health and Social Care

## This unit covers:

- The purpose and role of research in health and social care
- The research methodologies relevant to health and social care
- How to identify a suitable topic and produce a plan for a research proposal
- How to conduct research and present the findings
- How to evaluate a research project
- The implications of and ethical issues related to using research in health and social care

Health and social care services are always searching for more effective, economic and efficient ways to care for individuals. Good, evidence-based research is the foundation of this.

This unit aims to give you both a theoretical understanding of research and the opportunity for practical application. You will be able to understand its purpose, the methodologies available to use, ethical issues and implications of research in the field. You will then have an opportunity to design, plan and carry out basic research. You will also gain the skills to evaluate research.

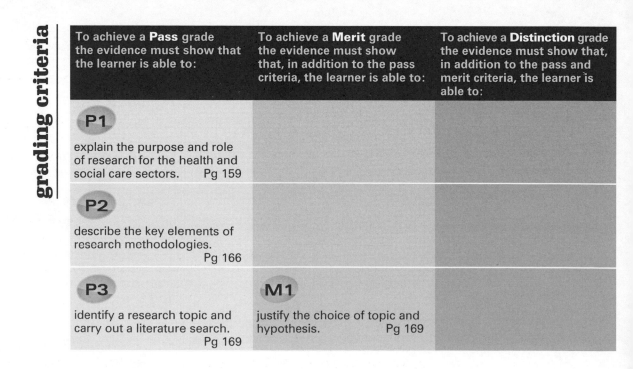

| grading criteria | To achieve a **Pass** grade the evidence must show that the learner is able to: | To achieve a **Merit** grade the evidence must show that, in addition to the pass criteria, the learner is able to: | To achieve a **Distinction** grade the evidence must show that, in addition to the pass and merit criteria, the learner is able to: |
|---|---|---|---|
| | **P1** explain the purpose and role of research for the health and social care sectors.     Pg 159 | | |
| | **P2** describe the key elements of research methodologies.     Pg 166 | | |
| | **P3** identify a research topic and carry out a literature search.     Pg 169 | **M1** justify the choice of topic and hypothesis.     Pg 169 | |

## grading criteria

| To achieve a **Pass** grade the evidence must show that the learner is able to: | To achieve a **Merit** grade the evidence must show that, in addition to the pass criteria, the learner is able to: | To achieve a **Distinction** grade the evidence must show that, in addition to the pass and merit criteria, the learner is able to: |
|---|---|---|
| **P4** carry out the primary research and collect and record appropriate data. Pg 176 | | |
| **P5** present and report findings in a relevant format, identifying sources of bias or error. Pg 183 | **M2** review the research methods chosen in relation to the results obtained, any sources of bias or error and ethical considerations. Pg 193 | **D1** discuss how the methodology of the research project could be altered to reduce bias and error. Pg 193 |
| **P6** discuss the findings of the research in relation to the original hypothesis. Pg 183 | **M3** analyse the findings of the research in relation to the original hypothesis. Pg 183 | **D2** analyse the purpose and role of research in the sectors, drawing on the piece of research undertaken. Pg 194 |
| **P7** outline any possible improvements to the research, referring to any relevant implications and ethical issues. Pg 194 | **M4** discuss the possible implications that the research results may have on current practice. Pg 194 | |

# The purpose and role of research within health and social care

## Purpose

Research, especially when done properly, takes time, effort, money and resources. So why go to all the effort? Below are four reasons why, but it is important to understand that the overall purpose of research is to study and investigate in order to discover new facts or information for use.

## Identify need

One reason for research is to identify need. Need is described as a requirement, often differentiated from 'wants'. As a service provider in health and social care, be that as an individual, or an organisation, you need to know what individuals need. By researching needs of individuals, it may be found that there are similarities or trends, allowing service providers to know collective needs of either geographical group (i.e. local needs) or a particular type of service user (i.e. by age, sex, disability, condition or impairment).

## Provide further knowledge

Another reason for research is to provide further knowledge. Think about the knowledge and understanding that we had 10 years, 20 years, 100 years or 500 years ago about health and well-being and the causes of illness. Society did not know for example, that washing hands prevented the spreading of disease, the dangers of asbestos, how to perform key hole surgery, how to create 'test-tube' babies, or how the transmission of HIV/AIDS occurred. All these discoveries and this 'new' understanding has developed because of research. Who knows what knowledge and understanding could be gained in the future? Cures for HIV/AIDS, cures for cancer, how to prevent growing old! It is only through research that this is possible.

## Gaps in provision

A further reason for research is to highlight gaps in provision. Service providers want to meet the needs of all individuals and match this with provision. Research can identify needs and investigate why people are not using a service; it may be because the service doesn't exist, or because people aren't aware of the service, or because barriers exist, deterring or stopping access. This research would allow a service to see where there are gaps in their provision and to make amends to this.

## Plan provision

Allowing services to plan provision is the final purpose for research in health and social care. Research allows us to improve the provision of services – More services? Fewer services? Different opening times? Staffing? Training needs? Physical resources? It will assist services to develop long-term plans.

# Role

Once we know the purpose of research in health and social care, the reason for undertaking it, it is also useful to look at how it can be used: what is its role?

*remember*

Research can be a long, costly process – you need to be clear on its purpose before you start!

Figure 22.1 Planning provision

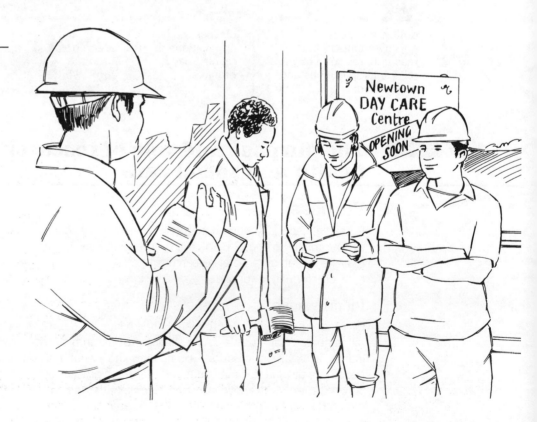

## Inform

Service providers may use the research to inform policy or practice, allowing service providers to change the way they operate. Society is constantly changing and facing new threats and challenges, and hence policy and practice needs to reflect this. As this is being written, many towns in England are suffering from flooding due to the heavy rain. People in authority have to make decisions on drinking water, on sewage, on care for those with disabilities or impairments, etc. They do not always have a 'foolproof' guide on how to approach the issue, but by referring to research their decisions will have been informed. Hence, in the example situation, the impact of the floods is minimised.

## Extend knowledge

It can also be used to extend knowledge and understanding, be that of the service, employees, management structures, treatments, clients, access, etc. Once that knowledge base has been extended, it allows for services to improve practice. It is imperative that all services are continuously reviewing practice. Localities change, lifestyles change, demographics change, infrastructures change, and hence society needs to know and understand about this so that practice can change. For example, even 10 years ago, the issue of MRSA was not highlighted as it is now. Because of research into its prevalence and how it is spread, practice has now changed, e.g. within hospitals there are now 'hand-wash stations'.

## Aid reflection

Whether due to a training course or not, all health and social care staff would benefit from reflecting on their practice and skills. Being aware of new research and developments will aid reflection. For example, if a nursery teacher read new research on the difficulties children with ADHD experience at nursery, they would hopefully reflect on this and then incorporate this into their teaching of children with ADHD.

## Monitor progress

Sometimes changes in practice may already have occurred, maybe past research indicated that this was the best option, but how can it be checked that the desired effects are taking place? Research allows progress to be monitored. For example, a new system for home care is put into place ensuring that people have assistance at a time which is more convenient to them. This was changed in the hope that complaints would be significantly reduced. Research could take place to ensure that this is indeed happening. If complaints were reducing, then the changes have been successful. If complaints were not falling, maybe timing was not the key issue, maybe it was something else, maybe the skills of the staff themselves?

Research also allows practitioners and policy makers to examine topics of contemporary importance. Currently, there is a debate about the impact on the smoking ban; will it stop people from starting smoking, will it help smokers to give up, what are the effects the ban will have on businesses, etc. Research can help all agencies concerned gather the facts about a contemporary topic to ensure there are limited negative effects.

Ultimately, it is hoped it can be seen that research in health and social care is extremely important. It allows policy makers to plan the best services and for practitioners to provide the best care. Many examples of research can be found in journals or on government websites.

*activity*
**INDIVIDUAL WORK 22.1**

Design a presentation to show to others in your class (you could do this as a display or as a PowerPoint) outlining the purpose and role of research in health and social care.

**P1**

Department of Health
www.dh.gov.uk
Department of Children, Schools and Families
www.dfes.gov.uk
National Institute of Clinical Excellence
www.nice.org.uk/
British Journal of Nursing
www.info.britishjournalofnursing.com/
British Journal of Social Work
www.bjsw.oxfordjournals.org/
British Medical Journal
www.bmj.com

# Research methodologies relevant to health and social care

## Types of research

Choosing the right research **methodology** can make or break a piece of research. Using an inappropriate method can result in obtaining invalid or erroneous results. The following section will help you to choose the most appropriate methodology.

### Quantitative and qualitative research

**Quantitative** research is defined by Bandolier, a website on evidence-based research in health care:

> 'Quantitative research generates numerical data or data that can be converted into numbers.'

And **qualitative** is also defined:

> 'Qualitative research is used to explore and understand people's beliefs, experiences, attitudes, behaviour and interactions.'

Simplistically, quantitative data answers the 'how many?' question, qualitative helps to answers the 'why?' question.

Primary data is data collected by the researcher themselves whilst secondary data is research collated and presented by another researcher. Good research is often based on a combination of both, as they can 'back up' each other. This is often referred to as **'triangulation'** and will be covered later.

### Primary research

#### *Questionnaires*

A questionnaire is a selection of questions designed by the researcher to be answered by the participant.

Figure 22.2 Undertaking
questionnaires

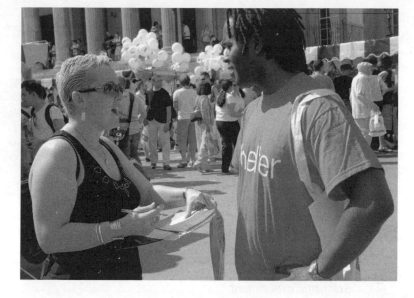

### *Interviews*

Interviews are when there is dialogue between the researcher and the participant.
Interviews can be face-to-face, over the phone, or increasingly, using instant messenger
services on the internet. Usually only one person is interviewed, but it can be that
groups are interviewed together. Interviews can be structured or unstructured.
Structured allows the researcher to have pre-determined questions.

Table 22.1  Advantages and disadvantages of questionnaires

| Advantages | Disadvantages |
| --- | --- |
| Can send to a large number of people. | Postage costs can be high. |
| Can be a relatively cheap way of finding information. | Response rates can be low. |
| The researcher could collect straight away. | Respondents may not always understand, and cannot ask the researcher. |
| The written answer allows the researcher to thoroughly evaluate answers. | It can take a long time to get all the questionnaires back. |
| Easier assessment can be achieved through the comparison of answers to specific questions. | Respondents may not always answer truthfully or seriously. |
| Reminders can be sent out to participants who have not returned their questionnaire. | A dissimilar style of language or text may not be inclusive. |
| Questionnaires can be anonymous. | People who do not have English as their first language, have alternative communication methods or have learning difficulties may be excluded. |
| Can use open or closed questions. | |

Table 22.2  Advantages and disadvantages of structured interviews

| Advantages | Disadvantages |
| --- | --- |
| Researcher and/or participant can stick to the task. | Cannot probe an interesting answer. |
| Allows for easier comparison between answers. | The flow of the conversation can feel a bit 'automated'. |
| Useful for inexperienced interviewers. | May only receive short, one word answers to questions. |

Unstructured interviews do not have a prescribed set of questions to be asked. This allows the researcher to have a more open discussion about the topic.

Table 22.3  Advantages and disadvantages of unstructured interviews

| Advantages | Disadvantages |
|---|---|
| Researcher can be as flexible as they wish. | Researcher and/or the participant can go off task. |
| Interesting answers can be explored. | More difficult for researcher to note answers. |
| Confusing answers can be explained. | More difficult to compare interview data. |

**Link** See Unit 1 in Health and Social Care Book 1 for the communication skills needed when interviewing.

### Scientific experiment

Scientific experiments are often associated with the 'sciences', however, they can be of great use in health and social care as many of the treatments/interventions have to be scientifically tested. Indeed the National Institute of Clinical Excellence is an independent organisation who advises on the best available evidence of effectiveness and cost effectiveness; this is usually, but not exclusively, based on scientific experiment.

Table 22.4  Advantages and disadvantages of scientific experiments

| Advantages | Disadvantages |
|---|---|
| It can be easier to establish cause and effect, as the researcher is able to control or remove different variables. | Research in a controlled environment, i.e. a laboratory, is different from a real environment. A laboratory may be too 'artificial' an environment? |
| Experiments can be replicated and repeated to improve confidence in the results. | The laboratory does not always take into account 'surprise' factors. |
| Experiments can often produce data in qualitative format. | Scientific experiments may not always be the best way to study human behaviour as humans are conscious, thinking beings not passive, inanimate beings. People may react differently in different social situations. |

Figure 22.3  Performing interviews

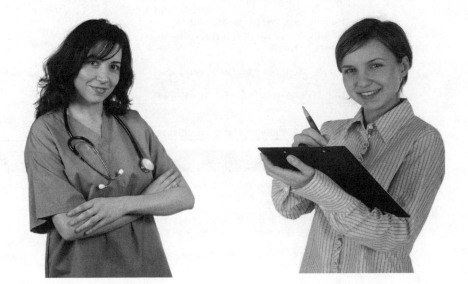

### Formal and informal observation

Observations are when the researcher observes behaviours/actions of individuals.

Observations can either be formal or informal. Informal observations are more unstructured or exploratory. Researchers usually have little knowledge of the population and their behaviour. The main purpose of informal observation is to create hypotheses to be tested later. Formal observations are more structured or systematic. It is similar to the structured interview described above, but in this case, questions are not asked, instead, particular types of behaviour are looked for, and counted.

Observations can also be direct or indirect. Direct observations are where the researcher participates in the behaviour, e.g. plays with the children in the nursery. Alternatively, observations can be indirect, this is where the researcher is a non-participant, e.g. simply observes the children playing in the nursery.

Observations can also either be covert or overt. Covert observations are where the researcher observes without the consent of the individuals concerned; this may achieve a truer picture, but could be ethically problematic, as essentially the researcher is 'spying' on the participants, and they may feel deceived. Overt observation is where the researcher has explained their research and gained permission from the participants to observe them. However, by the participant having knowledge of being observed, there may be a risk that their behaviour is modified.

Therefore, it can be seen that observations can be a combination of three types (formal/informal, direct/indirect, covert/overt).

Table 22.5 Advantages and disadvantages of observations

| Advantages | Disadvantages |
|---|---|
| These can be useful as the researcher is able to see the individual in their natural environment; it can often therefore reveal a more truthful representation.<br><br>In covert observation, 'researcher bias' can be removed, i.e. respondents will not behave how they think they should in front of the researcher.<br><br>Observations can be done on more than one individual at one time.<br><br>The process may be video-taped or recorded.<br><br>The researcher is able to observe body language, which can sometimes reveal more than what is said. | There are many ethical issues with observations as, in essence, you are 'watching' individuals, especially covert (ethical issues will be covered later in the chapter).<br><br>Watching and accurate noticing of behaviour traits and recording of information all need to be done simultaneously; this can be a difficult skill to master.<br><br>To perform covert, direct observation, the researcher may have to 'become' one of the group; this can be difficult as some groups may be difficult to 'infiltrate', e.g. drug users.<br><br>The data collected can often be too unstructured.<br><br>Observing is subjective; what one researcher may feel is 'significant behaviour', another researcher may not.<br><br>The use of recording equipment may be problematic – practically and ethically.<br><br>In overt observations, participants may modify their behaviour to present a better image. |

Figure 22.4 Observing
behaviour

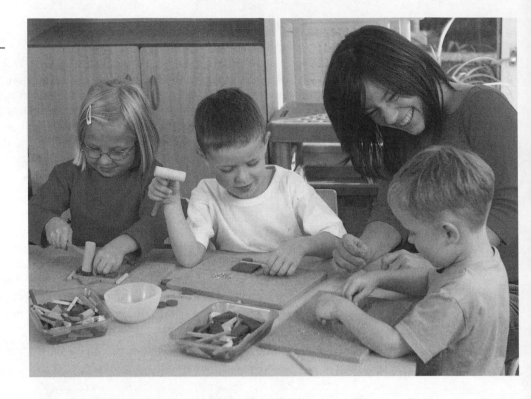

## Secondary research

### Internet

Increasingly so, the internet is becoming more and more useful as a source of
**secondary research**. The internet is a worldwide network of computers; it allows for
information to be available to view and also to be transferred via electronic mail, online
chat facilities and file transfers. It is very likely that you yourself have used the internet
to research information for your assignments. This means that a wide source of research
findings are now available to view and to be transferred.

Table 22.6 Advantages and disadvantages of the internet

| Advantages | Disadvantages |
|---|---|
| A massive amount of research is available to view. | Not everyone is computer literate. |
| Computers and internet access are available in most educational establishments, libraries and in many people's own homes. | There are no regulatory systems in place to control what is placed on the internet. |
| Research from anywhere in the world can be viewed. | Sometimes, research from other places in the world isn't relevant. |
| Research can be found in a matter of seconds. | Sometimes, research can be dated. |
| Research which is found, can be saved, viewed later or printed off. | Unless the specific web address is known, it can sometimes take a very long time to find what is required. |
| Search engines (e.g. Yahoo, Ask, Google) can be used to help find what is wanted, if specific details are not available. | Sometimes, there is just too much information to view. |
| Encyclopaedias, dictionaries, newspapers, government agencies, etc. are all available online. | |
| There are many online libraries of research e.g. ERIC. | |

### Journals

A journal is a publication which is published periodically, e.g. weekly, monthly, three monthly, annually, etc., therefore it is different to a book which is usually a one-off publication. Journals usually have collections of different works from different authors which the editors believe meet the standards required. There are many journals that are published which have research findings included, e.g. *British Medical Journal*, *British Journal of Nursing*, *British Journal of Social Work*.

Figure 22.5 Using secondary sources

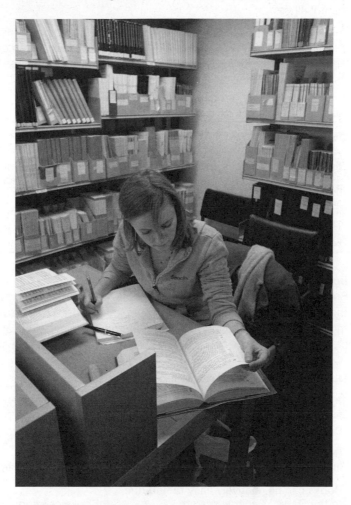

Table 22.7 Advantages and disadvantages of using journals

| Advantages | Disadvantages |
|---|---|
| Articles in journals often have to meet high standards to be published. | Journals are not always accessible in terms of availability; libraries do not always stock them. |
| Many research reports are peer reviewed to ensure high standards. | Journals are not always accessible in terms of cost. |
| Due to being published at intervals, research reports are often contemporary and 'hot off the press'. | Journals are often very academic and written to a very high standard, hence they may not always be easy to read and understand. |
| They are a trusted source of research findings, the standards associated with them have earned them prestige. | The referencing system is not always clear and hence they can be difficult to search. |
| | There can be long delays from submission to publication. |

### Media

The media can both *influence* society and also *reflect* society. The media includes television, newspapers, films, radio, magazines, etc. Therefore researching the media can provide an indicator of society, as the media can mirror society. For example if you wanted to understand society's views on mental illness, by examining films portraying people with mental illness, newspaper reports of people with mental illness, television characters suffering from mental illness, a picture could be gained of how society views mental illness.

Further, the media can be used as a knowledge source in terms of news articles, documentaries and report investigative journalism. These can often report the facts which may be useful for research. Researching media coverage can establish whether issues are believed to be serious or trivialised.

Table 22.10  Advantages and disadvantages of using the media

| Advantages | Disadvantages |
|---|---|
| The media can be easy to access.<br><br>Past media can be easy to access in archives, on the internet, etc.<br><br>The media is relatively cheap to use. | The media can be biased politically and can represent personal views and hence may not always be a representation of society, may be just an individual.<br><br>The media can often be sensationalist and/or distort the truth. |

### Books

Books are a traditional source of information and facts. The written word is one of the oldest forms of communication. People have used rock, clay, bark, etc. to record thoughts or information in the past. Due to technological advances and the development of printing, books are now a widespread and easily accessible source of information.

Table 22.11  Advantages and disadvantages of using books

| Advantages | Disadvantages |
|---|---|
| Books can be cheap.<br><br>Books can be borrowed for free from libraries.<br><br>Books can be relatively easy to find due to the Dewey Decimal system.<br><br>Information can be photocopied. | Not all books are available in every library; some need to be ordered in.<br><br>There are copyright laws on books limiting what can be copied.<br><br>Books can soon become dated.<br><br>Books can only represent the views of the author/s. |

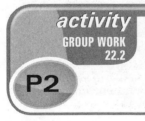

*activity*
GROUP WORK
22.2

P2

Working in small groups, each individual chooses one or two research methods. Produce an outline on one sheet of A4. Try to include a description of the method, their strengths and weaknesses. When all methods have been completed, collate them all for a 'book on research methods'.

British Psychological Society
www.bps.org.uk
Sociology central
www.sociology.org.uk/index.htm
Sociology online
www.sociologyonline.net
British Journal of Nursing
www.info.britishjournalofnursing.com
British Medical Journal
www.bmj.com
NICE
www.nice.org.uk
SCIE
www.scie.org.uk/index.asp
ERIC
www.eric.ed.gov

## case study

Fig.22.6

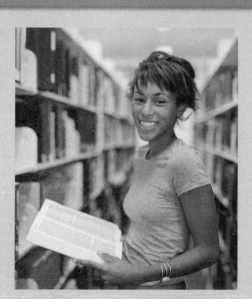

Sehrish has a **research question** of 'What are the reasons students study Health and Social Care?' She would like to triangulate (see glossary) her ideas and include both primary and secondary research as well as get information from both students and staff.

## activity
### INDIVIDUAL WORK

1.  Do you have any ideas for Sehrish?  What research methodologies could she use?
2.  Justify your choices.

# Identifying a suitable topic and producing a plan for a research proposal

## Topic and hypothesis

Identifying a suitable health and social care related topic is as broad as it is limiting. When you are choosing your research topic, it may be wise to also consider any career options you are considering, university courses you may consider, other subjects you are studying which may help, any interests you have, and possibly the resources available, both in terms of **primary research** opportunities and secondary research opportunities.

Although by no means exhaustive, here are some areas that are available to study:

You could choose a research topic around a service user:

- Age: infant, child, teenager, adult, older person
- Condition: A person with a disability, with an impairment, with a physical health condition, mental health condition, a learning difficulty, etc.

You could choose a research topic around a service provider:

- A health care establishment – GP, hospital, dentist, optician, pharmacy, clinic, a nursing home, etc
- A social care establishment – a residential care home, a day care centre, domiciliary care, fostering/adoption services, counselling services, etc.
- An early years establishment – nursery, playgroup, school, breakfast club, after school club, summer schools, au pair/nanny services, etc.

You could choose a research topic around a possible future career:

- Nurse
- Midwife
- Teacher/teaching assistant
- Nursery teacher/assistant
- Child carer
- Social worker
- Care assistant
- Occupational therapist
- Dental assistant.

You could choose a research topic around a health and social care issue:

- Met needs
- Unmet needs
- Access
- Barriers
- Discrimination
- Communication
- Health
- Health Promotion
- Health Education
- Health and safety
- Lifestyle choices
- Staff

- Teaching strategies
- Care strategies

Think of any issues that might have been highlighted in the other units you have studied in your BTEC Health and Social Care Course.

---

**_activity_**
**INDIVIDUAL WORK 22.3**

**P3**

**M1**

1. Make a list of five issues you may like to investigate in some way. Choose one idea and perform a literature search on this.
2. Finalise your topic and **hypothesis**. Justify your choice of topic and your hypothesis.

---

Once you have decided, the next stage in your research would be to perform a literature search to find out what research is already available on the said topic.

It may be the case that you have a broad interest, but cannot narrow it down; in this case, the use of a literature search may be helpful. Say for example you had a general interest in the 5-a-day campaign, and you would like to research something in that area but you are unsure what, and you wouldn't want to duplicate research that has been done before. It would be a wise decision to perform a literature search. Here you may find information already found out on the amounts of fruit and vegetables eaten, by age and gender, you may find research already undertaken on reasons why people don't eat fruit and vegetables (availability, cost, convenience). You may find research already undertaken on campaigns to increase the consumption of fruit and vegetables, however, you may see a gap in the research. For example, is there research on the difference

Figure 22.7 What shall I choose?

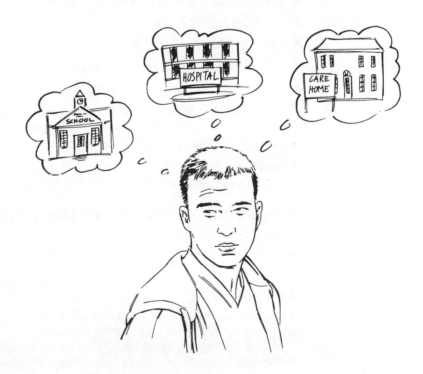

between teenage boys and teenage girls? Is there research on the cost and availability of fruit and vegetables in school canteens?

Performing a literature search allows you to become more knowledgeable on the subject, not repeat research that has already been done, see where there are omissions (gaps) in the topic and introduce your research project clearer. Hence you can justify your research project more confidently.

When choosing your research topic, it is also important that you consider the suitability of a topic with reference to ethical issues. Although this will be covered in more detail later in the chapter, it is worth considering **ethics** *before* you choose your topic. When considering ethics, you need to consider whether the research topic is going to cause any harm or upset to the participants, will you need to get their consent, how will you protect the rights of participants (privacy, respect, etc.), will they have a right to withdraw, will issues be dealt with sensitively, will participants remain anonymous, how will information be kept confidential, how can you guarantee that data is recorded accurately and is a true representation of their views, etc? It will be far easier to deal with these issues now if they are considered at the outset, when the topic is being decided.

A further issue to consider when choosing a research topic is the formulation of a relevant, realistic hypothesis/research question. A hypothesis is a statement that, with research, can be proved or disproved. A research question is a question which aims to be answered by the research project.

Examples of hypotheses are:

- Violent behaviour is more likely to occur after the consumption of alcohol.
- The quantity and quality of sports provision within primary schools is inadequate.
- The support available in primary schools to children with special needs is inadequate.
- Children under twelve eat a more balanced diet than those over twelve.
- The provision of day care services within town A is unsatisfactory.

Examples of research questions are:

- Do health services meet the needs of people who are deaf?
- What are the differences in the teaching methods for gifted and talented students?
- Do girls in infant school have a better work ethic than boys?
- What are the different ways that schools teach literacy?
- What are the attitudes of people towards people with mental health problems?

It is important that you choose a hypothesis/research question that has a clear title which allows you to stay on track with your research. If the topic is too vague or too broad it can be difficult to prove/disprove/answer.

Although the choosing of a topic should not be affected by monetary factors, it is wise to considerer costs, as a budget may be required, even for printing, posting, copying, etc.

## Producing an outline of the planned research

Once you have decided what your research topic is, it is good practice to have a plan. This ensures that everyone knows what their responsibilities are (especially if it is a team conducting the research).

### Methodology

Firstly, it is important to plan the **methodology**. It is not enough to simply outline which type of research methodology or methodologies are to be used. It is useful to explain details too. For primary research, you will have to consider the numbers to be observed, interviewed, given questionnaires, experiments to take place. The location of where the research will take place is important as well as dates and times; indeed it may be that

**remember**
Choosing the right methodology is critical, as it bears significantly on the outcome of the research project.

appointments have to be made. It may be the case that printing, copying and other admin tasks need to be done. Maybe recording equipment needs to be booked.

One very important aspect to consider is to pilot the research methodology. Firstly, allow a small **sample** of people to run through your methodology. This allows for any mistakes or problems to be highlighted. Secondly, it allows the researcher to gain confidence in conducting the research. Mistakes can be costly both in terms of money and time, so getting as much as possible piloted is invaluable.

## Target group

It is also of great importance to be clear about who your target group and sample are. It is very important to be clear on who you will be including in the research. Firstly, you need to be clear on who the population to be asked is. Population is the general term for whoever it is that you want to generalise about – people in a town, users of a hospital, residents of a care home. However, it is often very difficult to have all of the population take part in the research (time, cost, resources, availability). Therefore, you may need a sample.

## Sampling

A sample needs to be representative of your population. For this to happen your sample needs to be large enough and similar enough to the population it is representing; this would allow you to generalise about the population.

Therefore, you need to ensure that your research title is clear on the population to be studied. Look at the following research hypotheses, and consider who would be included in the population.

- Children eat a better diet than teenagers.

- Children under 12 eat a better diet than those aged between 12–16.

- Children in year 6 eat a better diet than children in year 7.

- In Wakefield, children in year 6 eat a better diet than children in year 7.

- In Wakefield, children in year 6 eat a better diet at school than children in year 7.

- In the town of Pontefract, in Wakefield, children in year 7 eat a better diet at school than they do at home.

Figure 22.8 Population sampling

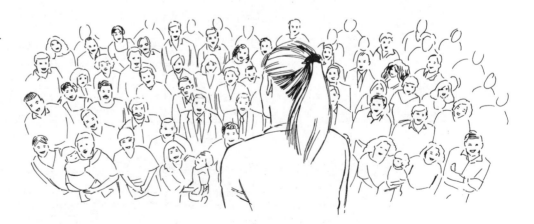

Hopefully, you have been able to see that the first hypothesis had too big and too vague a population to be studied, it would be very difficult to gain a representative sample for this. As the hypotheses get more specific, you should be able to see that, even if you are still not able to get all of the population to participate in your research, it should be easier to have a sample which is representative of the population.

Once you have an established population, and you are clear that a sample is needed, it is important to establish *how* you will select your sample.

Sampling means a smaller, representative part of the larger population. The first question you need to ask is, is your sample from the 'whole' population you are researching? It is incumbent on the researcher to clearly define the target population.

Sometimes, the entire population will be sufficiently small, and the researcher can include the entire population in the study. This type of research is called a census study because data is gathered on every member of the population.

Usually, the population is too large for the researcher to attempt to survey all of its members. So a small, but carefully chosen sample can be used to represent the population. The sample reflects the characteristics of the population from which it is drawn. Sampling methods are classified as either *probability* or *non-probability*.

In probability samples, each member of the population has a known non-zero probability of being selected. Probability methods include simple random sampling, stratified random sampling, cluster sampling and systematic sampling.

In non-probability sampling, members are selected from the population in some non-random manner. These include convenience sampling, quota sampling, and snowball sampling.

The advantage of probability sampling is that sampling error can be calculated. Sampling error is the degree to which a sample might differ from the population. In non-probability sampling, the degree to which the sample differs from the population remains unknown.

Figure 22.9 Sampling options

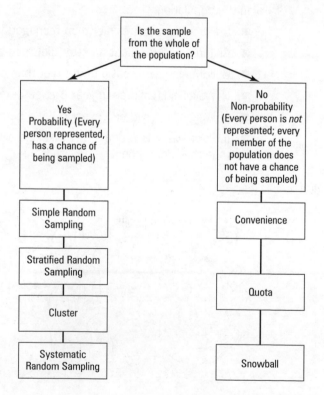

## Simple random sampling

This is the purest form of probability sampling. Each member of the population has an equal and known chance of being selected.

## Stratified random sampling

This is a commonly used probability method, which can help reduce sampling error. Subsets of the population that share one common characteristic, e.g. males and females, or managers and non-managers are selected and then chosen with relation to their actual representation in the population. Random sampling is then used to select a *sufficient* number of subjects from each stratum. '*Sufficien*' refers to a sample size large enough for us to be reasonably confident that the subset represents the population. This ensures that all the subsets are represented.

## Systematic random sampling

This is often used instead of random sampling. It is also called an Nth name selection technique. After the required sample size has been calculated, every Nth record is selected from a list of population members. As long as the list does not contain any hidden order, this sampling method is as good as the random sampling method. Its only advantage over the random sampling technique is simplicity. Systematic sampling is frequently used to select a specified number of records from a computer file.

## Cluster sampling

This is the entire population divided into groups, or clusters, and a random sample of these clusters are selected. Cluster sampling is typically used when the researcher cannot get a complete list of the members of a population they wish to study but can get a complete list of groups or 'clusters' of the population; e.g. users of clinics for a rare condition. It is also used when a random sample would produce a list so widely scattered that including them would prove to be far too expensive, for example, people who live in different postal districts in the UK.

## Convenience sampling

This is used in exploratory research where the researcher is interested in getting an inexpensive approximation of the truth. As the name implies, the sample is selected because they are convenient. This non-probability method is often used during preliminary research to get an estimate of the results, without incurring the cost or time required to select a random sample.

## Quota sampling

This is the non-probability equivalent of stratified sampling. Like stratified sampling, the researcher first identifies the subsets and their proportions as they are represented in the population. Then convenience sampling is used to select the required number of subjects from each subset.

## Snowball sampling

This is a special non-probability method used when the desired sample characteristic is rare. It may be extremely difficult or costly to locate respondents in these situations. Snowball sampling relies on referrals from initial subjects to generate additional subjects. While this technique can dramatically lower search costs, it comes at the expense of introducing bias because the technique itself reduces the likelihood that the sample will represent a good cross section from the population.

You then need to decide what your sample size will be. You now have your sampling frame.

A further important factor when planning your research is outlining your rationale. A rationale is the 'raison d'être' for the research. Why is it being done? Of what use will it be?

You may want to consider the rationale in two ways:

1. Why is this a problem within society?

2. Why will society be better because of this research? What will change? Could new health and social care services be planned because of it? Could monies be better spent?

Using the earlier example of researching the diet of young people in year 7, what could a rationale be for this?

1. ■ Obesity is a contemporary problem.

   ■ Many young people are deficient in nutrients.

   ■ A lot of money and resources are spent dealing with health problems as a result of poor diet.

   ■ The consumption of fruit and vegetables is a main factor in preventing cancer.

2. ■ More money could be spent better educating year 7 students on good diets.

   ■ More money could be spent educating teachers at schools about the benefits of year 7 students eating better.

   ■ Obesity and malnutrition could be reduced.

   ■ Money spent on health problems relating to a poor diet may fall.

## Time scales

Time scales are needed to ensure that you do not get behind in your research. Although it is tempting to jump straight into the research, it is wise to plan ahead. Plan time for all aspects of your project. As a rule of thumb, it may be wise to think in quarters: a quarter planning, a quarter conducting, a quarter analysing and a quarter writing up.

## Action plan

It is also a wise idea to have a specific action plan, outlining specifically:

■ what is going to happen?

■ by when?

■ by whom?

■ how?

> **remember**
>
> Good planning is essential. Fail to prepare, prepare to fail!

---

**case study 22.2**

### Natalie

Natalie is interested in sports provision in schools. Her hypotheses is 'The quantity and quality of sports provision in primary schools is inadequate.' To research this, she has decided to:

1. Interview headteachers.
2. Observe PE lessons in primary schools.
3. Perform a literary review of sport in schools.

This is Natalie's first project and she is a little unsure. She doesn't want the workload to get too demanding and wants to behave ethically.

---

**activity**
**GROUP WORK**

1. Design an action plan for Natalie.
2. Share your ideas with the group. Discuss how each of you would have approached this.

---

Although an action plan is an important guide to work to, it is not always the case that everything goes to plan, or indeed, it may be the case that better, more efficient ways to progress are identified. Good plans benefit from monitoring and modification. By keeping check on how the plan is developing, changes can be made as and when they are needed. It may be too late at the end of the research. Avoid thinking at the end, 'Well, if we'd have only realised that was happening, we could have intervened and dealt with it.'

## Resources

It is always advisable to use of a range of sources.

*remember*

Once your action plan is ready, you will be ready to start your research. Hence you will now need to have your primary and secondary resources ready. You will need to have your experiments set up, your interview questions and your recording methods ready, your questionnaires designed, copied and ready to distribute or your observation plan and recording methods ready. You will have your supply of secondary resources ready.

*i*

British Psychological Society
www.bps.org.uk
Sociology central
www.sociology.org.uk/index.htm
Sociology online
www.sociologyonline.net

# Conducting the research and presenting the findings

## Undertake the research

You should now be in a position to undertake your research; both **primary** and **secondary**. This can be time consuming, but time spent doing this properly will ensure your analysis and evaluation for your conclusion will be better. Make sure you keep a record of all your statistics and data.

It is good practice to pilot your research project before it goes 'live'. This will ensure that any errors are highlighted before it goes to participants. This could involve a teacher or a group of friends or family; it doesn't matter, as long as they have no more information or guidance than your 'real' participants would have.

It is important that when you undertake your research, at all times you must make sure you are safe. Wear appropriate clothing (especially if an experiment), always let people know where you are going, what time you expect to be back, leave telephone numbers and avoid dark, lonely places.

 You will learn more about Health and Safety in Unit 3 in Health and Social Care Book 1.

*Professional Practice*

When conducting your primary research, you are not only representing yourself but others. In this case, it may be your school or college, but in future, it may be an organisation and/or employment. Therefore it is good practice to act as professionally as you can. Dress smartly, be organised, be punctual, be friendly, be well mannered.

As you are undertaking the research, you may want to monitor and review your progress. Having a plan is good practice, but it is not fixed; you need to be flexible. For example, if you are not getting many responses from a postal questionnaire, you could review your research design and decide to send out reminder letters.

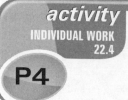

Using a topic and research methods of your choice, carry out primary research, recording appropriate data.

## Introduction

When writing your report, you should make sure that you include an introduction to your research project, outlining the key points and methodology. One thing to include is a summary of current research in the field. This is almost 'setting the scene' for the reader, outlining to them what is known already about the topic and justifying your choice of research topic.

## Method

A more detailed section outlining your method should be included. You should clearly outline your hypothesis or research question; this should make sense for the reader, as you will have previously outlined current research, or lack of, in the introduction. Next, you should outline your methodology; both what primary research and secondary research will be undertaken. This allows your reader to openly see how you will be collecting the data. It is useful to also outline how you will be recording the data: paper based, video recording, audio recording, using IT, etc.

A preferred method when researching is to always make sure you use more than one source of data; this is known as 'triangulation'. This describes a situation where more than one method is used in a study with a view to double (or triple) checking results. The idea is that one can be more confident with a result if different methods lead to the same result.

## Results

You should now be in a position to collate your results. If this is done poorly, it could severely affect the **validity** of your research. Whatever format your research is in you will need accuracy when compiling data. Below are some tips for compiling data from four different types of research.

When compiling secondary research, it is important to make sure:

- you work systematically through material, try to have some order, be it chronological or alphabetical
- there are clear, concise notes
- that if you are going to directly quote data, you make sure you record it correctly
- you record the author, title of the book, journal, etc., the year it was published, the publisher and the place of publishing; it is also important to have the page number. This is so that when you are presenting your data, you do not have problems sourcing it. Green (2000) has an excellent section on bibliographies and referencing
- you do not take valuable time reading whole publications unnecessarily – it may be an idea to read the introduction or conclusion first, to see if it is of use
- that headings, colour, underlining, etc. are used in your notes to make the data clearer
- plagiarising work is avoided at all times.

If you are compiling primary data such as questionnaires then you will need to consider:

- What the response rate is; does a reminder need to be sent?
- When it is felt that there are as many responses as you are likely to get (you can then start to collate the data).
- Adding/counting/accumulating responses.
- Sectioning into piles, e.g. male responses and female responses.

If you are compiling primary data such as observations, you should consider:

- Recording the date, time, participants observed and location.
- Writing up one observation before going on to the next one to avoid any confusion between observations.
- Writing the observations as soon as possible whilst they are fresh in your mind, not days later!
- Producing an audio/visual recording of the data. If you do, you may want to watch the data as soon as possible to ensure your interpretation of the data is as accurate as possible.
- Watching the data on numerous occasions to get a better feel and understanding for the data.
- Trying to organise your data into themes, e.g. certain types of behaviours observed.
- Organising your data quantitatively, e.g. the length of time a child will try a task independently before asking for guidance.
- Compiling 'flow-charts' of what you observed to allow you to do better comparisons.

If you are compiling primary data such as interviews, you may:

- Record the date, time, participants interviewed and location.
- Want to note one interview before going on to the next one to avoid any confusion between interviews.
- Want to note the interview as soon as possible whilst it is fresh in your mind, not days later.
- Produce an audio/visual record of the data, and if you do, you may want to watch or listen to the data as soon as possible to ensure your interpretation of the data is as accurate as possible.
- Want to watch or listen to the data on numerous occasions to get a better feel and understanding for the data.
- Organise your data, e.g. responses to questions.

Whatever your data source, always make sure you keep copies of your raw data for future reference. You must, however, bear **confidentiality** in mind and store data securely.

Once you have compiled your data, you will need to present your data. This could be done statistically or graphically; both of which may be aided by the use of computer software.

## Presentation of results – statistically

Although using statistics can sound quite daunting at first, the use of some simple statistical methods can aid your description of your data massively, and hence the understanding of a reader. Here are four ways you could use statistics, some of which you may be familiar with already.

Figure 22.10 Using
statistics

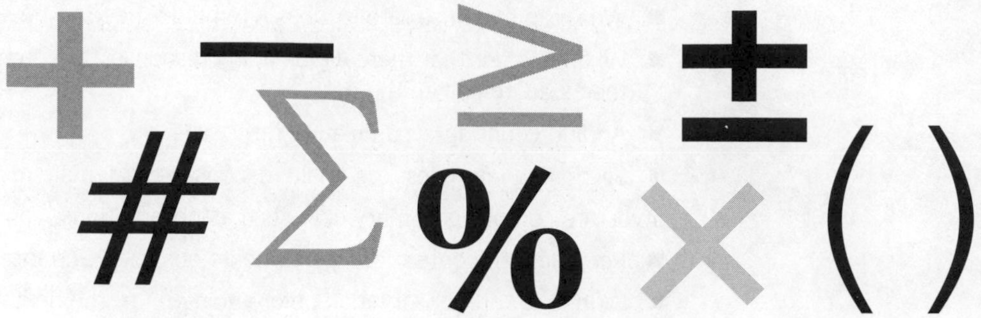

### Percentages

This is where the figure given represents that number out of 100. This would then allow for easier comparison.

For example, if you had a questionnaire result that 22 people out of 50 said they agreed; this could be put into a percentage. You would do this by dividing the number of responses by the total possible, and then multiplying that by 100.

$$\frac{22}{50} \times 100 = 44$$

Hence, 44% of responses agreed.

### Mean

This is an average of the total number.

For example, if you had ten responses of the ages that people first drank alcohol; this could be put into a **mean**. You would do this by adding all the responses together, and then dividing by the total number of answers, in this case 10.

Add (12, 13, 15, 19, 20, 16, 13, 12, 16, 16) = 152/10 = 15.2

Therefore, the mean age that people in your sample started drinking is 15.2 years.

### Median

This is another average, but this time, the average is the number in the middle, when all the numbers are in numerical order.

For example, if you had those same ten responses of first consumption of alcohol, putting them in numerical order would be:

Table 22.10

| 1st | 2nd | 3rd | 4th | 5th | 6th | 7th | 8th | 9th | 10th |
|-----|-----|-----|-----|-----|-----|-----|-----|-----|------|
| 12 | 12 | 13 | 13 | 15 | 16 | 16 | 16 | 19 | 20 |

Therefore, the middle number here would be between the 5th and 6th. If you have an even number in 'the middle', as in this case, then you need to add those two numbers together and divide by 2

$$\frac{(15 + 16)}{2} = 15.5$$

Therefore, the **median** age that people in your sample started drinking is 15 and a half years.

### Mode

This is another average, but this time, the average number is the one that is the 'most popular'.

For example, if you had those same ten responses of first consumption of alcohol, then the 'most popular' response was 16, as that response was said more often than any other, in fact three times.

Therefore, the modal age that people in your sample started drinking is 16 years.

Remember, the mean, median and **mode** answers could be the same; three different answers will not always be gained.

## Other methods of presentation

As with the use of statistics, presenting your results well can make a big difference to the understanding of your data. Remembering some simple rules when presenting your images, should help you.

■ Always give your diagrams a title.

■ Always label your axis, sections, columns and rows.

■ Use colour clearly, and remember that if photocopied in black and white, this will be lost, so you may choose to use 'patterns' instead of colour.

■ Only use diagrams if they aid understanding; do not put them in for the sake of it.

■ Only use diagrams that you understand; do not try to be fancy, especially if using computer software. The result could be not being able to understand the diagram yourself!

■ Choose the right format to display your information, e.g. avoid using tables, if a pie chart is better suited.

■ It is useful in graphs/diagrams to also give numerical totals.

■ Always state the units of measurements, cm, kg, years, months, etc.

■ Always state the numerical category; is it a percentage, out of 100,000 or cumulative?

■ Always note the source of the information.

Here are five ways data could be presented.

### Bar charts

Bar charts are a very simple and very clear way of displaying data. They can be used for either 'discrete data' or 'continuous data'. 'Discrete' data is where one set of data does not relate to the other. This is different to 'continuous' data where when one set of data is related to the other data.

Discrete data – when data is discrete, it is often advised to have each bar separated by a small gap. For example, in the bar chart below, Leeds has no relation to Hull, nor Hull to York, etc. and so they are separate.

Figure 22.11 Bar chart using discrete data

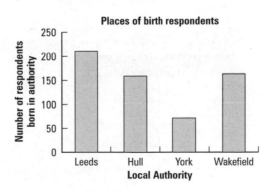

### Continuous data

When data is continuous, for example time, each bar does not need to be separated by a small gap. For example, in the bar chart below, Monday will 'run in' to Tuesday, etc., and hence, they can be close together.

Bar charts are also useful as you could have multiple sets of data displayed and they can be 'stacked'.

Figure 22.12  Bar chart using continuous data

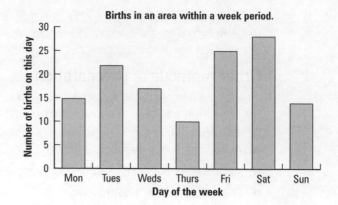

**Births in an area within a week period.**

## Histograms

According to Bland (1995), histograms are diagrams 'where the class intervals are on an axis and rectangles with heights or areas proportional to the frequencies erected on them'. What this means is that a histogram is different from a bar chart as it is the *area* of the bar that denotes the value, not the height. Histograms are used to represent continuous data and hence there are no gaps between the bars of a histogram.

An example of a histogram from 'GCSE Bitesize maths' is below and should you want more information on how to produce histograms, the GCSE bitesize website provides a detailed explanation of how to produce them.

As you can see, the 'age' classification is not uniform; 5–10 is different to 11–15 and is different to 16–17 and hence, the height needs to be altered to take account of this.

Figure 22.13  An example of a histogram

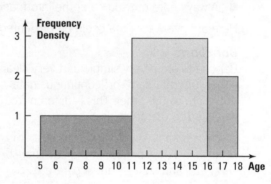

Table 22.11  Histogram data

| Age | Frequency |
|-----|-----------|
| 5–10 | 6 |
| 11–15 | 15 |
| 16–17 | 4 |
| >17 | 0 |

So because the class boundaries are different, the area is what represents the data, so that the height does not distort the impression of the data.

## Graphs

Line graphs in particular, are useful to show changes in a variable, particularly over a time period, so the data is continuous.

Figure 22.14  A line graph

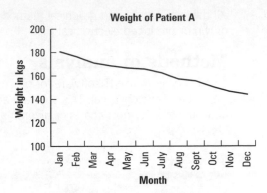

**Weight of Patient A**

## Pie charts

These use an image of a 'pie' to represent the total (sometimes 100 if data is displayed as a percentage), and each 'slice' of the pie to represent the quantity. Unless you have the use of computer software, pie charts require knowledge of angles (the total in a circle being 360) and percentages.

An outline of how to produce a pie chart manually is below.

Table 22.12  Pie chart data

|  | Number of children preferring the drink | As a percent of the total (72) | Multiplied by 360, to get the angle. |
|---|---|---|---|
| Milk | 36 | 0.5 | 180° |
| Fruit juice | 18 | 0.25 | 90° |
| Water | 12 | 0.16 (recurring) | 60° |
| Cordial | 6 | 0.083 (recurring) | 30° |

Figure 22.15  A pie chart

**Drink choice at lunchtime of 72 children in the nursery**

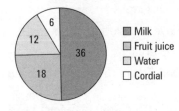

- Milk
- Fruit juice
- Water
- Cordial

## Table

These are a very simple way of displaying data. Further, because tables are essentially so simple, they can be used to include more data as can be seen below.

Table 22.13  An example of a table

|  | Age | Average amount of fruit and vegetables eaten per day | Smoker | Hours spent participating in activity/exercise per week |
|---|---|---|---|---|
| Robert | 54 | 5 | No | 5 |
| Susan | 53 | 7 | No | 4 |
| Peter | 28 | 6 | Yes | 12 |
| Adam | 25 | 4 | No | 10 |

All these statistical and graphical methods of describing your data can be manually drawn or produced electronically.

# Methods of analysis

If you choose to use IT software for processing statistical information, then a good start would be Microsoft Excel. This software allows you to perform most statistical analysis and will produce most charts or diagrams for you. A more advanced piece of software is SPSS.

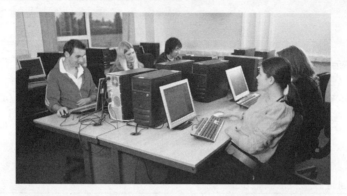

Figure 22.16 Using IT to process statistical information

These methods, whether manual or electronic will help you to draw conclusions, especially if it allows you to make comparisons. However, you do need to be aware of potential **bias** and error when using these. Bias and error will be considered in more detail later, but in terms of analysis, you would be wise to check certain aspects to minimise bias and error.

For your statistics:

- Have you written all your figures down correctly?

- Have you double checked your calculations?

- For larger scale calculations, it is wise to check early sums, to ensure that your final calculations, which may be based on earlier sums are not incorrect.

For your graphs:

- Have you plotted all your graphs accurately?

- Is everything labelled clearly and accurately?

- Don't claim there is a trend in data, unless you can clearly show it.

- When looking at graphs, possibly in your secondary research, have you noticed any manipulation of the data? Maybe the graph is skewed? Look at the following:

Figure 22.17 Same data, different graphs

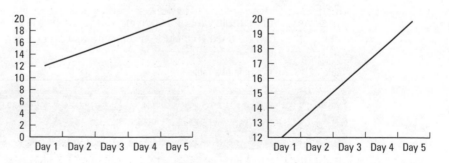

These two graphs both show the same data, but the increase looks much more substantial in the second graph. This is because of the way the y axis (the vertical axis) has been organised.

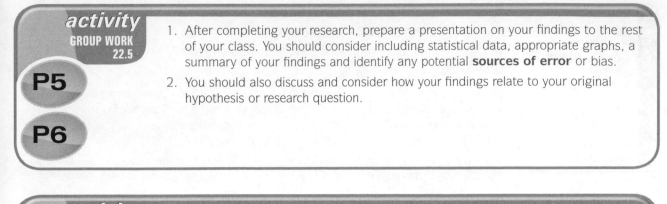

**activity**
**GROUP WORK**
**22.5**

**P5**

**P6**

1. After completing your research, prepare a presentation on your findings to the rest of your class. You should consider including statistical data, appropriate graphs, a summary of your findings and identify any potential **sources of error** or bias.

2. You should also discuss and consider how your findings relate to your original hypothesis or research question.

**activity**
**INDIVIDUAL WORK**
**22.6**

**M3**

Once you have given your presentation to the rest of the class, reflect on your research findings and analyse them in more depth in relation to the original hypothesis.

## Ethical considerations

Once you have completed presenting and analysing your data, you have an ethical consideration: that you do not use or misuse your results. Ethics will be considered in greater detail later in the chapter.

See the section Ethics.
GCSE bitesize
www.bbc.co.uk/schools/gcsebitesize/maths/
SPSS
www.spss.com
Statistics online
www.statistics.gov.uk

## Evaluating the research project

### Evaluation and conclusion

To evaluate is to look back and reflect on the project and to judge its successes and weaknesses. This is not only useful for your current project, but it also allows you to reflect and learn for future projects.

A good starting point when evaluating is to compare findings with the hypothesis or research question; after all, that was the whole basis of the research.

- Have you proved or disproved your hypothesis?
- Have you answered your research question?

If you haven't, then essentially, your research project has not been as successful as hoped. You may at this stage have clear ideas as to why you haven't. However, if not, then it may be worthwhile reflecting and considering each stage of your research project and considering any potential weaknesses.

In your final report, it will be wise to discuss your findings; simply, what did you find out? This will form the bulk of your report and will include:

- evidence, in the format of your statistics
- evidence, in the format of your graphs
- analysis, in the format of your interpretation of the data
- conclusions of your findings.

You also need to consider the relationships of the results to current research. Consider the literature search that was performed initially – do the findings from your research reinforce or contradict their position? If they reinforce the literature search, then evidently, they strengthen the validity of that perspective.

However, if it contradicts the current research, you may want to consider why. Possible considerations are that the current research is now flawed, maybe:

- the current research was not performed recently and is outdated
- the current research did not take into account factors which you have
- the secondary research is invalid – there is no guarantee that the author of that work has performed the research without error or bias.

Possibly it is just because the research projects are different:

- your research may be based on a group with different cultures/lifestyles
- your research may have been based on another locality
- your research may have used a sample population that was a different age.

Or it may be that it was *your* research that was flawed. Hence, you would need to identify limitations of your research project. Possible considerations are:

- the hypothesis/research question was poor
- the research project was designed poorly
- timescales were inadequate
- planning was poor
- research methods were inaccurate
- response rate was low
- the primary research was flawed
- the secondary research was flawed
- researcher bias occurred
- ethical issues arose
- statistical analysis was poor
- graphical presentation of data was poor
- interpretation was inaccurate
- **reliability** was poor
- validity was poor
- sources of error occurred
- sources of bias occurred.

By thoroughly analysing your project, you will have confidence in your conclusions, your own learning and hopefully, confidence for your next project.

This should lead to consideration of potential areas for further development of research. Once conclusions have been made; thoughts could then be turning to how this could be investigated further to aid more in-depth understanding of your findings – why, how, when, how many, what, where, etc.?

Figure 22.18 What next?

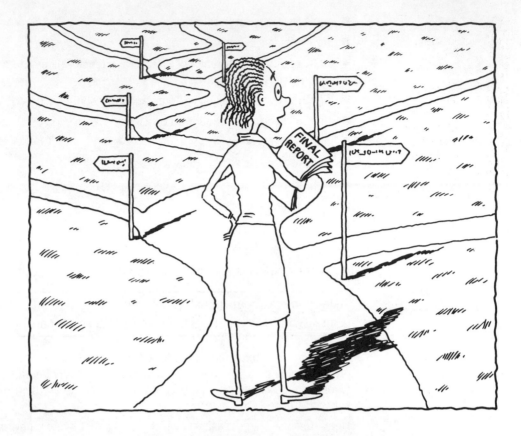

If you disproved your hypothesis or failed to answer your research question, thoughts may turn to how this could be investigated further to aid further understanding – why not, what other possibilities are there, were any factors ignored, etc.?

For example, if research was done on the hypothesis: 'The quantity and quality of sports provision within infant schools is inadequate' and it was disproved; what potential areas for further research could there be. Possible suggestions could be:

- The quantity and quality of sports provision within junior schools is inadequate.
- The quantity and quality of sports provision within high schools is inadequate.
- The opportunities for participation in sport outside of school hours are inadequate.
- The role of the parents is the key determinant in the exercise a young person participates in.
- Opportunities for exercise do exist for young people, but they fail to access them.
- It is the attitudes of young people themselves which determines the exercise they do.

Each of these examines a new potential factor.

When considering the research project, it is important to consider important aspects other than just the result of the project. It is important to consider the implications of the research project.

Firstly, it is important to consider the implications for human rights. Human rights are defined by the Oxford Dictionary as 'rights which are believed to belong justifiably to every person'. Therefore, the research project should not affect any of these rights. If this were looked at in terms of the Human Rights Act 1998, then research could not have any impact on a person's:

- right to life
- right to prohibition of torture
- right to prohibition of slavery and forced labour

- right to liberty and security
- right to a fair trial
- right not to be held guilty of a criminal offence which did not exist in law at the time at which it was committed
- right to privacy, family life, home and correspondence
- right to freedom of thought, conscience and religion
- right to freedom of expression
- right to freedom of assembly and association
- right to marry
- right to protection of property
- right to education
- right to free elections
- right to the rights and freedoms set out above without discrimination on any ground.

**To learn more about Human Rights see Unit 2 in Health and Social Care Book 1 (Equality, diversity and rights in health and social care).**

Also, the research needs to be considered in terms of any potential sources of bias and error. According to the Oxford Dictionary, bias is described as 'inclination or prejudice in favour of a particular person, thing, or viewpoint'. Everything has a bias; everything is written or done with a purpose.

Here are some generic aspects which could affect bias and error:

- Sample size – was it big enough, was it representative enough, did it have the right geographical, demographical make up?
- Sampling method – have all in your sampling frame had an equal chance of participating?
- Research methods – how could your choice of methods have affected your results?
- Pilot study – was one undertaken?
- Secondary data – were the sources accurate, reliable, free from bias, up-to-date?

Here are some specific aspects that would affect bias and error for specific research methods:

In terms of primary research:

- In an interview, the interviewer may have opinions or beliefs that affect the questions that are asked, or the answers that it is decided are worthy of noting. The participant may also answer differently, due to the presence of the researcher. This is often known as 'interviewer bias'.
- In an observation, the observer may have opinions or beliefs that affect what they are looking at, or the behaviour that it is decided are worthy of noting.
- With a questionnaire, the designer may have opinions or beliefs that affect the questions that are included, or the way they are phrased. For example, the question 'do you agree that there are better sentences than capital punishment, which is a barbaric and outdated way to punish people, when many people often reform and society can not be confident of a 100% accurate verdict?' will obviously lead respondents to answer in one way i.e. yes. Also, were any of the questions poorly written so they may have been misleading or unclear?

In terms of secondary research, consider the following ways bias could occur.

- Newspapers will often have a political perspective. Also, the final decision of what to print will always take into account the editor's final decision and opinions, hence reports may be biased.

- Even a government report, which is supposedly respected and objective, may have a political bias. In fact, it may be that evidence, which goes against the government's own standpoint, may be omitted.

- Television/news reports may be biased as these may be affected by firstly, the victims/interviewee's interpretation, secondly, the reporter's interpretation and thirdly, the time devoted to their coverage, etc. By devoting time to a news report on the royal family, it assumes that that is the news story that people are interested in, or indeed should be.

- A diary, which may be believed to be 100% accurate would still have bias, the writer only noting what they felt was important.

- Statistics can often be presented in a way that may be biased, sometimes like mathematical magic! You may have heard the quote by Benjamin Disraeli (Twain:1924) 'there are three kinds of lies: lies, damn lies and statistics'. As shown in the graphs above, statistics can easily be biased. Further, sometimes a statistic is given, and often people take it at face value and believe it. If you read in a textbook '64% of young people would prefer employment rather than further education', you may believe this. However, I just made that up. Remember, 97% of statistics are made up on the spot!

A further implication to consider is that of ethical issues, e.g. **confidentiality** and data protection, and these will be covered in more detail in the last section. However, you need to consider the implications of ethics when evaluating your research.

## Recommendations

Following your research project results, evaluation and conclusions, authors should then be in a position to make recommendations based on their findings. One of the ways the research could be used is for practitioners in their work or policy makers determining health and social care research.

In the past, there have been many major changes to policy and practice from influential pieces of research. Here are some influential research reports and the changes they led to:

Table 22.14  Important research reports and significant outcomes

| Research report | Outcome |
| --- | --- |
| Beverage's report, 1942 | The basis for the Welfare State |
| The Acheson report, 1998 | The basis for the Labour Government's Social Policy during the Blair years |
| Macpherson report into the death of Stephen Lawrence, 1999 | Reform of the police service to remove institutional racism |
| Laming report into the death of Victoria Climbié, 2000 | Every Child Matters: Change for Children and then Children Act 2004 |

Therefore it can be seen how good research can be influential at the top levels of government and the civil service.

It will also have an impact on future research proposals and the funding that goes into it. For example, based on his research, Dr Andrew Wakefield claimed MMR jabs resulted in an increased likelihood of autism developing in children. This led to policy makers undertaking *further* research on the links between MMR and autism, as his claims were strongly contested.

A further example is the research on the potential dangers of mobile phone masts which has led to *further* research being commissioned to investigate this danger in more depth.

Office Public Sector Information
www.opsi.gov.uk
NHS
www.nhs.uk
Independent Inquiry in to Inequalities in Health Report (Acheson Report)
www.archive.official-documents.co.uk/menu/bydoh.htm
The Stephen Lawrence Inquiry (Macpherson Report)
www.archive.official-documents.co.uk/menu/byhoff.htm
Laming Report
www.victoria-climbie-inquiry.org.uk/

# The implications of and ethical issues related to using research in health and social care

## Implications

There are a variety of implications of research. One implication is who commissions research. To commission something means that an authorisation has been given and this may, but not necessarily, come with funding. Organisations that may be involved with commissioning research are numerous, but some larger ones in health and social care are:

- The Department of Health – these have a section on their website where they invite full research proposals.

- The Department for Children, Schools and Families – again, there is a section on their website with details of commissioning.

- Joseph Rowntree Foundation – is a charity based organisation which commissions research into poverty; its causes and effects.

An implication of who has commissioned research is whether this will affect the outcome or not. Will they be satisfied whatever the outcome? Would the sugar industry be happy if research they commissioned proved that sugar consumption is the key factor determining obesity in children?

A further implication of research is that of human rights. We all have rights; some of these were outlined earlier in the context of the Human Rights Act; but we also have implicit rights such as:

- confidentiality
- respect
- privacy
- choice
- quality care
- non-discriminatory practice
- right to complain
- dignity
- safety
- to be treated as an individual
- equality/equal opportunities.

Research should not limit or curb any of our rights. For example, research that monitored behaviour in the garden on summer days (gardening, sunbathing, reading, eating etc.), which involved watching over someone's garden fence, most likely is affecting people's rights to privacy, respect and dignity. Research that examined the treatment of young people in a consultation at a sexual health clinic may affect people's rights to confidentiality, privacy, quality care, dignity, etc. The implications of research on human rights therefore are important.

A further implication is regards the **validity** and reliability of a study.

## Validity

Validity is the extent that the data is a measurement of what was supposed to be measured; i.e. it is a true meaning/measurement. Think about research into unemployment, homelessness, sex crimes, prostitution, drug use, etc. Can any of these measures claim to be 'valid'? For different reasons (victims failing to come forward, denial, embarrassment etc.), they will probably not 'paint a true picture' of reality.

## Reliability

Reliability is when something will always behave in the same way, and hence something is unreliable when it will not always behave in the same way. This means that if the research was done again, with a different sample, at a different time, the results would be the same; it would be reliable. This implies that there are no external factors affecting the results, e.g. interviewer bias, weather, etc.

There are many aspects that can affect a piece of research's validity and reliability. One aspect is ethics. If the research is ethical, participants will be more likely to participate, to be honest and open, not feel rushed, trust the researcher and feel that their contributions will be represented fairly and accurately by the researcher. Therefore, this data would be more valid (true) and more reliable (the same if repeated).

A further implication would be on the consequences/benefits of the findings. If the research was performed soundly, is valid, reliable and ethical, then the consequences are that the findings will be published, be taken more seriously, be read, be respected, be used. The findings will be beneficial. However, if the work is not, then few of the above, if any will happen. In fact, the research may be destroyed or withdrawn. Therefore it can be seen, that the effects of publications are immense. Not only will it affect the short term status of current research, but it will also affect the long term status of the researcher. Because the standards of publishers, be it in books, journals or by organisations or the government, are extremely tough, being published gives a certain

Figure 22.19 Validity and reliability

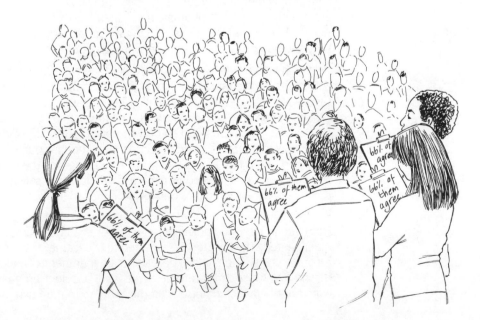

kudos to the research and the researcher. Hence the more works published, the greater the kudos. Further, there is a great sense of pride to be achieved if a researcher's published work has an impact on policy or provision.

Researchers also need to consider the implications of access to information. This could be both in terms of how it is gained initially and once the research is complete.

When aiming to gain access to information in terms of raw data, it can be difficult. It may even be the case that access to information is refused. This may be because the research puts confidentiality at risk, service users' safety at risk or may risk negative results from a competitor. One way to deal with this is firstly, to be ethical and secondly, make the participants aware of the purpose and methodology and thirdly, let the individual, group or organisation know that they have the right to review before any final work is submitted or published. If they can clearly see that the research is being done soundly, they will have more confidence and faith in the research and are more likely to give access to information.

When the research is complete, the researcher has to decide what information will have access to it and by whom. This has to incorporate the assurances given to the participants, how anonymous data has been made, and the importance of any data. The researcher needs to be very careful here not to become legally liable for any breach of confidentiality.

A further consideration is regards the vulnerability of client groups. Users of health, social care or early years services are by their very nature, in some way more vulnerable. This may be as a result of age (younger or older), health, disability, impairment, lifestyle, functioning, etc. Think how you would feel if you have been treated unfairly, deceived, had your details seen by people who shouldn't have, had your privacy invaded. Now think how that could affect someone who is already 'vulnerable'. The effects *could* be exacerbated. It may be the case that some people cannot make a fully informed decision for themselves and hence it would be exploitative not to deal with this by speaking to their parent, carer or legal guardian.

When dealing with client groups, researchers need to consider the topic of their research and consider whether it could be of a sensitive nature. Would it be ethical to try to interview people in a clinic for pregnancy terminations? As this is a sensitive topic, and the client group may be extremely vulnerable; most people would probably agree that is would be unethical.

This doesn't just apply to their current situation, but also from past events. Asking anyone, of any age, about terminations of pregnancy would be sensitive, as it is not known how the client group feels about the subject or whether this is a subject they are emotive about. At all times, the vulnerability of client groups must be considered. Researchers have to remember that participants are doing them the favour and hence they should be treated with respect and have all of their rights met.

Research with children also needs to be done cautiously. One famous experiment was completed by the famous psychologist Albert Bandura. He believed in a Social Learning theory whereby people, especially children, learn from the world around them. Three groups of children were each shown a film which involved adults abusing a Bobo doll (a doll that cannot be knocked down); however, all three films had different endings. One showed the adult being rewarded for the behaviour, one showed the adult being punished and the final one had no consequences for the adult. The three groups of children were then allowed to play with the doll themselves. The children who had seen the version where the adult was rewarded for their abusive behaviour, were more likely to hit the doll.

However, in the Bobo doll experiment, there has been criticism that the children were manipulated. The children were teased and became frustrated because they could not touch the toys. Some critics believed the experiment conducted was unethical because the children were 'trained to be aggressive'. Could it be guaranteed that these children would not be affected not only in the short term, but also in the long term?

Lastly, it should be mentioned that a good researcher should consider the vulnerability of participants when they are presenting them with the final research; they have to consider how it will affect them.

It should now be clear that research has a variety of implications.

# Ethical issues

The implications of ethical research are numerous. The Oxford Dictionary definition of ethics is 'the moral principles governing or influencing conduct; the branch of knowledge concerned with moral principles.' Hence, ethics are guidelines as to how society should behave, what is morally acceptable. Sometimes, it is clear what is 'unethical'. If you asked ten people whether it was acceptable to keep money that had been collected for charity, it is highly likely that most people would believe it to be highly unethical. Some other issues are more subjective. What about research involving animal testing? Some believe that this is ethical, as it is for the greater good; some believe this is wholly unethical.

## Confidentiality

There are many issues that need to be considered to produce good, ethical research and some will be covered here. One of the most important issues is that of confidentiality. Confidentiality means that information is not accessed by anyone who is not authorised to do so. Breaching confidentiality is unethical. If participants have allowed you access to information that they did not want to be made public, then to breach confidentiality is not only unethical, but also possibly illegal and may leave the researcher legally liable.

Confidentiality also applies to *after* the report has been published on two counts:

1. That the report does not include confidential information. That the 'raw data' (the questionnaires, the interview transcripts, the observation records, patient/client details etc.) are either destroyed or kept somewhere confidentially.

There are many ways that information can be kept confidential.

Table 22.15  Ways of keeping information confidential

| Paper based information | IT based information | Verbal based information |
| --- | --- | --- |
| Store tidily, use folders, etc. | Store tidily, use files, etc. | When in work, try to avoid conversing on stairwells, corridors, etc. |
| Never leave papers lying around. | Do not leave information on screen. | |
| Use filing cabinets that are lockable. | Avoid shared usage of areas. | When out of work, do not discuss work matters. |
| | Use passwords as much as possible. | |
| Avoid open lower ground windows. | Have password protected screensavers. | Use 'do not disturb' signs when meetings are in progress. |
| Make sure only authorised persons have access to papers. | If using removable hardware, e.g. USB sticks or disks, make sure they are password protected too. | Make sure only authorised persons have access to meetings. |
| | Make sure only authorised persons have access to files. | |

To ensure confidentiality is met at all times, researchers also need to be aware of data protection legislation; in particular the Data Protection Act 1998. This is a mandatory piece of legislation which all organisations that hold or process personal data MUST comply with.

The Data Protection Act contains 8 principles. These state that all data must be:

- Processed fairly and lawfully.
- Obtained and used only for specified and lawful purposes.
- Adequate, relevant and not excessive.
- Accurate, and where necessary, kept up-to-date.
- Kept for no longer than necessary.

- Processed in accordance with the individuals rights (as defined).
- Kept secure.
- Transferred only to countries that offer adequate data protection.

Source: Office of Public Sector Information

It is also ethical to consider the policy and procedures in place for research. By working to your own organisation's policies and procedures for research, this will ensure that the required ethical considerations are covered. Referring to the codes of practice (covered below) will also ensure ethical research is undertaken.

Ensuring the authenticity of all the work is not only ensuring validity, but is also ethical. Plagiarism will be avoided and recognition will be given where appropriate.

It is ethical to always ensure the inclusion of codes of practice on ethics.

Codes of practice are of use on three levels:

1. There may be a generic code of practice on ethics produced by the organisations, which ensures that all researchers belonging to that organisation are working to a set standard.

2. There may be a more specific code of practice on ethics that applies to that particular piece of research which ensures that all on that project are working to the same standards.

3. Codes of practices on ethics being used by researchers/organisations may be distributed to the participants so that *they* are aware of their rights.

One of the first codes of practice was the Nuremberg Code which was developed after the Second World War following revelations at the Nuremberg Trials regards unethical research carried out during the Nazi period in Germany. This set out ten conditions which must be followed closely for research to be ethical. Although these have now been updated and superseded by other codes, they are useful to look at to gain knowledge of ethical issues and to consider the importance of having codes and the horrendous consequences of not applying them. The online encyclopaedia Wikipedia provides a clear summary of the ten conditions.

The British Sociological Association has a code, namely, the 'Statement of Ethical Practice'. Similarly, the British Psychological Society has a 'Code of Ethics and Conduct'. Have a look at this to help you with ethics.

Although there are many examples of codes of practices available, especially on the internet, you may feel it necessary to produce your own. Some suggestions as to what *may* be covered in one which could be distributed to participants are below.

- What is the purpose of this research?
- What information could be sensitive? Solution?
- How will it be ensured that participants are not hurt/upset by the research?
- Will consent be gained from participants, or their parents, or guardians?
- Will participants have a right to review the report?
- How will confidentiality be ensured?
- How will participants' rights be met?
- How will it be ensured that participants' contributions are portrayed fairly and accurately?
- Will participants be aware of the right to withdraw?
- How will equality of opportunity be ensured?
- Will participants be kept anonymous in the report?
- How will it be ensured that participants are respected throughout?
- If I do not cover the above ethical issues, what could happen?

If you show participants the research purpose, design, plan and ethical outline, they are more likely to be 'on board'. Bailey et al (1995:19) provide a more detailed guide to producing your own ethical code.

The role of the media needs to be considered in terms of their ethical impact regards the publication of research. They have a responsibility to portray the research fairly and accurately. However, sometimes reports are distorted or trivialised. Therefore, researchers need to be aware of this, and in some respects, be prepared for misrepresentation.

## Use and misuse of data

Another ethical issue is that of use and misuse of data, e.g. statistics which inform practice. Being sensible and responsible with data is ethical. Before being released, consideration needs to be given to the consequences. The report by Dr Wakefield about the MMR vaccine has caused much controversy, which is still ongoing, and there are still doubts as to the accuracy of his findings. The outcome of this is that many parents have not had their children vaccinated against MMR using the triple vaccine or at all. Did Dr Wakefield misuse his data, or was he using them ethically to inform others of dangers? Bland (1995:4) quotes Altman's belief that 'bad statistics leads to bad research and bad research is unethical'. This is because it could lead to good therapies/interventions being abandoned and poor ones adopted. However, if good research has the potential to make changes in policy and provision for the better, then that is ethical.

> **remember**
>
> It is not just provision now that could be affected, but also provision for years to come, affecting future generations.

**activity**
**INDIVIDUAL WORK**
**22.7**

**M2**

**D1**

1. Consider your research methods; produce a report reviewing any sources of bias or error and ethical considerations.
2. Consider if you were to do the same research again, how you would alter the methodology to reduce bias and error in the future.

## Effects on policy and practice

As should now be seen, research reports have a massive effect on organisations. In health and social care, this could be from national level with government and organisations, regional level with Health Authorities, to local level with PCTs, Local Authorities, Local Education Authorities, etc. The impact of key reports is massive. You saw in Learning Outcome 4 some examples of key reports and their significant consequences.

The role of Social Care Institute for Excellence (SCIE), in their own words is to:

> improve the experience of people who use social care by developing and promoting knowledge about good practice in the sector. Using knowledge gathered from diverse sources and a broad range of people and organisations, we develop resources which we share freely, supporting those working in social care and empowering service users.

Therefore, for anyone in health and social care, this is useful to be aware of! Their website gives a full breakdown of their purpose and is well worth looking at. However, to summarise here, they were formed in 2001 to 'improve social care services for adults and children in the United Kingdom'. They help the 1.6 million people providing or planning social care, and 2.8 million people using social care services in the UK.

They work to:

- 'disseminate knowledge-based good practice guidance
- involve service users, practitioners, providers and policy makers in advancing and promoting good practice in social care
- enhance the skills and professionalism of social care workers through our tailored, targeted and user-friendly resources.'

Their values are that:

'We promise to:

- have a service user focus
- be independent in our research and findings
- promote empowerment and change
- be committed to equality and diversity
- be transparent
- be accessible in all our work
- be accountable to our stakeholders.'

Therefore the impact of SCIE research on policy can be seen to be vast. They currently categorise their research into:

- Adults' services
- Children and families' services
- E-learning
- Knowledge management
- People management
- Social work education
- Stakeholder participation
- Using knowledge in social care.

Therefore, they will work with and disseminate research to a wide range of partnerships and networks.

**Data Protection Act**
www.opsi.gov.uk
**On Bandura**
www.tip.psychology.org/bandura.html
**SCIE**
www.scie.org.uk/index.asp

---

*activity*
**INDIVIDUAL WORK**
**22.8**

**P7**

**M4**

1. Produce a ten point action plan of possible improvements to your research, referring to any relevant implications and ethical issues.

2. Think about the research you have done and the results you have gained. Imagine they were published; discuss the possible implications they may have on current practice.

---

*activity*
**INDIVIDUAL WORK**
**22.9**

**D2**

Consider your thoughts for Individual Activity 22.1 where you considered the purpose and role of research in the health and social care sectors. Develop your answer now, by analysing your ideas, drawing on the piece of research undertaken.

*Progress Check*

1. What are the purposes and roles of research in health and social care?
2. Outline the differences between quantitative and qualitative research and primary and secondary research.
3. Describe four methods of collecting primary research.
4. Describe four methods of collecting secondary research.
5. What are the mean, mode, and median of these numbers: 8, 7, 25, 9, 12, 9, 14?
6. Identify different ways data could be presented and outline some of the factors you would consider for each of them.
7. Outline some of the ethical issues relevant to health and social care research.
8. Outline some potential sources of error and bias in health and social care research.
9. Describe what is meant by validity and reliability?
10. What is the role of the SCIE?

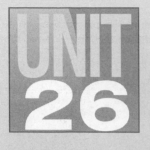

# Caring for Individuals with Additional Needs

## This unit covers:

- Why individuals may have additional needs
- Models of disability
- Current practice with respect to provision for additional needs
- Current legislation with respect to individuals with additional needs

All humans have needs, these range from basic physiological needs including food, shelter, warmth, to more complex needs relating to personal growth and development. In order to be happy and fulfilled these needs must be met.

Although all people have human needs, some require additional support to meet their needs, achieve their goals and live as independently as possible. For some people obtaining food, managing their daily lives and building friendships can be difficult because they have an underlying condition which has an impact on them. This could be a result of many different causes including: physical disability, learning disability or a mental health problem. The additional needs that an individual may have vary from time to time, they may have a disease or condition in which the level of support needed will fluctuate. For all health and social care workers knowledge of the reasons why such needs should arise, how they are identified and how best to support individuals who have them is essential. It is also important to be familiar with issues that people with such needs may face daily, which can include coping with a condition, difficulties accessing services, possible discrimination and social isolation.

| To achieve a **Pass** grade the evidence must show that the learner is able to: | To achieve a **Merit** grade the evidence must show that, in addition to the pass criteria, the learner is able to: | To achieve a **Distinction** grade the evidence must show that, in addition to the pass and merit criteria, the learner is able to: |
| --- | --- | --- |
| **P1** describe reasons why individuals may experience additional needs. Pg 202 | | |
| **P2** describe models of disability and how these may impact upon individuals. Pg 207 | **M1** compare two models of disability in terms of how these may impact upon individuals. Pg 207 | **D1** evaluate two models of disability in terms of explaining the concept of disability. Pg 207 |

grading criteria

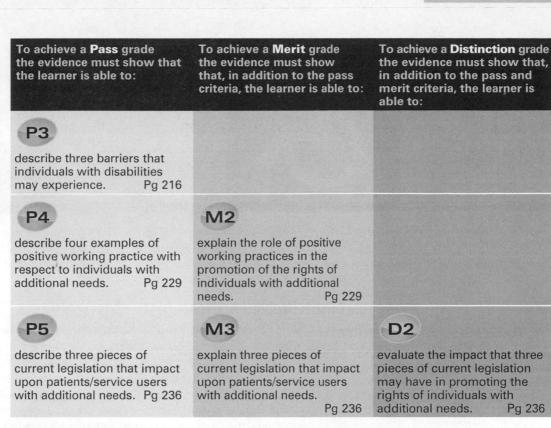

| To achieve a **Pass** grade the evidence must show that the learner is able to: | To achieve a **Merit** grade the evidence must show that, in addition to the pass criteria, the learner is able to: | To achieve a **Distinction** grade the evidence must show that, in addition to the pass and merit criteria, the learner is able to: |
|---|---|---|
| **P3** describe three barriers that individuals with disabilities may experience. Pg 216 | | |
| **P4** describe four examples of positive working practice with respect to individuals with additional needs. Pg 229 | **M2** explain the role of positive working practices in the promotion of the rights of individuals with additional needs. Pg 229 | |
| **P5** describe three pieces of current legislation that impact upon patients/service users with additional needs. Pg 236 | **M3** explain three pieces of current legislation that impact upon patients/service users with additional needs. Pg 236 | **D2** evaluate the impact that three pieces of current legislation may have in promoting the rights of individuals with additional needs. Pg 236 |

*grading criteria*

# Why individuals may have additional needs

In order to offer support and to provide it at the correct level, it is essential to understand why additional needs arise and to examine the means by which they can be addressed and services that may be available.

## Additional needs

The additional needs that an individual may have could be due to

- Physical illness or condition.
- Mental health problems.
- Learning difficulties/disabilities.

There are also many conditions which may have all three physical, mental and learning difficulties present and therefore significantly impacting on an individual's lifestyle.

## Physical illness or condition

These terms refer to conditions which have an impact on the body and the functioning of the body. Often when disability is considered it is wheelchair users and the physically disabled that immediately spring to mind. The symbol for disability reflects this.

There are obviously many conditions that can be physically debilitating. Most do not have any impact on an individual's intellectual ability, for example:

- Arthritis.
- Spinal cord injuries.
- Motor Neurone Disease.

There are some physical illnesses and conditions affecting the brain or injury to the brain that may have an impact on intellectual ability. Conditions affecting the brain can result in deficits which leave the individual with memory loss, the inability to retain information, inability to think clearly, confusion, disorientation and possible loss of consciousness.

Figure 26.1 The symbol for disability

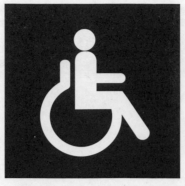

Many physical disabilities are unseen, for example blood disorders, visual impairment, hearing impairment. A physical disability may be particularly difficult to cope with, as the body may not be able to respond in the way the individual would wish. This can result in feelings of frustration and anger.

## Mental health problems

Mental health problems affect the way individuals think, their mood and behaviour. Mental problems are now increasingly common in society and are a major reason for individuals being unable to work, build relationships and lead a happy and fulfilled life. What causes such problems is often not clear and there may be a number of reasons, including a response to events in an individual's life, continued stress, lifestyle factors, links to drugs and alcohol and a genetic predisposition. Mental health problems are often hidden by individuals, they may be viewed as a stigma and something to be ashamed of. This is often because there is a lack of understanding regarding the impact that mental health problems can have and also how they can be managed. Mental health problems would include depression, anxiety disorders, personality disorders. The number of cases of depression has increased significantly in recent years and it is believed that depression and other mental health problems will be a major cause of disability in the future. Figures from NHS Direct reveal that 15% of the population of the UK will experience a bout of severe depression in their lives.

## Learning difficulties/disabilities

Based upon data from the Department of Health (DOH 2001), there are approximately 210,000 people with severe learning disabilities in England, with 1.2 million people with mild to moderate learning disabilities. The term 'learning disability' was introduced in the early 1990s by the department of health, to replace the term mental handicap. It means that an individual that has a learning disability may have difficulties learning new skills, communicating, handling complex information and living independently.

### What causes a learning disability?

The following are some reasons why learning disabilities could occur:

- Birth trauma: lack of oxygen before or during birth.

- Genetic conditions.

- Accident: traumatic brain injuries can result in learning disabilities.

- Exposure to chemicals which can damage the brain and brain development.

The learning disability may limit intellectual ability, and the ability to manage complex information and situations. An individual with learning disabilities may also have major communication problems. This is because they can have difficulties processing information. Processing information can involve:

- receiving information
- using information
- storing information in the memory
- remembering
- retrieving the right pieces of information
- communicating more information.

Some information can get lost or confused in the person's brain and it is much harder for them to make sense of it. Learning disabilities can also result in further confusion, as the person may understand information but may find it difficult to express this, which gives the impression that they do not understand. All these things can make learning, and following on from this, life in general, difficult to manage and extremely challenging.

Learning disabilities do not go away but individuals can build on their strengths. If the learning disability is not severe it is sometimes possible for people to improve, quite dramatically, the way that their brain processes information. It is also important to note that sometimes people who have a learning disability are also highly creative.

The level of learning disability may sometimes be described as mild, moderate, severe or profound, but this approach is not always helpful as it does not focus on what the individual can do – they may have many strengths and abilities. The term 'learning difficulties' is also used by some who do not like the negativity associated with the word disability.

The impact of physical, mental or learning disability on an individual will clearly be dependent on the nature of the condition and any possible deficits that the individual will experience as a result.

Some conditions are quite complex both in terms of how they occur and the impact they have on the human body.

## Genetic disorders

A genetic disorder is a disease which is due to abnormalities in the individual's DNA (deoxyribonucleic acid), the building blocks of the gene. The genes carry hereditary information from both parents. In many genetic diseases the child will not inherit the disease unless both parents pass down a defective copy of the gene, but they may become a carrier of a defective gene.

Figure 26.2 Genetic pattern of inheritance

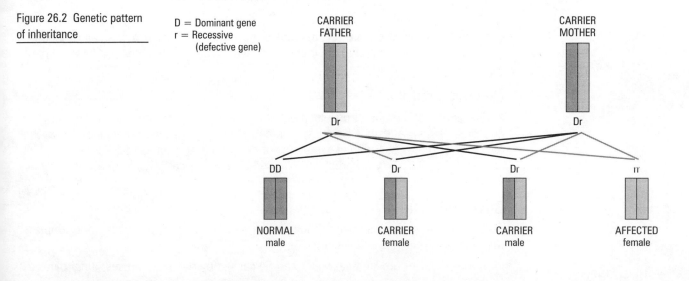

The problems can arise from a small mutation in a single gene or an extra chromosome or even a missing chromosome.

Examples of genetic disorders include:

### Sickle cell disease

This is a disorder which impedes the ability of the red blood cells to carry oxygen throughout the body.

### Cystic fibrosis

This primarily affects the respiratory and digestive systems – caused by a defective gene. The protein produced by this gene helps fluid move in and out of cells; if it is faulty, this process does not work effectively. The result is the formation of a thick mucous outside the cell. The cells of the lungs are badly affected by this problem.

### Down's syndrome

This is a chromosomal condition where there is an additional chromosome (Chromosome 21). An individual who has Down's syndrome usually has learning difficulties, a characteristic facial appearance and poor muscle tone.

Figure 26.3 Down's syndrome

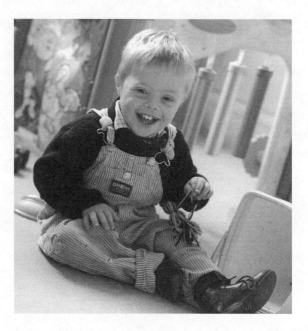

Other inherited disorders are called multifactorial. There might be very small variations in genes which when linked to environmental factors can trigger disease – for example many cancers, heart disease.

## Developmental

Autism is part of a group of developmental disorders known as the autism spectrum disorders (ASDs). Autism is the most common of these disorders, others include Asperger's. The most common symptoms of autism are difficulties with social interaction, problems with verbal and non-verbal communication, and unusual, repetitive activities.

## Environmental

Additional needs can arise due to the need for specific working practices, for example when an individual has an infection.

Infectious diseases are illnesses which can be caused by bacteria, viruses, fungi parasites or prions. Some infectious diseases can be easily transmitted from one person to another. When supporting an individual with an infectious disease it is necessary to know whether the disease can be transmitted and how. With this information additional precautions such as full isolation or additional personal protective equipment (PPE) can be taken. It is important to note that health and social care workers should always follow **standard precautions**, as an infection can be present but initially undetected. It is essential that health and social care workers follow the infection control policy specific to their work area.

## Stroke

A stroke (cerebral vascular accident, CVA) is possibly the most common cause of a severe disability. An estimated 250,000 people have disabilities caused by a stroke. (www.stroke.org.uk/information)

It most commonly affects the over 65s but all people are potentially at risk. A stroke occurs when the blood supply to part of the brain is cut off or reduced significantly. When this occurs, brain tissue dies. As the brain controls the rest of the body, so damage to the brain will result in a deficit in the areas of the body controlled by that part of the brain. An individual may experience hemiplegia – paralysis on one side of their body, an inability to communicate, or slurred speech.

## Attention deficit hyperactivity disorder (ADHD) and attention deficit disorder (ADD)

ADHD and ADD are conditions which result in problem behaviour and poor attention span. Children find it hard to control their behaviour. They might be impulsive, restless and inattentive. Children can have problems learning and socialising. The causes of ADHD are not clear. Possible causes are thought to be brain injury, chemical imbalance in the brain, genetic links, environmental factors and possible links to diet.

## Other causes of additional needs

Table 26.1 Examples of conditions which may trigger additional needs

| Reason why additional needs are present | Example | Possible problems | Possible additional needs |
|---|---|---|---|
| Sensory impairment | Visual impairment | Unable to see | Modify home, guide dog, Braille books, talking books |
| Accident | Road Traffic Accident (RTA) resulting in spinal damage Quadraplegia Paraplegia | Unable to walk, unable to undertake personal care, continence problems, depression | Wheelchair, assistance with personal care, modifications at home, adjustments at work |
| Illness | Cancer, arthritis | Pain, depression, limited mobility, problems with personal care | Pain relief, drug therapy, surgery, physiotherapy modifications to home |
| Developmental | Autism | Reduced ability to communicate, unpredictable behaviour | Educational support, quiet environment |
| Infectious diseases | Hepatitis C | Lethargy, virus carried in the blood | Counselling, information, re-infection control |
| Progressive illness | Multiple sclerosis, motor neurone disease | Increasing levels of weakness, unable to perform tasks | Counselling, mobility aids, modifications to home |
| Mental health problem | Schizophrenia, depression, personality disorders | Unpredictable behaviour, self-harm, harm to others | Drug therapy, counselling, close observation |

There are so many reasons why an individual may have additional needs, and these needs may change over time. The most important point is that individuals' needs should be identified and assessed and the support required planned in partnership.

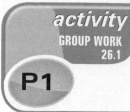

activity
GROUP WORK
26.1

**P1**

Divide into small groups. Each group list two reasons why individuals may experience additional needs, identify the possible needs the individuals might have.

# Models of disability

## Disability and dependency as a social construct

To understand the impact of disability and how best to support individuals who may experience this, it is helpful to examine how disability is viewed within our society and what has shaped this view. This is sometimes referred to as a social construct:

'**social construct**, a social mechanism, phenomenon, or category created and developed by society; a perception of an individual, group, or idea that is "constructed" through cultural or social practice'.

Source: Webster's Dictionary

## Impairment, disability, handicap

The idea of a social construct is very important when disability and dependence are examined because views about disabilities are heavily influenced by the society in which an individual lives. Also as society changes, so can social constructs. For example, wearing glasses is socially acceptable and not considered as a disability, but wearing a hearing aid is very different. Why is this the case?

In western society for most of the last century the way disability was viewed was based around dependence and independence. Having a disability might have meant that an individual could be separated from society. The situation would be regarded as a personal tragedy', (Barnes and Mercer 2003) for the individual resulting in a life of dependence, in which they are the passive recipient of care delivered by family, friends, service providers and policy makers. The disability was something to be dreaded as it dominated and blighted the individual's life. They would no longer be free to determine their own futures and plans but be dependent on others.

By exploring the language and the theory it is possible to analyse views and perceptions.

## The language

Think about the words associated with, or used to describe disability.

These words are not very pleasant. They are used as insults and put downs. Even terms and phrases such as 'the disabled' can depersonalise an individual.

In more recent years there has been a significant change in views and attitudes and an increase in the voice of the disabled people's movement. This has resulted in many changes, including a debate about the term 'disability', what it means and how it is applied. The language used to describe people with disabilities is very important. It is helpful to look at how the language has developed towards the latter part of the last century.

The World Health Organization (WHO) published classifications in 1980: 'International Classification of Impairments, Disabilities and Handicaps', known as ICIDH. The WHO identified three concepts and defined them as follows:

Impairment – 'any loss or abnormality of a psychological, physiological, or anatomical structure or function'. In other words problems with one functioning of the body.

Disability – 'any restriction or inability (resulting from an impairment) to perform an activity in the manner or within the range considered normal for a human being'. Limitations on the body caused by the impairment.

Handicap – 'any disadvantage for a given individual, resulting from an impairment or a disability, that limits or prevents the fulfillment of a role that is normal for that individual'. The handicap is the negative impact of the impairment and disability on the social roles of one individual. (WHO, 1980 cited in Barnes and Mercer 2003).

The impairment refers to the part of the body that is not functioning and the disability is limitations caused by the impairment, for example if a person has a hearing problem, the impairment is the deafness, the disability is the communication difficulties. The key part of these definitions is emphasising the difficulties that disabled people may face with day-to-day activities. Many people were supportive of these definitions when they were first published but the disabled groups were not happy. They felt that within these definitions the idea that the impairment causes both the disability and handicap presented a totally medical focus and does not highlight the importance of social and environmental factors for an individual.

As early as 1976 the disabled people's movement was developing strength and had produced their own definitions of impairment and disability:

Impairment – 'Lacking part or all of a limb, or having a defective limb, organ or mechanism of the body'.

Disability – 'The disadvantage or restriction of activity caused by a contemporary social organisation which takes little or no account of people who have physical impairments and thus excludes them from participation in the mainstream of social activities'.

(Union of the Physically Impaired Against Segregation (UPIAS) 1976)

As the disabled people's movement grew bigger to include a complete spectrum of disabilities, not only physical disabilities, the definitions were broadened in the following way and published by the Disabled Peoples International (DPI 1994, cited in Barnes and Mercer 2003).

Impairment – 'The functional limitation within the individual caused by physical, mental or sensory impairment'.

Disability – 'The loss or limitation of opportunities to take part in the normal life of the community on an equal level with others due to physical and social barriers'.

Faced with pressure from a range of sources the WHO changed the definitions in 1999 and produced ICIDH-2 which advocated the following approach to definitions and classification of disability. All individuals can experience health problems and as a result a degree of disability. Therefore disability is something that is applicable to everyone to some extent. By focusing not just on the cause of the disability but the influence it can have on the lives of individuals, the whole concept of disability is much broader. In a lifetime many people may have a health problems which could (albeit temporarily) disable them in some way. In terms of the three aspects of the original WHO definition the impairment remains pretty much the same, but disability is replaced by limitations on activities at the individual level; and handicap with restriction on participation in society. (www.who.int/classifications).

The word handicap is now considered to be an unacceptable term. All the definitions can be confusing and there is still much debate occurring as to what is the acceptable definition. Today the debate is whether the correct term is Disabled People or People with Disabilities. The discussion over language and terminology is sometimes thought to be excessive but language can be powerful and many of these words have very negative meanings.

The important point is to have an open mind, see the person and avoid categorising people on the basis of a label.

# Models

## 'Medical Model' (or individual model of disability)

In this model the disability is viewed as the most significant and defining factor for the individual. It is the disability that is the focus and this influences choices that are made. Medical professions and associated groups provide the diagnosis and the possible treatment options. The aim is to rehabilitate, and make the person fit in to society if possible. This model focuses on what the person can't do. It makes them the problem. People think about the disability and look for a medical cure and don't look at how the society is failing to accept the disability, accommodate the individual and include them as an equal. In fact in this model there are no demands on society to create a place for individuals with disabilities. When an individual has a disability they are considered in need of help that can be given by the health professionals. They are given a diagnosis, which can act as a label, defining them as an individual. Other people will consider the individual, often viewing the medical diagnosis as the most significant factor. The medical model creates a dependency culture, a paternalist approach in which people feel sorry for people.

This model can reinforce segregation and put up barriers that prevent a more inclusive approach by emphasising the following:

- The individual has a problem.
- The individual cannot fulfil the usual roles in our society, and may be excused from
  - work
  - relationships
  - parenting.
- The medical profession determine the treatment.
- The individual is not independent and is in need of some sort of support.

## The social model

The social model of disability looks at the situation from the other way round – it is society which is unable to adequately support individuals who have different needs due to their impairment or **chronic illness**. Disabled people face discrimination. This discrimination is a result of a society which is unable to accommodate the individual needs. Looking at the way in which society can pose barriers for disabled people changes the focus on to the shortfalls of the environment and society. It is possible that systems and structures within the society can be changed. Disabled groups argue that it is society that disables people with impairments. Disability is created in addition to the impairment. This is the basis of the social model of disability (sometimes called social barriers model of disability). The language and the way in which terms are used are vitally important in the social model.

This model can give people an opportunity to take a radically different view to the way they look at their disability and the world in which they live. Having a disability does not have to be looked at from a completely negative stand point, marking out the individual as some sort of failure or weak flawed person. This model can unite disabled people and give a sense of community as opposed to isolation and segregation. Ultimately this will be good for the wider community. Within social model a degree of dependence is not necessarily negative as many people are dependent on others for certain things.

*remember*

Would anybody like a friend who was only there out of pity?

Table 26.2 Comparing two models of disability

| Medical (individual) model | Social model |
|---|---|
| Personal tragedy theory | Social oppression theory |
| Personal problem | Social problem |
| Individual treatment | Social action |
| Medicalisation – everything is orientated around the medical diagnosis and treatment | Self-help – empowerment, give people control over their situations |
| Professional dominance | Individual and collective responsibility |
| Expertise – the professionals have all the answers | Experience – lived experience of people with disabilities |
| Individual identity – isolation and segregation | Collective identity – can be part of a bigger group |
| Prejudice | Promoting anti-discrimination |
| Care – delivered to the individual with the disability | Rights – what does the person want? They have rights and freedom like everyone else |
| Control – all the control is with the professionals | Choice – people have choices |
| Individual adjustment | Social change |

Source: Adapted from Barnes, Mercer, Shakespeare (1999)

Looking at the table, it is possible to summarise the key points from the models. Firstly the medical model – the individual is a victim who has experienced a personal tragedy about which people are sorry and sad. The individual will have many personal problems requiring individual treatment. The medical profession diagnoses the disability and prescribes the treatment – they are dominant and they are the experts. The individual with the disability is isolated by their condition, they may be segregated or excluded from the mainstream and viewed as different. People may be aware of prejudicial attitudes. The individual requires care, they have minimal control, social policy supports a system in which the individual can be given care, and it is up to the individual to adjust and accept what is offered.

Contrast this with the social model which asserts that it is social structures and systems which are disabling people – they isolate and exclude and therefore oppress individuals. The problems lie with society, and not merely the individual; they require social action in order to engender change. The experience of disability is important in this model: social circumstances, family life, relationships, finances, in fact a whole host of issues which are significant to everyone. The experiences of disabled people should be utilised in order to obtain accurate information and ideas from which everyone can learn. By having a collective identity the people with disabilities can be more powerful and influential, therefore challenging the dominance of the medical profession but also working with it to ensure the best outcomes for individuals. Disabled people can face discrimination and this must be recognised and stopped. Rather than being the passive recipients of care, people have rights and choices. Involvement in political movements can help to promote rights and ensure that disabled people have a voice and can make their own decisions. Hopefully by becoming more powerful as a group, people with disabilities will be able to instigate change.

For many people the level of the disability might prevent them from participation in major social change and some argue that the social model is unrealistic, but the advocates of the social model are keen to point out that the key message is that all people have the right to respect and a good standard of living. The social model is not in direct opposition to the medical model, it is simply another way of looking at a situation.

If a person is in hospital as a result of their impairment or chronic illness, the medical model will be more dominant because this is an **acute** care setting. But once they are discharged from hospital why should this model continue to dominate? The continued emphasis on the limitations and the problems for the individual leads people to accept the dominance of the medical profession. In order to challenge the medical model, the power and influence of the medical profession has to be recognised. This view does not reject the importance of medical interventions at part of a holistic approach to supporting an individual with a disability.

Figure 26.4 Medical model of disability

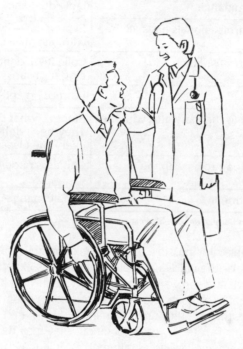

Figure 26.5 Social model of disability

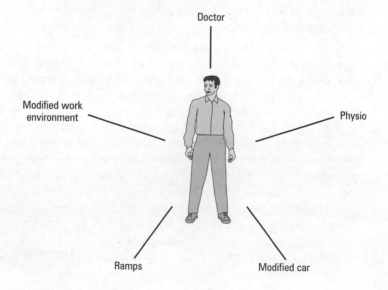

## Normalisation

This involves the moves to integrate disabled individuals into society, stopping the development of large institutions and supporting people to live in local communities. This approach was promoted in the latter part of the twentieth century amongst the Learning Disability services. Although it is viewed as an extremely positive step and a potential example of shifting the services from a large medically-led institution into the community, there was criticism from some parts as once again the whole process was led by professionals and not by the service user groups. The pressure was on people with learning disabilities to conform. This approach reinforces the idea that everyone has to fit into society, as opposed to adjustments being made and differences supported. Society decides what is normal and sets a benchmark against which people will be judged; there is no challenging of this idea.

Some people have conditions which make it virtually impossible to neatly integrate. They may look different, or act differently to the majority. Rather than the desperate attempts to make everyone fit in, it would be better to educate people to accept the differences. Most people do not want to live in a world where everyone is the same.

## Holistic approach

This involves examining the situation from a range of perspectives. What is the disability, how does it impact on the individual, what environment do they live in/work in, what are their leisure activities and what relationships are important to them? What services can be offered? How can they be funded? The individual with the disability should be at the centre of decision making.

Figure 26.6  Impact on services

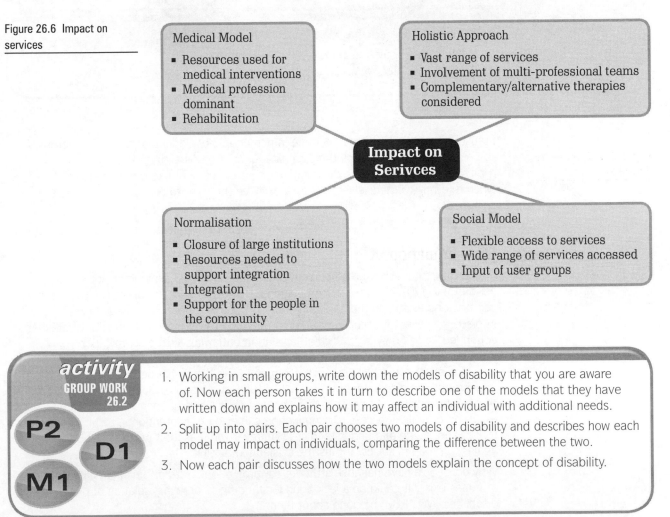

Medical Model
- Resources used for medical interventions
- Medical profession dominant
- Rehabilitation

Holistic Approach
- Vast range of services
- Involvement of multi-professional teams
- Complementary/alternative therapies considered

**Impact on Serivces**

Normalisation
- Closure of large institutions
- Resources needed to support integration
- Integration
- Support for the people in the community

Social Model
- Flexible access to services
- Wide range of services accessed
- Input of user groups

*activity*
GROUP WORK
26.2

P2
D1
M1

1. Working in small groups, write down the models of disability that you are aware of. Now each person takes it in turn to describe one of the models that they have written down and explains how it may affect an individual with additional needs.

2. Split up into pairs. Each pair chooses two models of disability and describes how each model may impact on individuals, comparing the difference between the two.

3. Now each pair discusses how the two models explain the concept of disability.

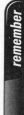

# Effects of disability

The effects of disability on the individual will obviously depend upon the nature of the impairment that the individual has. The individual might not be able to walk without a mobility aid, they may not be able to receive information in a standard format, requiring instead Braille, audio, large print. In other words individuals may have impairments which result in the need for additional support, but they can be disabled further by the society and other people's responses to the disability.

## case study 26.1   Mary

Mary has Multiple Sclerosis (MS) and now requires an electric wheelchair to mobilise. This has been difficult for Mary as she has always been an extremely active person. She is trying to cope with her condition and get used to the wheelchair. Today she tried to go to her local shop in the wheelchair but was unable to travel along the pavement easily as a number of the neighbours have parked their cars across it. When she arrived at the shop she couldn't reach what she wanted. A young shop assistant appeared momentarily, looked nervously at Mary then went into the back of the shop.

## activity
### INDIVIDUAL WORK

1. Identify the barriers that Mary encountered.
2. What impact could this have on Mary's confidence?
3. What can be done to improve this situation?

Statistics from the UK reveal that one in five people of working age are considered to be disabled as defined by the Disability Rights Commission and the Government. Many people with a long-term condition or illness may not use the term disability when referring to themselves, but they do have the right to be protected against unfair treatment.

(www.drc-gb.org/library, accessed August 2007)

## Discrimination

Prejudicial attitudes towards people with a disability are present within society. If people act on their prejudices then discrimination occurs. In the latter part of the twentieth century, oppression on the basis of gender or race was unacceptable and laws were in place to prevent it occurring; but discrimination towards individuals with disabilities continued. It was only in 1995 that legislation outlawing such discrimination was introduced with the passing of the Disability Discrimination Act. Discrimination against individuals with a disability can occur in many ways. It can happen directly, by depicting impairment in a disparaging way, belittling the individual or by labelling and implying that they have no identity other than the disability. It can happen indirectly, due to social exclusion or difficult access. Discrimination can also be unintentional, resulting from a lack of knowledge and understanding. Whatever the reason, if people are discriminating against a group in society it must be challenged at all levels.

Why do people have negative attitudes towards people with disabilities? Why do these attitudes exist? It could be a lack of understanding or ongoing isolation of people with disabilities. What can be done about them?

### Societal attitude

Many of the obstacles that individuals with disabilities face are results of the attitudes people have and which are reinforced by our society. Western society promotes the able body, often beautiful and youthful as the standard, so as a result many disabled people are immediately separated from the mainstream.

The reluctance to accept the disability by both the person with the disability and other members of society results in exclusion socially and in the workplace. On the basis of the disability people generalise about the person and assume they may have multiple problems including understanding; most people have heard the expression, 'Does he take sugar?'

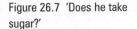
Figure 26.7 'Does he take sugar?'

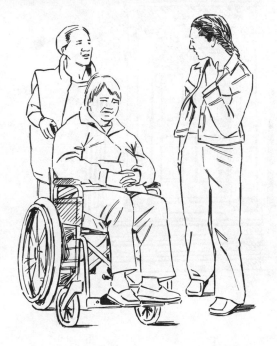

If people have positive attitudes, focusing on what can be done to address particular needs, then this can completely change the outcome for people who have a disability. It has been disabled groups who have led the challenge to the views of disability. This has not been easy as people often respond positively to people with disabilities if they are thankful and show a stoic approach.

Disabled people who achieve what an able bodied person might take for granted (job, marriage, parenthood) are held up as heroes by our society because they have triumphed over their 'bad' situation. For many disabled people this will not be possible but they do want and need the respect from other members of our society, this is often denied and discrimination continues. It is possible for these barriers to be overcome and for the non-disabled person to see the disabled person as an individual similar to them in most ways, this first step is recognising the barriers

## Barriers to access and opportunities

The following barriers have been identified. Look at each one and give an example of how this could occur and a means of overcoming this barrier.

### Architectural

For the majority of people, moving in and out of buildings is not something that is given any thought. It is taken for granted that this will be possible. On the rare occasion that this is not possible, for example a lift is broken or a car park is full, this might pose a minor inconvenience but gaining access to the building is still possible. For many disabled people access to buildings is something that requires thought and detailed planning. Many beautiful buildings have been designed to look good and meet the needs of the majority of the population. This approach is no longer acceptable; it is now a requirement that all new buildings meet the standards of access outlined in the Disability Discrimination Act 1995 and that 'reasonable adjustments' are made to existing buildings to allow access to all.

Figure 26.8 Architectural discrimination

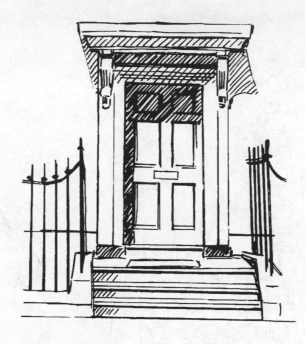

### Cultural

In some languages there is no one word for disability. Disability is subjective and the way it is viewed can vary. Some people do not consider that they have a disability even though they may have limitations due to physical, mental health or learning disabilities. In some cultures any sort of disability within a family could be hidden due to shame and negative feelings. In other cultures there is a much more relaxed approach. The cultural and the attitudinal are closely linked.

### Attitudinal

Attitudinal barriers are considered to be the most powerful barrier of all. Ingrained negative attitudes are hard to change and potentially pose a whole range of barriers for people with disabilities and are very difficult to legislate against. The best architecturally designed building can be rendered inaccessible if the receptionist has a dismissive attitude. Attitudinal barriers can emerge from disabled and non-disabled individuals.

Attitudinal barriers can include:

- Viewing people as inadequate due to their disability.
- Patronising people.
- Feeling sorry for the person.
- Viewing the individual as superman/woman for overcoming their disability and living independently.
- Asssuming there are multiple problems. One disability leads to another, e.g. in assuming that if someone is a wheelchair user they may also have difficulties understanding.
- Stereotyping.

- Anger – disabled people obtain extra benefits
- Scepticism that the disability actually exists if it is not obvious.
- Apprehension. Afraid to do the wrong thing, so keeping away from people with disabilities is easier.

### Removing attitudinal barriers

Attitudinal barriers can result in discrimination and exclusion; it is also difficult to challenge them because they might not be explicit. The best way to tackle these sorts of barriers is by not focusing on the disability and by trying to avoid preconceived ideas about what a person can and can't do.

There are now many support groups which are led by people with disabilities. Such groups can give advice and support to all. Promotional materials and websites can be excellent ways of getting information to a broad range of people.

Table 26.3 Dos and don'ts to minimise attitudinal barriers

| Do | Don't |
|---|---|
| Give people the opportunity to speak for themselves. Make eye contact and address the conversation to the person with the disability even though they may have a support person with them. | Assume that all people with a hearing impairment can lip read, or people who are blind can read Braille. |
| Ask people politely if they require assistance. | Pretend to understand someone. |
| Greet people with disabilities in the same way as you would usually greet individuals. | Don't use terms that evoke feelings of superiority, and pity. |
| Talk about people not broad groups – the disabled. | Touch wheelchairs without asking permission. |
| Give verbal information to people who are visually impaired and describe locations using a clock face or left and right. | Interrupt or attempt to finish off sentences for people who have speech impairment. |
| Be friendly and accepting, be honest and say if you are unsure about how to respond. | Assume that a person's ability to express themselves is an indicator of their intellect. |

Figure 26.9 Example of minimising attitudinal barriers

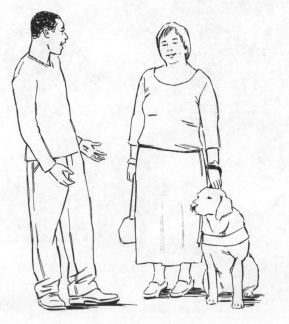

Figure 26.10 Example of attitudinal barriers

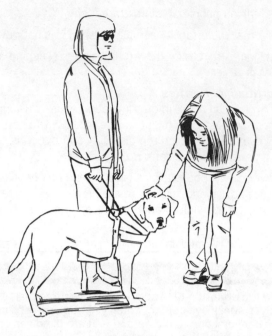

### Educational

There are many different views as to how compulsory education should be offered to children with disabilities and whether they should attend main stream schools or schools specifically aimed at meeting the needs of a child with a disability. There are many arguments for and against. One of the key arguments as to why children with disabilities should be educated in mainstream schools is to build understanding and acceptance of differences and to improve integration and mixing of children from the local communities. If children are segregated and isolated at school the message given to the child is that they are different in some way from other children. It has to be stated that it can be very difficult for a child with a disability within a mainstream school, as they may

Figure 26.11 Compulsory education

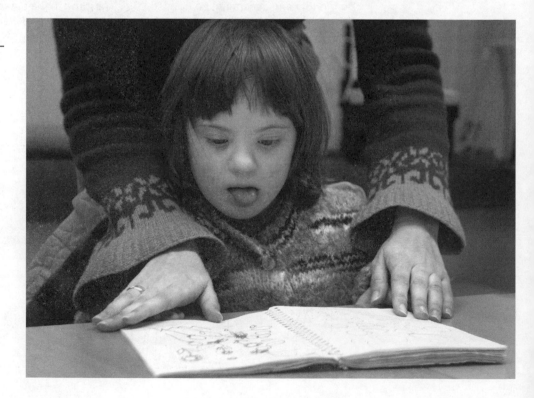

feel isolated and different from their peers. There is a policy which supports inclusion, but parents and local education authorities may handle the situation in a number of different ways with sound arguments on all sides. As with any issue relating to children it is hoped that the principle of always acting in the best interests and welfare of the child is the factor that determines where the child is educated.

Beyond the age of 16 education is offered at colleges and universities. Following the introduction of the Disability Discrimination Act all HE and FE educational institutions have the responsibility to ensure full access and facilities to support all learners. All universities now have information and guidance for students with disabilities or particular learning needs.

### Employment

Within western society, work is a means through which people are judged. Work brings status and respect, power and influence. Many people with impairments are excluded from the workforce. In Britain 60% of disabled people are classified as economically inactive, (Christie, Mensah-Coker, 1999). There are more disabled people at the lower end of the employment ladder – the less skilled. It is often difficult to overcome negative attitudes. Employers might have issues of access, potential additional resources being needed, physical appearance. There is now legislation in place to address this but current statistics do not show a significant improvement in the occupational opportunities for individuals with disabilities.

There has been criticism of working arrangements for individuals with learning disabilities who have been undertaking meaningless work for token payments. There has been a request for this to stop, as it is demeaning for individuals to be given work of this nature.

Charities, voluntary groups and self-help groups can offer useful advice and possible support to assist people with employment opportunities. The National Autistic Society is a national charity which offers a specialised employment service, the aim of which is to assist people with autism and Aspergers syndrome to obtain employment.

## case study 26.2     Mike

Mike (aged 31) has cystic fibrosis. He looks healthy and there are no obvious signs of his condition. He works out at the gym once per day. Mike is employed in a mobile phone company as a software designer. His colleagues think he is a fitness fanatic as he doesn't drink and is always taking tablets. He is off work twice a year for 3 weeks at a time as he has a course of intravenous antibiotics to clear his lungs of developing infections. His work colleagues are becoming resentful regarding Mike's sickness record. A job promotion was advised within the company and although Mike met the requirements in terms of qualifications and experience he was not short-listed for an interview.

## activity
### INDIVIDUAL WORK

1. What is cystic fibrosis?
2. Why is exercise important for Mike?
3. Why is Mike at risk of chest infections?
4. Can Mike take any action when he finds out he has not been short-listed for the interview?
5. What advice would you offer to Mike and his employer regarding the regular sick leave that Mike requires?

### Social and recreation

Social interaction can be difficult for disabled people. Some people try to hide disabilities or withdraw from society because it is too complicated, they might feel embarrassed or uncomfortable. However, it is possible for able-bodied and disabled individuals to work together, learn together and enjoy recreation time together. One example is the 'CandoCo' dance company which consists of disabled and non-disabled dancers. 'Our focus is on dance not disability, professionalism not therapy' (www.candoco.co.uk, accessed 24/08/07). This approach reinforces the view that for an activity people should be taken on their merit and suitability, and not on preconceived notions regarding what a certain person's capabilities might be.

## case study 26.3   Alicia

Alicia (aged 23) is interested in music, and listening to live music, and is considering going to a festival. She is a wheelchair user. Her family are not very happy, her mother is extremely worried that it is not safe and her brother thinks she will make a fool of herself.

### activity
**INDIVIDUAL WORK**

1. How would you support Alicia?
2. Do you feel attending a music festival is possible for her?
3. If so, how would you support her to get to a festival and to hopefully enjoy the music and the festival experience?

### Environmental

The environment and the transport systems can pose major barriers to participation for many people with disabilities. It can be extremely difficult for wheelchair users to get on and off public transport systems although attempts have been made to improve this. It is possible to modify some cars to suit individuals' specific needs in relation to their disability. Many people may be eligible for a mobility allowance as part of their benefit payment from the Government. This might enable them to use this to get a car. 'Motability' is a car scheme for disabled people through which a modified vehicle is leased or bought over a period of time. A car can bring a great deal of independence but for many people with disabilities driving is not an option. Motorised wheelchairs and scooters are available and are more common place now on the pavements of towns and cities. Having the confidence to use a motorised wheelchair or scooter will depend upon the patience and tolerance of other road and pavement users.

### Personal

The individual can often create their own barriers. This may be due to the trauma of coming to terms with an impairment if the onset is sudden. It may also be in response to attitudinal barriers from other people, which can damage confidence and lower **self-esteem**. Peer group support may be important in this situation and there are many self-help groups and disability rights groups which are led by disabled people.

### Financial

A major impact of disability on an individual can be on their financial situation. As the statistics have shown, people with disabilities are often not able to work, or are in lower paid employment. For many people they would like to work but cannot obtain suitable employment. As a result they are in a 'poverty trap' where the only jobs available are so lowly paid it is not worth them taking the job. Financial considerations are very

Figure 26.12 An example of how transport is adapted for people with disabilities

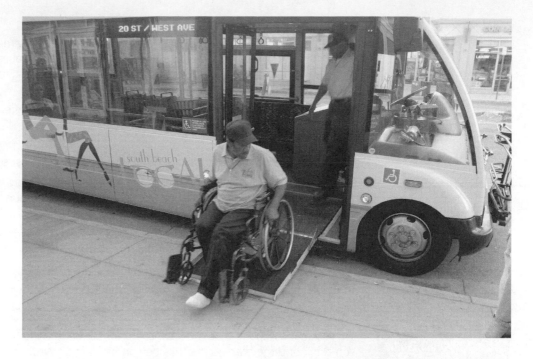

important because if equipment is required along with modifications to the home, things can become very expensive. It is often possible to obtain funding for special equipment but the funding may not be sufficient to obtain the latest version or exactly what the individual would like.

## case study 26.4 — Beth

Beth is 19 and she requires a wheelchair. When she went to get her wheelchair she didn't like what she was offered. She wanted something small and light, not big and clunky. She asked what the options were but was told that resources are tight, there is not much money around and she would have to make do with what was available. She was very upset. Her father decided to buy her one privately.

## activity
### INDIVIDUAL WORK

1. Find out how people access equipment in your local area.
2. What are the options for funding?

Financial support is available for individuals, the arrangements can be complicated and there are different allowances depending upon specific circumstances and the age of the individual.

Directgov –public services online
www.direct.gov.uk/DisabledPeople/
The Citizens Advice Bureau
www.citizensadvice.org.uk

Financial support is arranged in a number of different ways:

- Disability Living Allowance (DLA). This is for people who are ill, disabled (physically or mentally or both) or who are terminally ill. An individual may be eligible for this allowance if they have problems caring for themselves or difficulties walking or both. This benefit is for people up to the age of 65.

- Attendance Allowance. If a person is over 65 they may be eligible for Attendance Allowance. This is aimed at people who have an illness or disability and need help with personal care.

- Incapacity Benefit is aimed at people who can't work because of illness or disability.

It is now possible for people to receive direct payments, if they have been assessed by the local council and deemed to be in need of care and support services. This will allow people to arrange their own care.

Money to support the costs of the equipment to help with independent living or the modification of home equipment and fixtures and fittings may also be payable.

The Independent Living Fund helps severely disabled people to live independently rather than live in a care home. The money is payment towards personal care and domestic care.

**activity**

**INDIVIDUAL WORK 26.3**

**P3**

Think about someone that you have cared for; or know; who has additional needs. Can you think of three barriers that this person has faced? Write them down on a piece of paper.

# Current practice with respect to provision for additional needs

Positive working practice is all about placing the individual who requires support in the centre, and planning and delivering any support and care based upon their specific needs. Many of the issues which were examined in Unit 2, in Health and Social Care Book 1, are at the core of positive working practices. One of the important points to remember is that individuals who have additional needs may not be in a position to promote their own rights and choices and they are undoubtedly more at risk of having their rights overlooked or deliberately denied. Therefore the subject of positive working practice is particularly significant.

**Link**

See Unit 2 (Equality, Diversity and Rights in Health and Social Care) in Health and Social Care Book 1.

## Guidance

Implementing positive working practice requires guidance, as what one person considers acceptable may not be the same as another. In order to achieve this, systems and structures need to be in place at organisational, local and national levels. To establish guidance and set standards, care councils, **codes of practice** and charters and policies have been developed.

### Social care councils

The aim of social care councils is to regulate and monitor the social care sector monitoring the conduct of workers and the training that they receive. The need to establish social care councils was identified within the Care Standards Act 2000 and similar pieces of legislation in Northern Ireland and Scotland. The care councils are responsible for codes of practice, the setting up and maintaining of the Social Care Register and the education and training of staff.

**England**
The General Social Care Council
Tel: 020 7397 5100
www.gscc.org.uk
**Northern Ireland**
Northern Ireland Social Care Council
Tel: 02890 417600
Email: info@niscc.n-i.nhs.uk
www.niscc.info
**Scotland**
Scottish Social Services Council
Tel: 01382 207101 Information service: 0845 6030891
Email: enquiries@sssc.uk.com
www.sssc.uk.com
**Wales**
Care Council for Wales
Tel: 029 2022 6257
Email: info@ccwales.org.uk
www.ccwales.org.uk

The purpose of a social care council is to promote the interests of individuals who are in receipt of care. The council requires all social care workers to follow a code of practice and deliver care of the highest standard. It identifies the type and level of training required for social care workers. It is hoped that social care councils will be open, inclusive organisations that work closely with service users.

## Codes of practice

A code of practice is a set of principles or standards; it outlines values and ways of working, which cannot be ignored. Such a code is essential in certain areas of work and amongst many professional groups. In the health and social care sector it is necessary for individuals to be working at the same high standards and to have shared goals and standards of work.

Within the health sector there are codes of practice (or codes of professional conduct) for a number of professional groups, for example the nurses' Code of Professional Conduct, which is written by the Nursing and Midwifery Council.

*The NMC code of professional conduct: standards for conduct, performance and ethics (NMC 2004)*
This document outlines what is expected of a nurse and what standards of work must be met. It addresses subjects such as confidentiality and provides guidance as to how to respond in certain situations. The Code of Conduct highlights the importance of always acting in the best interests of the individual, protecting their interests and promoting their rights. This should be the guiding principle in the actions of any health and social care worker.

A code of practice has now been introduced for the social care sector within the UK. This is the first UK code of practice for social care workers and employers and is similar in its aim to the nursing code of conduct, outlining standards of practice. The code of practice will help the social care workforce to deliver care which is of a high standard and protect the public from poor practitioners and poor employers who do not meet the standards agreed. The code of practice states the responsibilities of employers and of social care workers. The need to introduce a code of practice was identified in the Care Standards Act 2000, and the Care Councils of the four countries of the UK have worked together to produce the document. Most people have welcomed its introduction as it simply states the values of the social care sector and stresses the importance of honesty and integrity for all people involved in this area. The code applies to all workers at any level within social care. It is crucial to note that it does not contain anything which is not immediately achievable by either a worker or an employer.

A requirement of the code of practice is the setting up of a Register of social care workers. This register will be used to make sure that all individuals involved in social care are appropriately trained and are following the code of practice. Failure to follow the code of practice will result in the worker being reported to the Care Council and possibly removed from the register and not being allowed to work in this sector. At present only social workers and social worker students can be on this register (please note that social worker is an official title and the only people allowed to use this are individuals who have undergone full social worker training at an approved educational institution). The plan is to eventually include all social care workers at all levels. In order to work in social care settings they must be on the register.

The expectation is that employers will make sure the code of practice is implemented into the workplace. It is also necessary for the code of practice to be reviewed. It will be possible for an employer to raise concerns regarding an employee to the General Social Care Council, to seek advice and possible investigation. This process will send a message to employers and staff, that working in the health and social care sector requires the right level of skill and the right attitude.

Figure 26.13 Example of a code of practice document

1. As a social care worker, you must protect the rights and promote the interests of service users and carers.

2. As a social care worker, you must strive to establish and maintain the trust and confidence of service users and carers.

3. As a social care worker, you must promote the independence of service users while protecting them as far as possible from danger or harm.

4. As a social care worker, you must respect the rights of service users while seeking to ensure that their behaviour does not harm themselves or other people.

5. As a social care worker, you must uphold public trust and confidence in social care services.

6. As a social care worker, you must be accountable for the quality of your work and take responsibility for maintaining and improving your knowledge and skills.

Source: The Code of Practice, www.gscc.org.uk/Good+practice+and+conduct/Codes+of+practice, accessed 01/09/2007

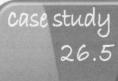

## Graham

Graham was worried about his sister. She lives in a residential care home which caters for people with learning disabilities. Although generally speaking most of the staff were kind and friendly, Graham had some reservations. His sister would often be in bed at 8.30 pm, her usual going to bed time at home had always been around 11pm. He visited on Saturdays and Wednesdays. On Saturdays he always brought her chocolates, fruit and magazines to look at but by Wednesday there was never any evidence of any. On more than one occasion he saw another resident wearing his sister's clothes.

**activity**
**INDIVIDUAL WORK**

1. What should Graham do?
2. What role does the General Social Care Council (GSCC) play in this situation?
3. How would the Code of Practice be used?

In response to the Care Standards Act, and as part of the process of tightening up of the rules regarding the provision of social care inspection agencies have been introduced across the U.K. the single independent inspectorate for social care in England; it is an amalgamation of a number of inspectorates.

Commission for Social Care Inspection (CSCI)
Tel: 020 7979 2000
www.csci.org.uk
Care and Social Services Inspectorate Wales (CSSIW)
Tel: 01443848450
www.csiw.wales.gov.uk/index.asp
Scottish Commission for the Regulation of Care
Tel: 01382207100
Social Services Inspectorate Northern Ireland
Tel: 02890520500

The primary remit is to inspect social care providers (public, private and voluntary). These inspections can take place unannounced so there is no opportunity to hide any bad practice. The care setting is judged against national minimum standards which are produced by the Department of Health (these are guidelines against which a judgment is made regarding the standard of the service). The inspection teams also take the Code of Practice for Social Care Employers into account when inspecting a care service and enforcing care standards.

Ideally individuals who use social care services themselves should be part of the inspection team. The inspection team interview all people involved in the social care setting, most importantly the service users. The inspectors produce a report and organisations that meet minimum standards are put on a register of services. All these changes mean that providers of social care are much more accountable than they were previously. The care that is being delivered is monitored closely. Hopefully this will eradicate the providers of sub-standard or inadequate care, however there are many people who feel there is still much to be done to improve standards of care.

Figure 26.14 Inspectors can
arrive unannounced

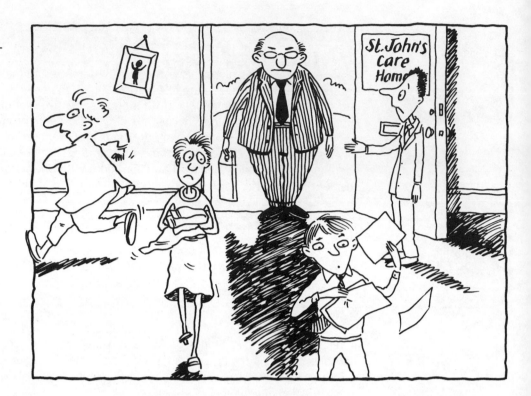

The inspectorates can handle complaints regarding care homes and council social
services. It is vital that any complaints procedure is open and easily accessible with
no fear of reprisals from any individual who has made a complaint. Anyone wishing
to make a complaint about a care home is advised to contact the service provider
initially. It is a requirement of the Care Standards Act that all service providers should
have a complaints procedure. If an individual is unable to complain directly then the
inspectorates can deal with the complaint.

Table 26.4  Commission for Social Care Inspection (CSCI)

| | Advantages of inspection | | |
|---|---|---|---|
| Service user | Close monitoring of care and services provided by external agency | Raising of standards | Route for complaints |
| Care providers (managers and workers) | They know what is expected of them. Opportunities for training and development | Standardisation of practice across the UK | **Whistle blowing** by staff is possible. Feedback to managers to raise standards |
| General public | Clear information | Confidence in a system which protects vulnerable groups | Route for complaints |

The National Minimum standards for adults 18–65 can be found at NMS – Care Homes
for Adults 18-65.

According to information from the Disability Rights Commission, many young adults are living in care homes which are not designed for their age group.

'8,000 young adults are living in care homes designed primarily for a different client group, usually older people'.

Source: www.drc-gb.org/newsroom/key_drc_facts_and_glossary/
disabled_people_living_in_inst.aspx

## Charters and policies

Guidance for health and social care workers is also provided within charters and policy documents. A charter gives details on the rights and standards that can be expected from a particular service or organisation. Find out if your organisation has a Charter of Rights. Charters for service users may be displayed within an organisation and it can be referred to if the rights are not upheld and standards are not met.

Policies are documents, which state the required process or procedure within an organisation or workplace. There are usually a great number of policies within an organisation. A policy will contain details of standards that must be met and provides procedural guidance and requirements for training.

**Figure 26.15 Charters and policies**

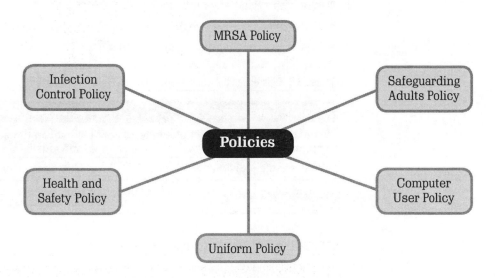

It is the responsibility of the health and social care worker to follow the policies of the organisation that they are working for, and it is the responsibility of the manager of an organisation to ensure that policies are in place, up-to-date and followed by staff, and that training is provided where necessary.

### Positive working practice – making it happen

From the discussion of the models of disability it is easy to see that the prevailing view of disability can have an impact on the way that services are offered to people.

Strange as it might seem, the health and social care services can sometimes discriminate against the very people they are attempting to support. This can be through a lack of understanding of complex chronic conditions, lack of resources, inexperience of working with individuals with specific needs (for example learning disabilities), established structures and systems which are inflexible. With recent legislation, which will be discussed in the next section, and a number of government papers which have had involvement and consultation from service users, steps have been taken to minimise these problems. Increased regulation, a culture of openness and accessible complaints procedures should also help to reduce these problems. At an individual level all health and social care workers can examine their own practice and identify if they need education and training and ask whether they be satisfied with the level of care they are delivering if it was their family or themselves on the receiving end.

### Needs-led assessment

Prior to 1990 individuals would be assessed to determine whether they might be eligible for existing services but the *NHS & Community Care Act 1990* introduced a change in emphasis. Instead of looking at how the individual would fit into the care sector, the needs of individuals would be identified and assessed and a decision would be made as to how the care sector could support the individual. On the basis of the assessment a plan of care would be developed, this needs-led approach introduces a more flexible way of planning care which is geared around the individual. Needs-led assessment is viewed as the key to high quality care. Before services can be arranged it is necessary for all individuals to have an assessment of their needs. This will usually include a discussion between the individual and the social services worker, and it may also involve a GP. The individual is encouraged to bring a relative, carer or someone who can speak up on their behalf. It is important that the individual has had a chance to think about their needs and what support they feel is necessary to enable them to go about their day-to-day lives.

The sort of questions that are asked at a needs led assessment are:

- What do you think your needs are?
- Are you having any problems?
- What help do you have at the moment?
- What help do you think you might need?

Table 26.5 Differences between needs- and service-led assessment

| Needs-led assessment | Service-led assessment |
|---|---|
| What does the person require in terms of support? | What can the service offer to the individual? |
| What are the individual's priorities? | 'One size fits all approach' |
| Individualised care package developed | Where is the capacity currently available? (Where can the person fit in?) |

## Person-centred planning

As the title suggests, similarly to need-led assessment, this is about the person who requires the care being the most important influential person in the planning and decision making process. If the individual lacks the mental capacity to make any decisions due to major brain injury or end stage dementia, then possibly family members, friends, carers and an independent advocate in the event of a crucial decision will also be involved (the Mental Capacity Act 2005 provides guidance for such cases). Person centred planning includes the following:

- Active involvement in the assessment, possible self-assessment.
- Integrated and multi-disciplinary assessment.
- Holistic and thorough assessment of all needs, listening to the individual and if possible getting to know them.
- Appropriate sharing of information.

## Empowering

This is all about giving people influence and control over their lives. In order to achieve this it is necessary to work with the individual who will be using the service, by engaging with them to find out what they want. This approach can also mean that service users can shape the services for the future.

'It is often the most isolated and the least identifiable of users – the ones who are never heard – who have the sorts of experience which can be most valuable.'

(Thornton and Tozer, 1995)

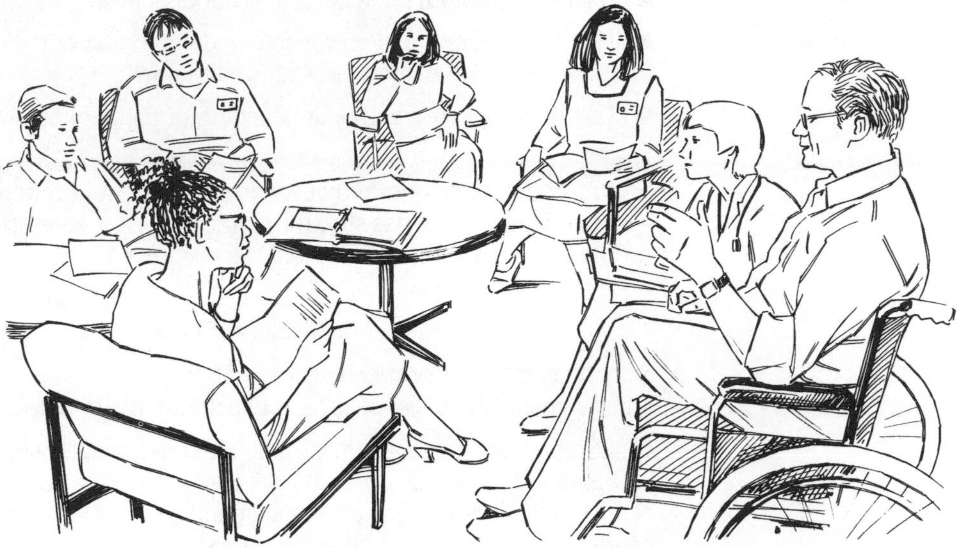

Figure 26.16 The role of health and social care workers is to support the individual.

Health and social care workers may think of their client group, and identify needs on the basis of the group that they fall into. However many service users may have nothing in common with each other and no shared ideas or values, they would not think of themselves as part of a bigger group – people with learning disabilities, or a disabled people.

Researchers have discovered that it is a mistake to assume that the views coming from one group of service users will be similar. It is in everyone's interests that the services provided are flexible and acceptable to all. It should be acknowledged that to involve people in their own care and to give them the power to make decisions and implement changes which affect them and which may in the long-term affect others will require a range of approaches.

## Expert Patients Programme

This is a programme introduced by the Department of Health in response to the increasingly knowledgeable groups of patients and service users.

'An observation frequently made by doctors who care for patients with long-term chronic disease is "my patients understand their disease better than I do". Many patients are, indeed, "experts" in their own right, as they have gained the life skills to cope with their chronic condition'

Source: DoH, 2006

The hope is that by training individuals to take responsibility for their own conditions, confidence in managing their daily lives will increase. There are now many courses being offered each year. This programme is led by non-clinical (non-professional) groups. It is aimed at people who have long-term conditions. It is predicted that chronic disease will be the biggest cause of disability in the future. According to DoH figures there are already 15 million, possibly 17.5 million, people with long-term conditions in England (DoH, 2006).

It is called the Expert Patients Programme (EPP) but it is aimed at users of health and social care services.

The Expert Patients Programme aims to teach people to:

- Work in partnership with health professionals to manage their condition.
- Share responsibility and communicate effectively.
- Have an accurate and reasonable understanding of their condition and the impact it is likely to have on their lives and their family.
- Use their expertise and understanding of their condition to be in control of their own lives.

Recent research has shown that the Expert Patient Programme is achieving positive results. 'Our research has shown that the EPP may be a useful addition to current services in the management of long-term conditions.'

Source: Rogers, Anne, 5 March 2007,
The National Primary Care Research and Development Centre.

Individuals have confirmed that they felt an increase in energy levels and small improvements in quality of life and improvements in self-esteem.

This Programme is proving invaluable for some people, helping them with problem solving and finding out information, creating networks and links to self-help groups. It is not suitable for all people as many people might feel uncomfortable discussing their condition in this way, but for some people it is very effective.

## Integrated practice

Many people develop long-term chronic conditions, and with an ageing population the expectation is that this will increase. In the past people would not have access to support and resources until their condition had deteriorated and they required interventions from the health services. Now there has been recognition of the fact that supporting people in the early stages of a condition is as important as later when there is progression of the problem. The support and the resources that the person might require at different stages will be totally different, as health and social care needs are increasingly complex and there are often many professionals and support systems involved in the delivery of care to the individual. The need for health and social practice to be co-ordinated and integrated is obvious. An individual with a long-term condition such as Parkinson's Disease, may be managing their condition with initially minimal support but this may change. Key workers, specialist nurses and other health and social care professionals can play a vital role in these situations. They can be flexible and available for the individual if required. They can offer advice, information and listen to concerns, and in doing so maintain independence and wellbeing for longer.

**remember**

The key points of this approach are:
- Encourage and increase self care.
- Offer services within the community.
- Access to specialist services.
- Health and social workers should work with individuals to plan ahead and anticipate support required to minimise problems.
- Co-ordination of services.

## Communication methods

People who have difficulties with communication including speaking and hearing can benefit from access to aids which can enable them to communicate. Hearing aids and glasses (spectacles) are perhaps the most common aids to communication that people come across. Any person that wears glasses knows how important they are and what a difference they make to the individual's ability to see and therefore communicate. The importance and usefulness of communication aids cannot be underestimated, but it must be the right communication aid for the individual. Imagine wearing glasses that were not suitable – wrong prescription or ill-fitting?

Figure 26.17  A hearing aid

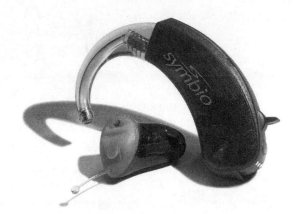

*remember*

It is essential to make sure that communication aids are:
- Correct for the individual.
- Fully functioning.
- Clean.
- Regularly reviewed and checked.

There are also more complex electronic devices which allow voice output, and computers which can be adapted specifically for an individual's needs. These will be discussed under the heading 'Assistive Technology'.

Aids to communication are not always about devices and technology. Sign language, modified sign language or relatively simple methods such as charts, pictures, symbols, letters or words are just as effective.

### Makaton

Makaton is a means of communication for individuals with communication and learning disabilities, and involves using signs and gestures to support the spoken word and symbols to support the written word. For many people signs are easier to understand as they represent pictures and can transmit a message much more readily than words. People may use the signs initially, then as their language develops they may drop the signs. Makaton also uses symbols to assist people with the written word. Important information can be produced using these symbols and this can mean that people can have information, instructions and messages in a format that they can easily understand. It can be used to produce warning signs or to give details regarding a certain task. Using signs and symbols can help speech and language to develop, but for some this may not be possible. A health and social care worker using makaton would sign and speak at the same time. Makaton is used throughout the world in more than 40 countries.

### Assistive Technology

Assistive Technology (AT), sometimes also called Adaptive Technology, refers to equipment and devices, which can be used to help with communication and other everyday jobs which an individual might not be able to perform due their impairment. Many severely disabled people can communicate using this technology and initiate tasks. Without this aid they would not easily be able to make themselves understood and could be completely dependent on other people. AT can significantly transform the life of an individual by making possible tasks which most people take for granted and by giving independence and freedom.

AT can range from simple changes to a computer keyboard, to much more complex equipment which allows a change in air pressure (when the individual takes a short breath in or out) to operate a switch. It could be a gadget to enable an individual to open a jar, or pick up a pair of socks, or get into the bath. It is also the term used for software that enables speech recognition and voice output.

Figure 26.18 Example of Makaton symbols

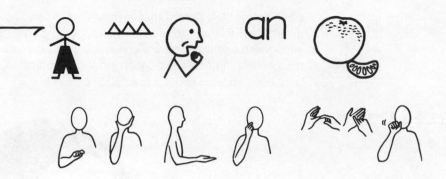

This whole area is set to develop further for a number of reasons. As the population ages many more people will look to AT to help them remain independent and less reliant on other people. AT could be used to assist people with personal care, and this may be advantageous in many ways. Firstly, although AT may have high costs initially, the costs of employing a carer may be considerably more. Also the benefits of relying on a machine rather than a person cannot be underestimated. Everyone uses gadgets every day and there is no negativity or stigma associated with this. The increased use of AT amongst groups of people with disabilities would be easier to accept than perhaps support from someone else. These sorts of systems can utilise the wireless connections and the rapid changes that are taking place in computer development in both hardware and software. Advances in design and technology generally and improvements in the field of electronics mean the potential for AT is huge.

Another significant change in the way support can be offered to individuals is via improvements in environmental controls and communication systems from an individual to the outside world. This has been referred to as 'Telecare' and involves using telecommunication systems to monitor and create a link between an individual and the support systems they may require from time to time. Such systems allow people to live independently but trigger the need for further support should it be required. For example an individual may have a sensor in their home which would alert a service provider that an intervention is required. Even simple things such as the ability to talk to someone on the phone and discuss anxieties can be enough to solve a problem and again avoid the need for further intervention or inappropriate hospitalisation. Telecare includes common systems which many people already make use of, such as a social alarm system, a reminder system, home security, sensors to monitor gas or security breaches.

## Coping strategies

The way individuals cope with disabilities will depend on many factors:

- Was it a sudden change in condition?
- What was their psychological state prior to the onset of the disability?
- Relationship and support of family and friends – studies have shown that support but not over-protection is important and the need to retain similar expectations of the individual.
- Impact on career and educational opportunities.
- Availability of support groups and networks.
- Resources and finances.
- Ability to assert own wants and needs.

### Developing coping strategies

Consistent with the growing strength of the disabled movement there are now many more self-help groups and forums for people with disabilities. Sharing concerns with people who can empathise, not sympathise, can often be very important and can give people a different perspective and reduce feelings of isolation.

www.disabledinfo.co.uk
www.1voice.org.uk

Figure 26.19 Coping strategies

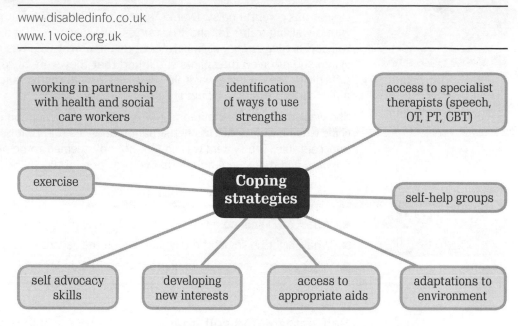

## Self advocacy

This involves an individual speaking up and speaking out in order to make choices about their lives (Ward, 1995). **Self advocacy** is all about choices and influencing the services that are provided. Although a person with a disability may require assistance and support from others, they are still in control of their own life and destiny.

Even people who cannot speak due to the nature of their condition can be "self advocates" but another person may be required to accurately interpret what they say. An ideal spokesperson for an individual who cannot speak might be another person with a similar disability, as they may be in a better position to understand what is being communicated. Self advocacy can be difficult for many people. Some people do not wish to upset people who are delivering care to them and there are risks associated with asserting your own views.

People with disabilities can form service user groups in order to participate and influence the care services that are being offered to them. They can have the most valuable contributions to make when it comes to planning and reviewing services. It seems obvious, but involvement in decision making and policy planning was not considered to be possible for many disable people until relatively recently.

Preparing to become an effective self-advocate:

- Acknowledge the disability.
- Be aware that other issues might affect the ability to be an effective self advocate, such as feeling frustrated, getting angry, low self-esteem.
- Identify needs and plan ahead.
- Know rights and responsibilities.
- Negotiate, make plans, agree decisions
- Obtain support from peers.

**remember**
Learning self advocacy skills can be important and useful, and working as part of a group can definitely help.

Self advocacy groups for people with learning disabilities
www.peoplefirst.org.uk

<table>
<tr><td>

**case study**

**26.6**

</td><td>

## Dolma

Dolma has cerebral palsy. Dolma, uses a wheelchair sometimes and also mobilises with a walking frame for short distances. She was prescribed some orthotic splints to keep her legs and feet in correct body alignment when using her wheelchair. When she received the splints she found that they were uncomfortable and difficult to use, but she was told there was no alternative and she would have to make do and that she would get used to them.

She was so upset she shouted at the person on the reception desk of the orthotic clinic when trying to discuss her situation and was told that her behaviour was unacceptable. The system was so big, nobody seemed to be able to give her any answers and there were no alternative providers of the splints.

</td></tr>
</table>

<table>
<tr><td>

*activity*

**INDIVIDUAL WORK**

</td><td>

- What can Dolma do now?
- What might be some of the limitations on the service?
- What can the service do to improve the situation for her?

</td></tr>
</table>

## Self-esteem and self image

Self-esteem is considered to be of great importance in terms of how people cope with life's challenges. Building self-esteem and a positive self image can require certain steps. It requires self acceptance and self love. The support of others: family, partners, friends is undoubtedly of great importance in terms of self-esteem. Equally, if people are sending a negative message reinforcing what a person can't do, this can damage self-esteem and reduce confidence. It is important for all individuals to take care of themselves, showing themselves respect.

Self-esteem can be damaged by many things, the following are some examples:

- Not having basic needs met adequately.
- Having feelings ignored or denied.
- Being put down or humiliated.
- Feeling views are unimportant.
- Being overprotected.
- Being given a label.
- Being constantly reminded of what is not possible and of limitations.

Self-esteem and self image are often linked together as the view that a person has of themselves will obviously have an impact on their self-esteem. If somebody feels that they do not look good or that other people might think that then they will not feel good about themselves.

It is easy to see that disabled people can experience a lowered self-esteem as they may experience many of the above and there is obviously no quick fix solution. Hopefully the growth of the disabled people's movement will highlight some of these issues at a strategic level, challenging media images and at a personal level accessing support and working on building confidence and self-esteem may help.

### Tips for building confidence and self-esteem

There are many self-help books which give lots of information on how to build self-esteem. Many suggest: avoid generalising that everything will go wrong, change the mindset and look at the situation from another angle. Remember positive situations and feelings and develop assertiveness skills. Other suggestions are:

- Display nice fun photos of yourself.
- Identify strengths.
- Share positive information.
- Try to avoid complaining too much.
- Remember everyone is unique and has their own particular qualities.
- Be kind to yourself.
- Develop interests.

Often simple things can help – positive relationships, meaningful work, friendly greetings. A major boost to self-esteem is often the response of others – for health and social care workers listening to people, giving people time and attention is important, it may boost the self-esteem of the individual and in doing so boost the self-esteem of the worker. This has got to be good for everyone.

Figure 26.20 Developing interests

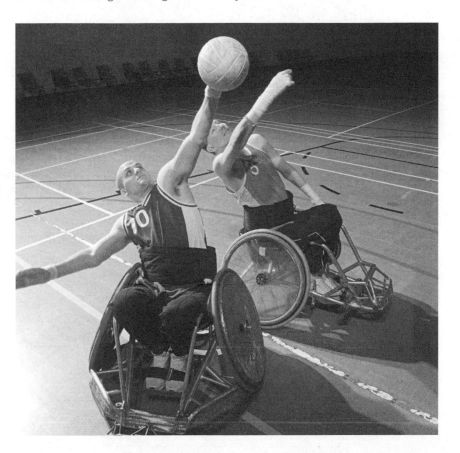

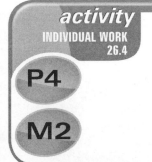

**activity**
INDIVIDUAL WORK
26.4

P4

M2

Thinking about people you have worked with who have additional needs, write down four examples of positive working practice that you have witnessed or that you think would help.

Now describe how these positive working practices play a part in promoting the rights of people with additional needs.

# Current legislation with respect to individuals with additional needs

## Legislation and regulations

In recent years an enormous amount of legislation has been passed which has a significant bearing on health and social care and in particular the rights of individuals who are in receipt of care. Although looking at legislation can be an onerous task that many people avoid as it seems to have limited relevance to day-to-day lives, for health and social care workers it is vital to both be familiar with and adhere to, the crucial pieces of legislation.

### Mental Health Act 1983

Most people who are in the psychiatric unit of a hospital or a mental health unit due to mental health problems are there because they choose to be as in the same way as if they had a physical health problems (they are called informal patients). A small number, approximately 15% (www.mind.org.uk), are there compulsorily – they are referred to as formal patients. The Mental Health Act 1983 allows individuals to be detained without their consent if they have severe mental health problems which they may not recognise in themselves and they are considered to be a danger to themselves and/or the public. The 1986 Mental Health (Northern Ireland) Order fulfills the same function for individuals living in Northern Ireland.

The Mental Health Act 1983 has various sections. Each section provides information and guidance regarding specific situations relating to management of an individual with a significant mental health problem. The term 'sectioned' is used within health and social care settings to describe the procedure for a compulsory admission to a psychiatric unit. As this means that the person will be denied their freedom, this process must be undertaken following stringent rules to ensure mistakes are not made and all actions are taken in the best interests of the individual (and/or other members of the public).

The following are some of the sections of the Mental Health Act 1983:

- Section 1 gives definitions of mental disorder.
- Section 2 describes the situations in which people can be admitted to hospital compulsorily, providing specific timeframes in which assessment must be undertaken.
- Section 3 describes the provisions for admission for treatment, again there are specific guidelines regarding timescales.
- Section 4 is regarding the emergency admissions.
- Section 5 is about the detention of a voluntary patient for a period of assessment.

There are sections which deal with taking people to a place of safety. There are also a number of sections which deal with admission to hospital which is linked to criminal proceedings.

Many people who are in receipt of health and social care may have some degree of mental health problems but the Mental Health Act is not applicable as they are treated voluntarily and are not considered a danger to themselves or others.

The Mental Health Act 1983 is now over 20 years old and there have been many developments in the treatment and the way in which mental health problems are addressed. In order to ensure that it is consistent with other important pieces of legislation which relate to freedom, decision making, the rights of the individual and the general public, a Mental Health Bill has been written to confirm the legal position when complex situations arise. This Bill has caused a great deal of discussion and has only recently been agreed.

## Mental Health Bill

This will make changes to the Mental Health Act of 1983 and to link to the Mental Capacity Act 2005. The main aims of the Mental Health Bill are to simplify and bring up to date the definition of mental disorders and the reasons why individuals should be detained. Supervised community treatment is introduced and also the number of health professionals that might be involved in the care of individuals with mental health problems.

Another important part of this bill is the wish to make sure that people who have conditions which mean they are unable to care for themselves and might put themselves in a situation of danger are protected from being simply 'locked' away in a residential or nursing home setting with no review of their situation and no safeguards in place. Under the Mental Health Act 1983 if a person is detained they have the right to have their case and situation reviewed at regular intervals by a team of health professionals. This is not always the case for people with severe learning disabilities or dementia. It has been recently identified that it is possible for people to be 'locked away' with no means of redress or avenues for appeal. This Bill introduces safeguards to prevent this from occurring, or ensures that when it is necessary to deprive someone of their liberty due to the severity of their condition, guidelines are followed. These changes are very significant for hospitals and many residential or nursing homes, as units are often locked for health, safety and security reasons. If this is the case then each individual who is unable to leave (and therefore deprived of their liberty) will require a review of their situation and authorisation must be given to make sure that the restrictions are reasonable and it is in their best interests that they do not wander out of the building unsupervised.

## Mental Capacity Act 2005

This is a recent Act concerning the ability of individuals to make decisions about their lives.

In any single day people constantly make decisions, some are easy and straightforward, some can be quite difficult.

Identify an easy decision that you have recently made – I am going to the cinema.

Identify a difficult decision that you have recently made – I am leaving my partner.

Have you ever made a bad decision? Most of us have, even if it didn't really matter (choosing the wrong thing from a menu, not taking an umbrella).

Some people, due to the nature of their condition, for example dementia, traumatic brain injury, learning disability, may not be able to make decisions for themselves or may be making extremely dangerous decisions which could result in serious harm. This act provides a legal framework through which these situations can be dealt with and people who do not have the mental capacity to make decisions will be supported. This can include independent advocates and a court of protection if necessary. One of the major themes of this act is that wherever possible the individual themselves should be supported to make decisions. The emphasis is on promoting mental capacity, not jumping to conclusions that people have no influence over their lives once they develop a certain condition.

The five key principles of the Mental Capacity Act are:

1. People have the right to make their own decisions – inability to make decisions has to be proven.

2. People should be supported to make their own decisions.

3. People can make what might seem eccentric or unwise decisions.

4. Any decisions made for a person who does not have the mental capacity to make their decisions must be done in their best interests.

5. Any decisions made for a person who does not have capacity should be the least restrictive of rights and freedom.

## Disability Discrimination Act 1995 (DDA)

The Disability Discrimination Act 1995 was a major landmark piece of legislation that impacted on the lives of people with additional needs. This law replaced the Disabled Persons (Services, Consultation and Representation) Act 1986. The name itself clearly indicates what this Act is all about. There has been acceptance that people with disabilities do face discrimination, whether intentional or unintentional.

The Disability Discrimination Act was passed in 1995, and the aim of the Act was to end the discrimination that many disabled people experience. This act makes it illegal to discriminate against people with disabilities in relation to their employment, in shops or similar services for example restaurants and also in the buying or renting of a property.

Within the Disability Discrimination Act 1995 a disability is defined as 'a physical or mental impairment which has a substantial and long-term adverse effect on a person's ability to carry out normal day-to-day activities.'

Initially there was concern that the Act did not go far enough. Since that time the Act has been developed further with the passing of the following:

- Disability Rights Commission Act 1999.
- Special Educational Needs and Disability Act 2001.
- Disability Discrimination Act 2005.

The significant change is that mental illness is considered in the same way as all other mental and physical impairments. Also, progressive diseases are covered by the Disability Discrimination Act 2005 from the point of diagnosis and not just when the disease starts to have an impact on an individual's life.

Disabled people's rights are further protected in the areas of:

- employment
- education
- access to goods, facilities and services
- buying or renting land or property, including making it easier for disabled people to rent property and for tenants to make disability-related adaptations.

The Act now requires public bodies to actively promote equality of opportunity for disabled people. It also allows the Government to set minimum standards so that disabled people can use public transport easily.

### *Access to care services*

Most people would be surprised and shocked to find out that people with disabilities often find that they are disadvantaged when they visit hospitals and other care services. It seems contradictory that the place where health care is delivered is one of the places in which individuals can experience discrimination. In many cases the life expectancy of people who have a disability can be shorter due to a failure to access services or get the best out of the health service, rather than the underlying condition, which has caused the disability. The amendment of the DDA should address this point and ensure that people with disabilities can access health care in the same way as the rest of the population.

As part of the DDA 2005, a Disability Equality Duty has been introduced – this means that public sector organisations such as the NHS have a responsibility to ensure that there is equality for people with disabilities. Practical steps must be taken to stop discrimination. This may include some physical changes to the building or set-up of various clinics but also and usually most importantly, attitudinal changes. All staff must examine the services that they offer to people with disabilities and challenge the current practice if they feel there are any inequalities.

**Advice for hospitals and health professionals**

Do not focus on the disability – significant symptoms could be missed and serious illnesses not diagnosed. Take action quickly if concerned.

How to communicate – family, friends, carers, modified sign language (makaton), pictures, symbols. Get the input from carers or significant others as they may know the signs of distress.

Act in the individuals best interests and consistent with their wishes. The law relating to Mental Capacity is now in place.

Do not assume that a person has a poor quality of life due to their learning disability or other disabilities.

Obtain help from other social care and health services.

The Disability Discrimination Act requires that reasonable adjustments are made, this includes the way in which health services are offered to people.

Source: Adapted from www.mencap.org.uk/html/campaigns/deathbyindifference/goodpractice.asp

This Disability Equality Duty is very significant for the NHS as both a deliverer of services to the public and also as an employer. It should ensure that all individuals, especially people with learning disabilities, are getting full access to health services.

Key themes from the Disability Equality Duty include:

■ Eliminating unlawful disability discrimination and disability-related harassment.

■ Promoting equality of opportunity for disabled people, taking account of their disabilities.

■ Promoting positive attitudes towards disabled people.

■ Encouraging disabled people to take part in public life.

It does seem strange that people should encounter barriers when they are trying to access health care but this is the reality for many people.

There has been criticism of this act from disabled people's movement because it is not as strong a piece of legislation as they hoped it would be. Statistics show that it has had a minimal impact on the employment of disabled people. The fact that organisations can take cost into consideration when making reasonable adjustments provides a loop hole and they can argue that the cost is prohibitive and therefore the disabled person cannot be employed. There is also concern that the term 'reasonable adjustments' is just too subjective and open to interpretation.

## The Children Act 1989

This act promotes the rights of the child and puts the needs of the child first. Children have rights, views and opinions and they should be listened to. The Act states that children are ideally brought up in a family situation and they should not be removed from this situation unless there is a risk of danger or harm. This act changed the way that services for children were delivered by placing greater emphasis on the wants and needs of the child and the importance of preserving family structures if at all possible.

## The Children Act 2004

This Act builds on the earlier Act. A new Children's Commissioner has been established to promote the interests of the child. It advocates that local authorities should work together to support the following key aims for children:

■ Being healthy.

■ Being safe.

■ Being happy and realising own goals.

- Being involved and contributing.
- Financial security.

## Care Standards Act 2000

This Act introduced regulations for social care and independent health care services, (residential and nursing homes). Many of the changes introduced by this piece of legislation have been discussed earlier in this chapter. The Commission for Social Care Inspection (CSCI) was established as part of this Act. Social Care Councils have now been created across the UK along with a Code of Practice for social care workers. This act means that it is no longer possible for care homes to be unregulated and unmonitored. This should safeguard the individuals who live there. This Act is broad in its remit and covers the delivery of care in a range of settings. The aim is to ensure that care, wherever it is delivered, can be regulated and national minimum standards will be in place.

## Nursing and Residential Care Homes Regulations 1984 (amended 2002)

By April 2002, the Care Standards Act 2000 replaced the Registered Homes Act 1984.

See Unit 28, pages 264–275 on the role of the care worker in supporting older people, and legislation and regulations.

## Data Protection Act 1998

The original Data Protection Act was passed in 1984.

This Act gives individuals rights in relation to personal information about the individual. No personal data can be held unless there is an appropriate registration with the Data Protection Registrar. Individuals can find out what personal data is being held about them. Incorrect data can be corrected or removed from the computer system and they can be compensated if the data is inaccurate. For health and social care staff the important points to note are that they can be held responsible for maintaining the confidentiality of the data which they handle. If organisations hold personal data then they have to register with the registrar indicating what type of data is being held, who has access and how security is maintained.

This Act has eight data protection principles:

1. All information must be processed and handled according to this law.
2. It should be used for the purpose for which it was asked for.
3. The information should be accurate and just enough to meet the requirements for which it is being asked for.
4. It should be accurate and up-to-date.
5. It should not be kept for longer than it is needed.
6. Information should be processed and handled following the rights of individuals under this Act.
7. The information should be safe and secure and protected.
8. The information will not be transferred to another country unless the safety of the data can be guaranteed and the rights of the individual concerned will be protected.

The post of Information Commissioner was introduced as part of this Act. The role of the Commissioner is to make sure the Act is followed and to respond with advice should the situation arise. In any day in health and social care there is an enormous amount of information regarding individuals being obtained, reviewed and stored. This information should be protected and only shared on a need-to-know basis by the health and social care team involved in an individual's case and/or with the person's permission.

It is in everyone's interests to follow the data handling principles and ensure that confidentiality of information is respected as it protects both individuals in receipt of care and the staff who are supporting them

Core Services Improvement Partnership – Valuing People
www.valuingpeople.gov.uk

## The Department of Health White Paper 'Valuing People: A New Strategy for Learning Disability for the 21st Century', 2001

This document outlines how the Government intends to support people with learning disabilities, ensuring that they have the same rights and choices and access to resources as other individuals living in the UK. Input from people with learning disabilities, families, carers and people who work in this area is included in this document. The background to this paper acknowledges that people with learning disabilities are not given the same choices and opportunities as other people. They often do not have the means to express opinions and they have little if any choice over their lifestyle. Raising the general public's awareness of issues that people with learning disabilities may face and promoting integration of individuals into their local community are key objectives of this paper.

This document identifies the need for health action plans to be developed for all individuals with learning disabilities. Concerns were raised that the general health needs of individuals with learning disabilties are overlooked. People with a learning disability are far less likely to access health care screening programmes and participate in health promotion initiatives, this could contribute to poor health. Often when people with a learning disability have contact with the health service their learning disability may be viewed as the most significant factor and they may not be offered the same treatment as another member of the public. Individuals with learning disabilities are more likely to develop chronic health problems and to experience mental health problems. People with learning disabilities are more likely to have a vision impairment and many are reported to have a hearing impairment. According to research they are 58 times more likely to die before the age of 50 than the general population (DRC, 2006).

This report has triggered some major changes in the way people approach the area of learning disabilities. The need for people with learning difficulties to be involved in services they use and the strategies that are being developed to support them was identified – the motto is: 'nothing about us without us'.

In addition to being more influential in determining the delivery of services for people with learning disabilities, individuals are also encouraged to be actively involved in planning their own care and their futures. Another important point that has been highlighted is the availability of accessible information. Information is now being made available in a variety of formats. Fifteen years ago an assumption would be made that it wouldn't be necessary to produce information in an easy-to-read format because people with learning disabilities would not understand it. As with the population generally, there is a huge range of reading and comprehension abilities within a group of individuals who have learning disabilities.

Easyinfo – making information easier for people with learning difficulties
www.easyinfo.org.uk

## Human Rights Act 1998

This Act brings the rights and freedoms in the European Convention on Human Rights (Convention rights) into UK law.

The Act consists of a series of articles which state the rights that can be expected for all human beings in the UK. The introduction of this Act was seen as an opportunity to raise awareness that all people have the same rights. This is very important for people with disabilities as this was often not the case and they could be excluded from services provided to all other citizens. This Act is applicable to public authorities, in other words most health and social care settings would come under its remit.

### Article 2, the right to life.
This would not allow decisions to be made about an individual's treatment to be restricted because they had a disability. It should result in a more equitable allocation of resources within the health service. People could challenge a decision not to treat a disabled person due to their impairment (disability).

### Article 3, the right to protection against inhuman or degrading treatment.
The lack of respect and potential for humiliating treatment for people with disabilities can be addressed via this article.

### Article 5, provides for the right to liberty.
There is now provision to challenge an inappropriate restriction of freedom that might be imposed upon individuals with certain disabilities.

### Article 8, protects the right to private and family life, and Article 12, the right to marry and establish a family.
These articles are vitally important for disabled people as they strengthen the case for independent living and real choices over contraception and having a family.

### Article 10, guarantees freedom of expression
This may help disabled groups and also improve access to information.

### Article 14, prohibits discrimination against people, including disabled people, accessing services

See Unit 28, Understand the role of the care worker in supporting older people, Legislation and regulations.

## Carers and Disabled Children Act 2000

There is so much work undertaken by carers and often this is not acknowledged. A carer might prioritise the needs of the person they are caring for and not have much time left for themselves. Following consultation with carers it emerged that carers needed the ability to take a break once in a while knowing that the person who requires care will be cared for properly. This Act allows carers to be assessed for their own needs and grants powers to local councils to support carers.

A system has been introduced which involves vouchers being given to carers, putting them in the position of being able to organise a break which suits them and the person they are caring for. An alternative carer can be arranged more flexibly to allow the primary carer to have a rest without the worry of inappropriate care being given.

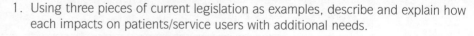

*activity*
**INDIVIDUAL WORK**
**26.5**

**P5**
**D2**
**M3**

1. Using three pieces of current legislation as examples, describe and explain how each impacts on patients/service users with additional needs.
2. Explain how each example may have an impact on promoting the rights of these people.

## European Convention on Human Rights and Fundamental Freedoms 1950; The Convention on the Rights of the Child 1989

The conventions of Human Rights and Rights of the Child state that human rights and freedoms that individuals expect are to be cherished, valued and protected. To live freely is the right of all the citizens of the countries that agreed the conventions. The rights of the child were highlighted and it was made clear that children require special care and protection. This affirmation of the importance of human rights is of great significance for disabled individuals of all ages as they may potentially be at risk of a denial of their human rights and fundamental freedoms that the remainder of the population may be able to take for granted.

**Link**

See unit 28, Understand the role of the care worker in supporting older people; legislation and regulations.

---

*Progress Check*

1. Compare the medical model and the social model of disability.
2. What is the social model definition of disability and impairment?
3. What does the term 'learning disability' mean?
4. What difficulties may a person with learning disabilities experience?
5. Give two examples of disabling conditions, identify causes of each condition and the potential problems that the individual could experience.
6. Explain the role of the Commission for Social Care Inspection (CSCI)?
7. Identify three examples of how the environment can pose barriers for disabled people.
8. What strategies could a health and social care worker use to support an individual coming to terms with a disability?
9. Is becoming an 'Expert Patient' a good idea? Explain you answer.
10. How can the Disability Discrimination Act support a disabled person who has been refused employment because the building might not be suitable?

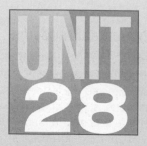

# Caring for Older People

## This unit covers:

- The ageing process
- The role of the care worker in supporting older people

People are living longer than they ever have before and the number of old people is growing fast. Nearly a third of people in Britain are aged over 50 and although some struggle, many enjoy an active and healthy life. This unit gives you an opportunity to explore and challenge ideas and stereotypical attitudes to ageing, to learn about and evaluate various theories of ageing, to understand why people are living longer and to investigate some of the more common physiological disorders associated with increasing age. It also gives you an opportunity to look at the role of care workers in promoting quality of life, choice and independence for older people, and to understand the issues presented as life draws to a close.

## grading criteria

| To achieve a **Pass** grade the evidence must show that the learner is able to: | To achieve a **Merit** grade the evidence must show that, in addition to the pass criteria, the learner is able to: | To achieve a **Distinction** grade the evidence must show that, in addition to the pass and merit criteria, the learner is able to: |
|---|---|---|
| **P1** describe the meaning of the term 'older people'. Pg 245 | **M1** explain why there are difficulties in defining the term 'older people'. Pg 245 | |
| **P2** describe one sociological/ psychological and one biological theory of ageing. Pg 248 | **M2** compare two theories of ageing. Pg 248 | **D1** use examples to evaluate the two theories of ageing. Pg 248 |
| **P3** explain potential effects of changes in demography on the older person. Pg 252 | | |
| **P4** describe potential influences on ageing. Pg 259 | **M3** explain potential influences on ageing. Pg 259 | |

**grading criteria**

| To achieve a **Pass** grade the evidence must show that the learner is able to: | To achieve a **Merit** grade the evidence must show that, in addition to the pass criteria, the learner is able to: | To achieve a **Distinction** grade the evidence must show that, in addition to the pass and merit criteria, the learner is able to: |
|---|---|---|
| **P5** describe the role of the care worker in supporting older people. Pg 266 | **M4** explain potential dilemmas for the care worker in supporting of older people. Pg 266 | **D2** use examples to evaluate the role of the care worker in supporting older people. Pg 266 |
| **P6** describe two aspects of quality and choice at the end of life. Pg 270 | **M5** analyse two aspects of quality and choice at the end of life. Pg 270 | |

# The ageing process

Ageing is brought about by **biological**, **sociological** and **psychological** changes that reduce an individual's life expectancy and ability to use their physical, social and intellectual skills; and increase their vulnerability to physical and mental ill health and disability, social isolation and so on.

## Attitudes

An attitude is an idea or feeling about someone or something. Attitudes can be positive and useful, for example the feelings most of us have towards babies and small children motivate us to care for them and protect them from danger. Similarly, most of us recognise that young people are our future, therefore we are prepared to invest time, money and effort into bringing them up and giving them an education.

Some attitudes are negative and destructive. How do you feel about the following ideas?

- A woman's place is in the kitchen.
- Men should not be allowed to work with small children.
- School children are a nuisance and should be banned from shops.
- Elderly and disabled people are a drain on health and social care services.
- Immigrants should not be allowed to live and work in our country.

Do you agree with any of them? Or do you think that such attitudes are negative and could cause offence to the people concerned? In addition to causing offence, if we allow negative attitudes to affect the way we behave, we act in a discriminatory way, which is illegal. For example, it would be sexist to refuse women the chance of a career and men the opportunity to be employed in what is traditionally seen as 'women's work'; it would be ageist to deny school children and elderly people access to services; it would be disablist to deny people who are disabled the right to use services; and it would be racist to prevent immigration other than for legal reasons.

 **Link**

You looked at discrimination in Unit 2 in Health and Social Care Book 1, and will revisit ageism shortly.

Many people have a negative attitude to ageing, which demonstrates a lack of respect for older people. Most negative attitudes toward older people relate to their characters and to their declining skills and abilities, for example their:

- intellectual skills, such as communicating, learning new things, thinking and reasoning
- social skills, such as interacting appropriately and maintaining relationships
- physical abilities, such as getting about and being independent
- ability to maintain their personal hygiene and appearance, such as dressing, washing, shaving, cleaning their clothes and using the toilet.

Our attitudes toward ageing and older people are implanted in us from a very early age. However, whilst ageing is to do with the body weakening and slowing down, it is important to remember that there is still a person inside the body who has an **identity**, a history and a wealth of knowledge, understanding, skills, experiences and wisdom.

Figure 28.1 Negative attitudes associated with ageing

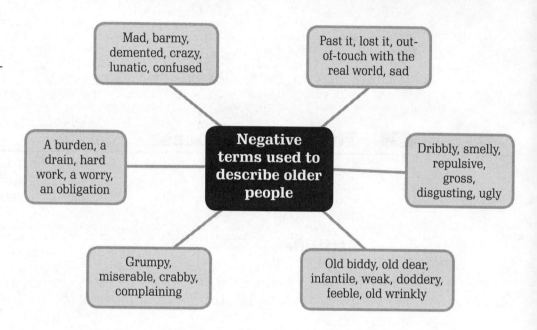

It is important that we develop a positive attitude to ageing and older people. Like Lena in the case study, the majority of older people lead relatively active lives and are as intelligent and good company as anyone else. For example:

- Today's average 70 year old is as fit as someone aged 60 a hundred years ago.
- Many people in their 70s and older are as capable of learning new skills as people in their 30s.
- Modern medicine and care means that people are growing older in better health and with a better quality of life than ever before.

Having a positive attitude to ageing shows that we appreciate older people as individuals and recognise the importance of their knowledge, skills, experiences and wisdom. It also allows us to be positive and realistic in the way we prepare for and approach our own old age.

The BBC website
www.bbc.co.uk
Age Concern, Cheshire
www.ageconcerneastcheshire.co.uk

## case study 28.1 — Lena

'I didn't realise what being old would be like when I was a young woman. But since I got into my seventies, things have really changed for me. For example, I have difficulty opening cans and bottles and things and getting dressed because of the arthritis but I've bought some special gadgets and they're very helpful.

My main worry at the moment is the toilet, you know, being caught out. However, I'll have to meet that problem when it comes; worrying doesn't help, I guess. A number of my friends have that problem and they'll be able to advise me what to do.

I can't walk so far these days because I get tired more quickly so it's usually just down to the shops and back a couple or three times a week. It can be frustrating and it takes me a long time but then I do stop to chat with lots of people, something I never used to have time for!

My memory plays tricks on me, for example I have problems remembering people's names but fortunately most of my friends are in the same boat so we just laugh about it and make names up! Actually, spending time with friends keeps me quite sharp. We laugh about the good old days, discuss what's going on in the world at the moment and we're learning to use the computer, slowly but surely! We're all widowed but some of us have families, all grown up and gone of course, and we all had jobs so you get some interesting things to talk about. When we're together I feel like I'm 21 again, not an old person at all!'

### activity
**GROUP WORK**

1. Identify the factors in Lena's life that are associated with her advancing years. How could these factors affect the way she may be described by someone who has a negative attitude to ageing?

2. Discuss the factors in Lena's life about which she speaks positively.

3. Discuss how you could use Lena's positive attitude to help someone who has a negative attitude toward ageing and older people.

4. Discuss how you could use her positive attitude to help someone who is worried about their:
   - declining intellectual skills
   - declining physical abilities
   - declining ability to maintain their personal hygiene and appearance.

## Stereotyping

Look at the negative terms used to describe older people that were mentioned earlier. Some of them may apply to one or two of the older people you know! However, it would be an overstatement to say that each term applies to all older people, in the same way that it would be an overstatement to say that all young people are binge drinkers and all middle aged people are looking forward to retirement. Grouping people together on the assumption that they share a characteristic is known as stereotyping. Stereotypical images of older people, for example that they are all confused, are damaging because they fail to present them as individuals. And denying people their individuality excludes them from playing a role in society for which they may be just as capable as younger people.

When working with older people care workers must:

■ have a positive attitude toward ageing

■ respect and promote the older people's individuality.

Many stereotypical images of older people present them as grumpy, frail, incontinent and, at best, demented. As you read earlier, ageing is brought about by biological, sociological and psychological changes (you will read about these shortly). However, the fact that we are all individuals means that changes affect us in different ways. It follows that any age-associated decline in ability and skills and increase in vulnerability affects different individuals at different times and to different degrees. Stereotypical images of older people that present them as vulnerable and lacking skills and abilities reinforce the idea that, for example, they are all incapacitated, have lost their independence and are a burden on society.

Our chronological age is related to our date of birth and the authorities use it to dictate when we can, for example, start school, buy tobacco, drive a car, get married, and, until recently, retire – women were deemed old enough to retire when they reached age 60 and men when they were 65. 'Old old' and 'oldest old' are terms often used to refer to people aged 75 plus and 85 plus respectively. Chronological age is the basis for the expression 'Act your age' but it takes no account of the way we feel. We all have days when we 'feel our age'; we also all have days when we feel on top of the world and, like Lena in the case study, much younger than our chronological age! Stereotypical images of older people that present them as tired and feeble reinforce the idea that they have no energy and persuade others into thinking that they are 'past their best' and no longer have any value.

Figure 28.2 Challenging the stereotypes

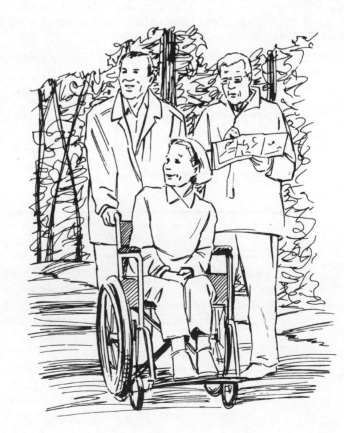

According to research on ageing:

- people in more affluent countries have a more positive view of old age compared with those in developing countries who see old age as a time for rest and relaxation and being looked after by their children

- old age is a stage of life, not something that just happens when someone retires or has their 60th, 65th or even 80th birthday. We are as old as we feel and whilst one person may feel 'old' at 60, someone in their 80s may feel quite youthful

- many people want to carry on working for as long as they are able to do their jobs well and not be forced to retire because of age-based restrictions

- younger people have different ideas about what makes for old age than the older generation, for example in one American survey, people aged between 18 and 24 thought someone was old at 58, while people aged 65 or older considered 75 to be old.

Although in general, attitudes to ageing and to older people are very positive, there are some interesting cultural differences to ageing.

Table 28.1 Cultural differences to ageing

| Country | Attitudes to ageing |
| --- | --- |
| Canada | Old age is a time for new opportunities and challenges, achieving ambitions and building close relationships with family and friends. Canadians have very positive attitudes to ageing and older people. |
| China | Old age begins at 50 and is a time for relaxing and accessing support from the family. There are mixed attitudes to older people, some negative, e.g. older people have too much time on their hands and some positive, e.g. older people are full of wisdom. |
| France | Old age is a time for staying young at heart, keeping the mind sharp and staying healthy, but whilst the French think that older people deserve respect, they worry about being a burden to their families when they are old. |
| India | Old age begins when a person's children get married or their grandchildren are born and is a time to live with and be cared for and supported by the family. Many Indians think that older people are full of wisdom and deserve respect; very few think they are a burden to society. |
| Japan | Old age is a time for good health, self-reliance and fulfilment through working. There are mixed views about older people – some Japanese think that older people are full of wisdom, deserve respect and are interesting to be around but a few also think they are a burden to society. |
| UK | Old age is a time for being independent and for becoming more active in the community, through part-time or voluntary work. Some think that older people deserve respect but others think that they spend too much time living in the past. Many think that older people are interesting to be around. |
| USA | Old age is a time for a new career, spiritual fulfilment and independence from the family. Americans have a very positive attitude to ageing and older people. |

HSBC Global Forum on Ageing and Retirement
www.ageingforum.org

## Ageism

You read earlier that discrimination occurs when people allow their negative attitudes to affect the way they behave towards others. Ageism is a form of discrimination. It happens when people are treated unfairly because of their age. Discrimination against older people is the most practiced from of discrimination and exists in many walks of life, for example:

- in the workplace, where they are harassed and bullied on the basis of their age; where the working environment prevents them from working to the best of their ability; and where the chances of being recruited for a job, promoted or trained are limited because of negative attitudes held about their skills and abilities. The Age Discrimination Act 2006 bans unfair treatment at work on the grounds of age. You will read more about this piece of legislation shortly.

- in their own homes or in care homes, where they are bullied, abused or neglected by carers and care workers.

- in education, where they are not given opportunities to learn or the support and encouragement to do well because it's assumed that their age affects their ability to learn. As you know, many people in their 70s and older are as capable of learning new skills as people in their 30s.

  'In youth we learn, in old age we understand.' Mexican proverb.

- in housing, where poorly designed, maintained and secured accommodation makes it difficult for them to carry out everyday living activities and puts their health, safety and security at risk.

- in the community, due to people's intolerance of their behaviour and lifestyles; where older people's opinions are disregarded or not asked for because they're considered to be 'past it', to 'have one foot in the grave'; and so on.

- in buying goods and services, for example where they are treated with impatience, ignored or not given appropriate help to see and choose goods, complete an order form or write a cheque; where they are refused insurance or access to a new credit card on the basis of their age; where they are exploited and persuaded into making unwanted purchases; and so on.

- in using health and social care services. The attitudes of health and social care staff affect the way older people are treated. For example, in the past the care of older people was not a priority and many were not resuscitated if they fell into a coma; many older people report that they are given second-class treatment, simply because they are not in a strong enough position to speak out and be heard; and inappropriate and unkind comments are made.

Figure 28.3  Ageism

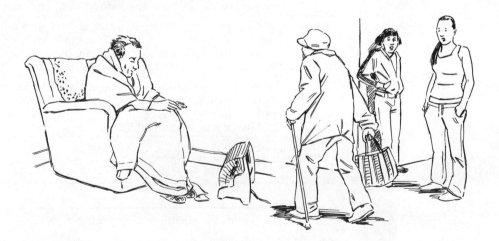

Ageism has tragic effects on older people. Bullying, harassment and exploitation cause a loss of self-confidence and self-worth and as a result, they become isolated, lonely and fearful of others. Unfair, unjust treatment that denies equal opportunities prevents them developing skills, finding employment and accessing services, which in turn leads to poverty, poor nutrition, poor housing and an unsafe living environment. Older people living like this have few chances of maintaining good health and wellbeing, and are deprived of any quality of life.

Age Concern
www.ageconcern.org.uk
Help the Aged
www.helptheaged.org.uk/
The BBC website
www.bbc.co.uk
Dept of Work and Pensions
www.dwp.gov.uk

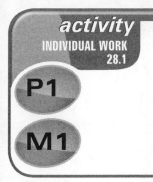

**activity**

**INDIVIDUAL WORK 28.1**

**P1**

**M1**

Interview a number of people from the range of age groups (children, adolescents, adults, older people) and from different cultural backgrounds in order to explore the meaning of the term 'older people' and explain why there are difficulties in defining it. Use your findings to write a report for the journal 'Working with Older People'.

## Theories of ageing

There are a number of theories that seek to explain the biological, sociological and psychological changes that cause an individual to age.

**Link**

Unit 4 in Health and Social Care Book 1 (Development Through the Life Stages) gives additional detail about theories of and changes associated with ageing.

### Disengagement theory

The disengagement theory suggests that older people make a positive effort to withdraw from their social life as a preparation for death. By doing so, they extricate themselves from their roles, for example of employee, father, church-goer; they restrict their social contacts, for example they stop spending time with friends and family; and they give up their traditional, normal ways of behaving, becoming gradually less and less sociable in the way they behave.

Society seems to facilitate older people withdrawing from life. For example, retirement and care homes cut them off from being active in the world of work and their community. And by conditioning younger people to take on their responsibilities and to fill the gaps provided by their withdrawal from society, it ensures a smooth transfer of power from one generation to the next. However, cutting older people off from society and removing their powers can be demoralising and reduce their self-esteem and self-confidence. Thus the disengagement theory is both a sociological and a psychological theory.

### Activity theory

The activity theory has a more optimistic view of ageing than the disengagement theory. It suggests that being involved with family, friends, neighbours, colleagues, etc. is positively linked with personal satisfaction and that the more social contacts, activities and positive attitudes an individual has, the better their quality of life.

As people become older, their social networks diminish and they have to give up certain activities. This can be frustrating, depressing and disheartening, and lead to social isolation and loneliness. To preserve a positive attitude and to compensate for the changes, the activity theory suggests that older people must have the opportunity of retaining and adding to their social networks and trying out and engaging in alternative activities that give them fulfilment and a sense of achievement. Like the disengagement theory, the activity theory is both a sociological and a psychological theory.

Figure 28.4 Staying active and preserving social networks

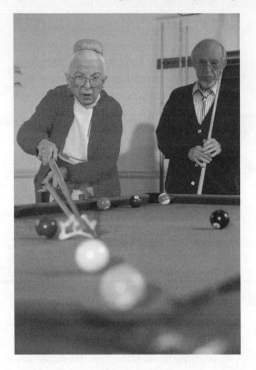

## Social creation of dependency

The social creation of dependency suggests that discriminating social policies, such as age-restricted retirement policies and opportunities to participate in the community, and poverty caused by low pension and income levels cause older people to become dependent on society.

The effect of these social policies is to single out and isolate older people. As a result, they feel stigmatised and stand out as being vulnerable and helpless, signalling a stereotypical image of being useless and inadequate. They then become the focus of negative attitudes, which in turn cause them to act in the way they think they are expected, i.e. they become increasingly dependent on family, friends, social care services and so on. Like the disengagement and activity theories, the social creation of dependency theory is both a sociological and a psychological theory.

## Genetically programmed theory

The genetically programmed theory is a biological theory that suggests that ageing is the result of the programming of **genes** to destroy cells after a given span of time or life. Different living organisms have different life spans but they each have a characteristic life span that is determined by their genetic programme. The genetically programmed theory predicts that organisms are programmed to die.

In addition to being genetically programmed, there are suggestions that ageing is also under the control of the nervous and endocrine systems.

## Disposable soma theory

The disposable soma theory is another biological theory. Unlike the genetically programmed theory, it predicts that organisms are programmed to live because of the body's ability to protect, maintain and repair **somatic cells** throughout the normal life span. However, if somatic cells deteriorate or become damaged, for example through mutations to their DNA, or when they are not maintained and repaired, tissues and organs become impaired, which brings about the characteristics of ageing.

The disposable soma theory suggests that cell damage and lack of cell maintenance is due to a lack of resources that the body needs for metabolism (the processes that occur within the body to maintain life), for example nutrients and energy. In other words, our lifestyle – the food we eat, the exercise we take – plays an important role in the ageing process.

You can read about metabolism in Unit 21.

## Gender differences

**Gender** issues, particularly those relating to being female, are also used to explain the ageing process. As opposed to sex, which is to do with being male or female, gender is to do with femininity and masculinity, both of which are defined by the social or cultural group in which we live. In other words, femininity and masculinity are **socially constructed concepts** and what makes for femininity and masculinity varies between different cultures.

Figure 28.5 'It's nice when workmen say "Good morning, mum", but it was nicer when they whistled.' Pam Brown, writer and poet

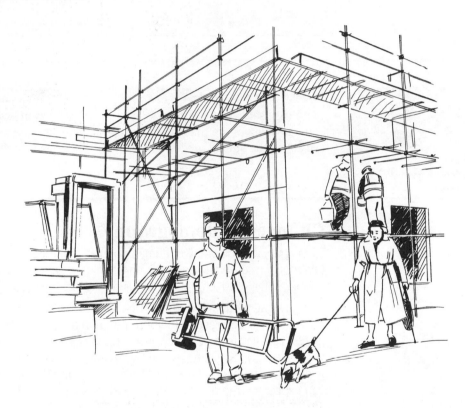

The female primary and secondary sexual characteristics diminish as women age, for example breasts and vagina shrivel and pubic hair is lost. In addition, masculine traits develop, for example voices may deepen, the clitoris enlarges, there is a growth of facial hair and head hair can become scant. This loss of socially constructed femininity and increase in socially constructed masculinity paints a picture of a genderless old woman, devoid of any physical attraction. As a result, older women are ignored and dismissed as obsolete despite their continuing ability and need to give and receive love and affection and to enjoy an active sexual life.

Many older women claim that they have become invisible and powerless because they have had to step aside for the slimmer, more attractive and desirable younger woman – despite female emancipation, society continues to judge women by their appearance. These women are forced by society into the category of 'old' and are the butt of jokes and stories about fat, ugly, obsolete older women, despite not feeling old but full of life, wisdom and ability.

*activity*

**INDIVIDUAL WORK
28.2**

**P2**

**M2**

Complete the following table to show your understanding of two different theories of ageing.

| Theories of ageing | Similarities | Differences |
|---|---|---|
| **Biological theory**<br>Name:<br>Description (P2 part): | | |
| **Sociological/psychological theory**<br>Name:<br>Description (P2 part): | | |

*activity*

**INDIVIDUAL WORK
28.3**

**D1**

Write case studies of two older people who you know in which you apply your understanding of the theories of ageing and evaluate the usefulness of each in explaining the ageing process. Remember to maintain confidentiality.

## Changes in demography

Demography is the study of human populations using statistics relating to births, deaths, health and disease and so on. Changes in demography have far-reaching effects on people, some of which this section aims to introduce you to.

Over the twentieth and into the twenty-first centuries, the population in the UK has aged due to a decrease in the birth rate and an increase in life expectancy. For example, in 1981, male life expectancy at age 65 was 14 years; it is predicted to increase to 22 years by 2051. Similarly, female life expectancy in 1981 at age 65 was 18 years and is predicted to increase to 24 years by 2051. In other words, in 2051, males aged 65 can expect to live until they are 87 and females aged 65 until they are 89. (*Population Trends 2005*).

Because of the drop in birth rate and therefore reduction in size of the working population, and because of the growth in numbers of older people, we can expect an increasing financial and **human resource** strain on the provision of, for example:

■ pensions, which are likely to decrease due to the need to pay more people for longer periods of time. This could affect the financial situation of many older people and consequently their ability to pay for basic needs such as nutritious food, fuel for cooking, warmth and hot water, telephone bills, and the maintenance of, for example, their homes and gardens and their appearance and personal hygiene.

■ health and social care, including nursing care, residential care, day care and domiciliary care (care at home). The older people become, the more they need and become dependent on health and social care. Strained resources along with a continuing increase in demand for services could therefore impact negatively on their health and wellbeing.

■ housing, for example residential homes, sheltered and adapted housing. A lack in provision could impact on older people with a range of physical needs such as movement, mobility and sensory needs; and socio-emotional needs, such as the need for relationships and interaction with others and the need to remain independent.

■ public transport, which could affect the quality of life for older people who do not have access to or are no longer able to use their own transport. Restrictions on the provision of public transport could also restrict older people's independence and ability to travel, go shopping, visit their GP, friends and family, and so on.

Figure 28.6 Demographic statistics and predictions for the UK

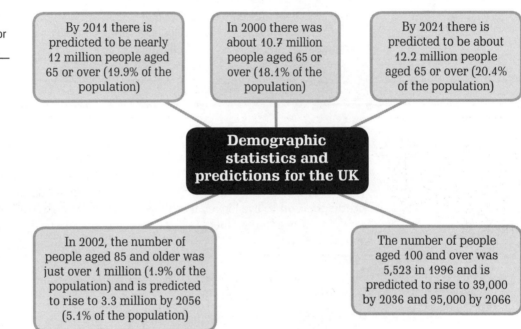

By 2011 there is predicted to be nearly 12 million people aged 65 or over (19.9% of the population)

In 2000 there was about 10.7 million people aged 65 or over (18.1% of the population)

By 2021 there is predicted to be about 12.2 million people aged 65 or over (20.4% of the population)

**Demographic statistics and predictions for the UK**

In 2002, the number of people aged 85 and older was just over 1 million (1.9% of the population) and is predicted to rise to 3.3 million by 2056 (5.1% of the population)

The number of people aged 100 and over was 5,523 in 1996 and is predicted to rise to 39,000 by 2036 and 95,000 by 2066

Family patterns have also changed quite dramatically over the last few generations. More and more people are choosing to live alone and changes in employment practices such as working away from home, and increased choice regarding where to live mean that family members are often spread around the country, if not the globe. In addition, a rise in the divorce rate, improved opportunities for women to work outside of the home and the decisions of both couples and singletons to delay having children mean that families are growing smaller.

The consequence of changing family patterns and smaller families is that the number of family members with whom older people have contact and on whom they can depend on for help, care and support has become much smaller. As a result, many become very lonely and socially isolated and others have to move into care homes.

## case study 28.2 · Yourtown District Council

Statistics collected by Yourtown District Council reveal that the number of older residents is likely to rise by 30% over the next two years. A service provision planning meeting has been convened between representatives of the Health and Social Services and Housing Departments, as well as from the local transport authority, which is heavily subsidised by Council Tax. Apart from increasing local taxes and the receipt of Central Government grants that reflect the rate of inflation, the council has no other means of raising its income.

### activity
**GROUP WORK**

In your group:

1. Discuss how council funds could be re-apportioned to take account of the needs of the growing number of older people. Assume that any increases in funding will be minimal and think in terms of priorities.

2. Discuss how the re-apportionment of council funds might impact on the lives of the people living in Yourtown.

There continues to be a difference in the life expectancy between males and females and in the health status of older men and women, with women expecting to live about three years longer than men and to enjoy better health than men as they advance in years. There are many theories as to why this is so, for example that women have a **genetic predisposition** to live longer, that they have a more positive attitude to and take better care of their health than men, that they are not exposed to the same stresses as men, and so on.

Whatever the reason, the upshot of different life expectancies and health status is that there are many more older women living on their own than there are older men, as the following statistics for 2001 show:

- nearly 50% of women aged 65 and over and 80% of women aged 85 and over were widows

- 17% of men aged 65 and over and 43% of men aged 85 and over were widowers.

    Source: Census 2001, Office for National Statistics, Mid Year Population Estimates, Office for National Statistics

Some people who become widowed choose to live alone. Whilst living alone is hard for older people of either sex, it can be especially hard for those women whose role has been the traditional one of homemaker and care giver. Although an increasing number of women are able to deal with the responsibilities associated with maintaining a house, car or garden, to handle personal and household finances, and to speak up on their own behalf, many are not and as a result neglect themselves and become socially isolated and deprived. They are also quite vulnerable, which puts them at risk of abuse and exploitation.

Some older people live with their children; others live in a communal setting such as a retirement village, sheltered housing or a care home. Communal living is expected to become more common, due, for example, to older people's children growing old themselves or because their children are not able or prepared to care for them in ways that are appropriate to their needs. In 2001, the proportion of women living in a care home was double that of men of the same age.

Figure 28.7 Communal living

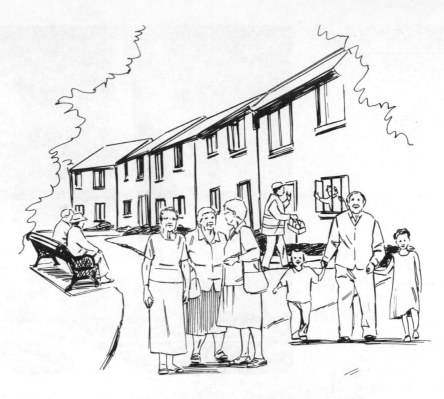

**Social exclusion** is caused in part by poverty, and poverty and old age go hand in hand. In the early 2000s, about a quarter of individuals on a low income were older people. Although the number of older people living in poverty is falling, at the time of writing, just over a fifth of all pensioners claim the Pension Guarantee Credit. By 2050 it is predicted that up to 80% of people aged 65 and over could be relying on means-tested benefits, which are only paid to the poor.

The eldest women tend to have the lowest incomes – the **median** gross weekly income of women over 80 was £109 in 2001–02, compared with an average weekly income of £189 for pensioners aged 75 and over and £203 for pensioners under 75.

Many old people whose income is just above the poverty threshold struggle to make ends meet. Holidays, meals out and visits to the hairdresser are usually out of the question. They survive by, for example, restricting their use of the phone, cutting down on heating, buying food that is reduced in price because it has reached its sell-by date and shopping for second-hand goods. As a result, their health and wellbeing is seriously threatened.

You read earlier that research shows that many people want to carry on working for as long as they are able to do their jobs well and not be forced to retire because of age-based restrictions. Although they are more likely to be self-employed, employment rates for older workers are beginning to rise:

■ for women aged 60 plus, it rose from 7.83% in 1998 to 9.85% in 2004

■ for men aged 65 plus, it rose from 7.30% in 2001 to 8.55% in 2004.

The Age Discrimination Act 2006 promotes rising employment rates for older people by:

■ banning restricted employment prospects for older people, for example rigid retirement and redundancy policies that are based on age

■ ensuring that employers take older workers' abilities, potential and experiences into consideration when allocating them jobs so that they can do them as well as possible.

The Age Discrimination Act 2006 also addresses the need for older workers to be given vocational training. Many have fewer qualifications than their younger colleagues but are likely to have been denied training on the basis that they were too old.

Figure 28.8  The older worker

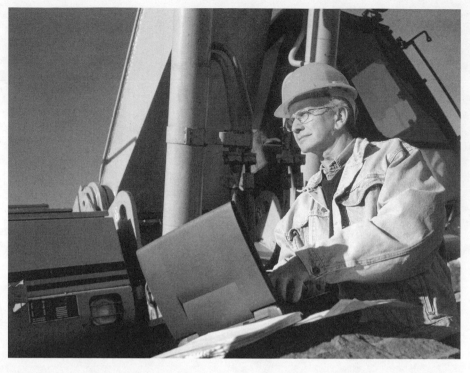

Employment in older age, whether full or part-time, enables people to supplement their pension, thereby reducing the strain on resources and enabling them to live the lifestyle they choose, stay in contact with people, keep up with changes in, for example, technology and employment practices, and achieve fulfillment and personal satisfaction. In addition, society benefits by having an experienced, wise workforce that is motivated, committed and reliable.

SENSE
www.sense.org.uk
National Statistics Online
www.statistics.gov.uk
Help the Aged
www.helptheaged.org.uk
The Tomorrow Project
www.tomorrowproject.net

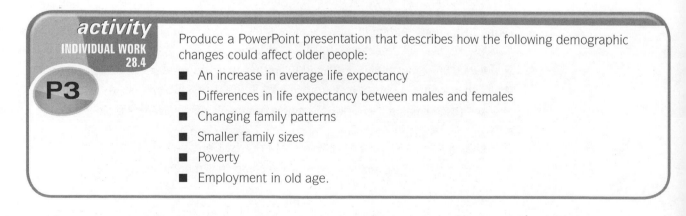

*activity*
INDIVIDUAL WORK
28.4

P3

Produce a PowerPoint presentation that describes how the following demographic changes could affect older people:

- An increase in average life expectancy
- Differences in life expectancy between males and females
- Changing family patterns
- Smaller family sizes
- Poverty
- Employment in old age.

# Increase in average life expectancy

There are a number of reasons why people are living longer than they used to. For example, improvements in living conditions have a significant affect on physical and mental health and therefore on life expectancy.

Figure 28.9 Improvements in living conditions that have contributed to an increase in life expectancy

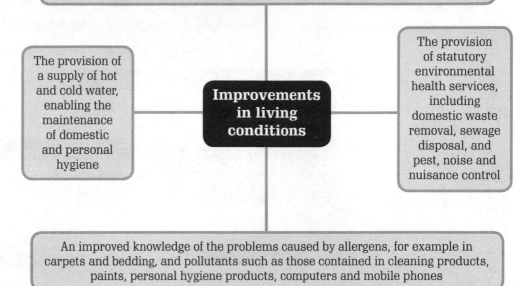

The replacement of rundown, overcrowded housing with decent accommodation that provides basic standards of comfort, such as privacy, warmth, ventilation, light and security and that has access to green spaces

The provision of a supply of hot and cold water, enabling the maintenance of domestic and personal hygiene

**Improvements in living conditions**

The provision of statutory environmental health services, including domestic waste removal, sewage disposal, and pest, noise and nuisance control

An improved knowledge of the problems caused by allergens, for example in carpets and bedding, and pollutants such as those contained in cleaning products, paints, personal hygiene products, computers and mobile phones

In addition, it has been shown that people live longer, happier and healthier lives if living conditions in their own homes, rather than in a care home, overcome the difficulties they face with daily living activities. To help promote the wellbeing of people with growing physical, emotional, social and intellectual needs, it is important that they have appropriate access to:

■ social, emotional and intellectual support, for example someone to talk to, and help when preparing food, taking medication and maintaining health, safety and security

■ physical support, for example aids such as adapted cutlery and crockery and raised toilet seats, adaptations such as ramps and grab rails, and equipment such as stair lifts and hoists.

Health care is not so much concerned with saving or prolonging people's lives. It is more to do with reducing the number of years that they spend diseased or disabled by treating conditions that cause pain and discomfort. In other words, the aim of health care is to improve quality of life. However, improvements in health care that improve quality of life indirectly increase average life expectancy and are due to developments in:

■ medical technology, for example of radiological scanners, which enable physiological disorders such as cancer, Multiple Sclerosis, Alzheimer's disease and Parkinson's disease to be diagnosed and treated

■ surgical techniques, to treat injuries, such as the correction of joint problems and the partial or total replacement of knee and hip joints; and disease, such as lung reduction surgery in the treatment of emphysema and the use of **angioplasty** as a treatment for heart attack

■ medicines, for example to treat chronic disorders such as stomach ulcers, blood clots, high blood pressure and inflamed airways; and to protect against age-related disorders such as dementia and cancer.

You can read about medical technology, surgical techniques and medicines in the diagnosis and treatment of physiological disorders in Unit 14 (Physiological disorders).

The Health and Safety at Work Act (HSWA) 1974 has had, and continues to have, a dramatic influence on the incidence of workplace injury, disease and illness. The table below identifies some of the areas in which a reduction in harmful working practices has led to a reduction in injury, disease and illness, and by extension, to an increase in average life expectancy.

Table 28.2  Comparison of workplace injury, disease and illness since the introduction of HSWA 1974

| Workplace injuries | 1974 | 2005/06 |
|---|---|---|
| Fatal injuries | 651 | 155 |
| Non-fatal injuries | 336,701 | 107,050 |
| Workplace disease | 1974 | 2004 |
| Deaths from pneumoconiosis | 453 | 214 |
| Deaths from asbestosis | 25 | 100 (large figure due to exposure to asbestos 30 to 40 years ago) |
| Workplace illness | 1990 | 2005/06 |
| Musculoskeletal disorders, e.g. back problems | 2,800 | 1,900 |

Source: www.hse.gov.uk/statistics/history/index.htm

You can read about legislation and guidelines that affect working practices, including the HSWA 1974, in Unit 3 (Health, safety and security in health and social care) in Health and Social Care Book 1.

Improvements in lifestyle over the last few generations have had a marked influence on longevity and the extent to which people can enjoy their final years.

Our knowledge of the effect of lifestyle behaviours, such as what we eat and drink, enables us to make informed decisions about how to live a long and healthy life. Such knowledge continues to grow, for example recent research suggests that:

- drinking red wine and cooking with olive oil, as in a Mediterranean diet, promotes good health and prolongs life, since both red wine and olive oil contain substances that protect against cancer and heart disease

- eating a diet that is rich in nutrients but low in **empty calories**, as opposed to one that contains large amounts of processed food, helps retain the characteristics of a younger body, such as flexible muscles, a healthy heart, weight and blood pressure, and low levels of blood sugar, body fat and cholesterol

- lifelong vegetarians live longer and have better health than meat eaters.

You can read about diet and health in greater detail in Unit 21 (Nutrition for health and social care).

It is also well known that physical exercise has a beneficial effect on health and longevity. An American study suggested that for each hour a person exercises, they get roughly two extra hours of life! Regular physical exercise:

- raises high-density lipoprotein (HDL) cholesterol, reducing the risk of developing coronary heart disease
- strengthens muscles, including the heart muscle
- helps to lower blood pressure, decreasing the risk of heart attack and stroke
- strengthens the bones, reducing the chance of developing osteoporosis
- reduces the chance of becoming obese or developing non-insulin-dependent diabetes (NID)
- has been linked with lower rates of certain kinds of cancer.

**Link** You can read about physiological disorders in greater detail in Unit 14 (Physiological Disorders).

Giving the brain a good workout, for example by learning new things, reading and participating in problem solving activities such as crosswords and sudoku puzzles, improves existing and creates new nerve connections within the brain. As a result, it improves mental agility, slows down the mental deterioration associated with ageing and is thought by some to slow the onset of dementia. Physical exercise, such as regular walking, has also been shown to help keep the brain in trim. Maintaining mental agility provides us with the means to live longer and enjoy a better quality of life.

Having a positive, 'can-do' attitude can also make for a happy, healthy final stage of life. Older people can develop a positive attitude by:

- maintaining good relationships with family and friends and others in their social support networks, for example the milkman, window cleaner and social care workers
- maintaining a measure of independence, whether they live on their own, with their family or with their peers in a care home
- learning new things
- being willing to adapt to change
- staying involved in their community, for example through voluntary work, worship with others and chatting to neighbours.

Figure 28.10 Keeping the brain in trim

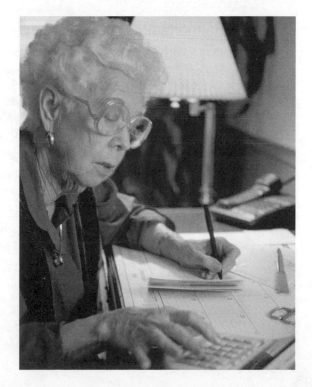

The Healthy House
www.healthy-house.co.uk
The Health and Safety Executive
www.hse.gov.uk
BUPA
www.bupa.co.uk
The BBC website
www.bbc.co.uk
The Welcome Trust
www.wellcome.ac.uk
The British Psychological Society
www.bps.org.uk

---

**activity**
**GROUP WORK**
**28.3**

**P4**

**M3**

In your group think about three famous, older people who are alive today.

1. Discuss why they are still alive.

2. Describe how they could be used in health promotion campaigns aimed at improving the life chances for the public in general.

## Age-related degenerative diseases

A degenerative disease is one in which the structure or function of tissues or organs changes for the worse over time. Degenerative diseases associated with growing older include Alzheimer's disease, osteoporosis, macular degeneration, hearing loss and prostate cancer.

### Alzheimer's disease

Alzheimer's disease is a form of dementia, a word which originates from the Latin word 'demens', meaning 'out of one's mind'. It is caused by a gradual loss of brain function due to a build up of clumps and bundles ('plaques' and 'tangles') of proteins both inside and outside the brain cells. These clumps and bundles gradually destroy the connections between cells that are essential for normal mental activity, leading to progressive memory problems, confusion, **disorientation** and changes in behaviour.

The impact of Alzheimer's disease can be far reaching:

- Progressive memory loss causes emotional difficulties such as frustration and anxiety. Confusion and disorientation cause alarm and agitation. Frustration, anxiety, agitation and alarm can, in turn, lead to unpredictable changes in behaviour.

- Memory loss can lead to self-neglect, which increases the risk of infection, weight loss and general physical deterioration; and increases the risk of accidents in the living environment.

- Changes in behaviour, particularly to those which are socially unacceptable, such as a loss of inhibition, rudeness, **paranoia** and violence, can lead to social isolation, loneliness and depression.

Patients with severe Alzheimer's disease can do little on their own and need full time care, either in their own home or in a care home. Although the disease progresses at different rates in different people, most patients die about eight years after first experiencing the symptoms, usually from an infection such as pneumonia that develops as a complication.

You can read more about Alzheimer's disease in Unit 14 (Physiological Disorders).

## Osteoporosis

Healthy bone consists of a thick outer shell and an inner, spongy mesh made from protein and minerals (particularly calcium). Old, worn out bone is broken down and absorbed by the body and new bone is created from fresh protein and minerals.

- In children and young people, more new bone is created than is broken down, making bones bigger, dense and very strong.

- In our mid-twenties, there is roughly the same amount of bone creation as there is bone breakdown.

- From our mid-thirties, bone loss begins to overtake bone creation as part of the normal ageing process.

In osteoporosis, a word which means 'porous bones', bone loss happens much more quickly than bone creation. This reduces the density of bones, making them weaker and as a result, joints become painful and bones are more likely to fracture. Hip and wrist fractures are the most common, but small fractures can occur in the **vertebrae**, causing a loss of height and a curved back (sometimes known as 'dowager's hump'). This makes it difficult to support the weight of the body and leads to long-lasting neck and back pain. The older a person is the less effectively fractures repair, which can lead to a permanent decrease in movement and mobility and an increasing dependence on others.

## Macular degeneration

Macular degeneration is a progressive disorder that affects the part of the **retina** known as the macula, the region for keenest vision. Although total blindness rarely occurs and **peripheral vision** is not affected, macular degeneration results in the loss of central, detailed vision, making it difficult to see straight ahead, for example to watch television, drive and recognise people; and to see detail, for example the printed word. In addition, vision can become distorted, making it difficult to make judgements about height and distance; the eyes can become sensitive to light; and lights and colours may appear which don't actually exist. Eventually, central vision is replaced by a black spot.

Age-Related Macular Degeneration (ARMD) is the most common form of macular degeneration and its incidence increases with age – almost 15% of 75 year olds are affected, in particular females. A diagnosis brings feelings of worry and uncertainty about the future, for example about carrying out everyday living activities, staying safe, getting out and about, remaining independent, maintaining relationships and taking part in social activities.

## Hearing loss

There are two types of hearing loss:

1. Conductive hearing loss, which is caused by problems such as middle ear infections, wax and fluid blockages, injury to the eardrum and rheumatoid arthritis that interfere with transmission of sound from the outer ear to the inner ear.

2. Sensorineural hearing loss, which is caused by a problem with the inner ear or with the nervous pathway from the inner ear to the brain, for example age-related hearing loss, injury to the ear due to loud noise, inner ear and **auditory nerve** infections, such as mumps and rubella, and disorders such as Ménière's disease, meningitis, MS, brain tumour and stroke.

Figure 28.11 Degenerative
diseases

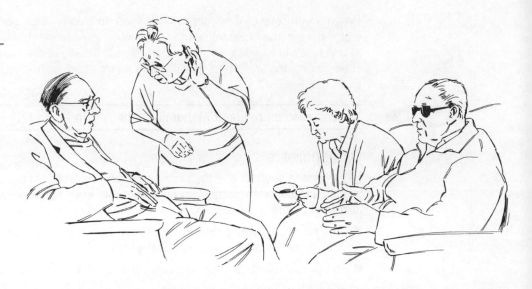

The biggest cause of hearing loss is age, due to progressive damage to and loss of **hair cells** in the **cochlea**. By the time they are 40, most people have lost some of their hearing; by the age of 80, most people have significant hearing loss, particularly of high frequency sounds such as children's and female voices, and of the letters s, t, k, p, and f.

Hearing loss has a huge impact on communication, because listening requires a great deal of concentration, which is physically and emotionally draining for the person concerned; and speaking may be difficult, because of difficulties in hearing one's own voice. As a result, relationships can become strained, socialising restricted and the person isolated and lonely.

## Prostate cancer

The prostate gland is situated at the base of the male bladder where it produces a fluid that mixes with sperm to form semen. Prostate cancer is an enlargement of the prostate gland caused by a tumour, which, if left untreated, may spread to other parts of the body. It is rarely found in men under 45 but its incidence increases with age and nearly three out of four men in their 80s have tiny specks of prostate cancer.

Prostate cancer grows very slowly and may never need treatment nor cause any symptoms. However, symptoms that can indicate its presence include:

- a need to urinate frequently, especially at night
- difficulty to start urinating, to hold back urine and painful urination
- a weak or interrupted flow of urine and blood in the urine
- difficulty in having an erection, painful ejaculation and blood in the semen
- pain or stiffness in the lower back, hips or upper thighs.

Like all degenerative diseases, prostate cancer causes anxiety for the future, particularly as it can be fatal.

The Alzheimer's Society
www.alzheimers.org.uk
National Osteoporosis Society
www.nos.org.uk
BUPA
www.bupa.co.uk
NHS Direct
www.nhsdirect.nhs.uk

Royal National Institute for the Blind
www.rnib.org.uk
Royal National Institute for the Deaf
www.rnid.org.uk
The Prostate Cancer Charity
www.prostate-cancer.org.uk

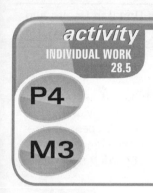

**activity**
**INDIVIDUAL WORK**
**28.5**

**P4**

**M3**

Talk to two or three older people to find out what factors have influenced their ageing. Use your findings to write a report that describes and explains the influences on ageing.

# The role of the care worker in supporting older people

## Role of the carer in supporting quality of life

Anyone who works with older people has a responsibility to help them maintain their quality of life. It is difficult to define the term 'quality of life' because it means different things to different people.

Figure 28.12  The meaning of quality of life

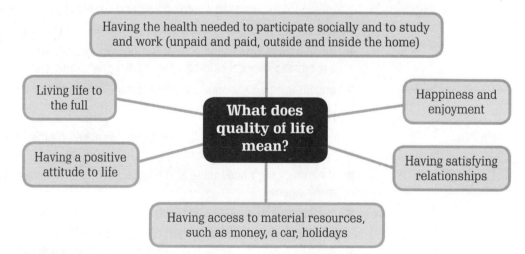

However we choose to define it, the quality of life for many people tends to decline as they get older, due to the progression of degenerative diseases, increased dependence on others, the impact on them of negative attitudes and discrimination, and so on. Perhaps the most significant way to help older people hang on to their quality of life is to give them an opportunity to make their own choices about how they want to live.

## Choices

We all need to be able to make our own choices – making choices helps us to stay in control of our lives; not being able to make choices can be frustrating and create dependence on others. Older people who need support have a right to choose how to live their lives, for example when to get up and go to bed; what and when to eat; how to spend their time and who to spend it with; and so on. They also have a right to be cared for in ways that take account of their choices, for example what their care involves and how it is to be given. The principles of care require care workers to support people's rights to make choices; and by encouraging them to make their own decisions, care workers help them stay in control and thereby maintain as much quality of life as possible.

You can read more about rights and the principles of care in Unit 2 in Health and Social Care Book 1 (Equality, Diversity and Rights in Health and Social Care).

## Respect

Respect is another requirement of the principles of care. We each have a right to be respected for our individuality, and we have a right to respect for our family and private life. By being considerate, polite and appreciative in their work with older people, care workers demonstrate respect for their wants, needs, likes, dislikes, preferences, beliefs, values, experiences, expectations, privacy and lifestyle, thereby supporting their quality of life.

## Motivation

Many older people lose quality of life because they lose the motivation and enthusiasm to, for example, participate in activities that they used to enjoy, maintain relationships with family and friends, learn new things or do something different. One of the roles of a care worker is to stimulate and inspire older people to maintain or regain their quality of life by:

- finding out what quality of life means to them – no-one should assume that their definition of quality of life is the same as that for other people
- finding out how they developed their quality of life, for example what they are interested in, what they enjoy doing and who they like to be with
- finding out what they would like to do to improve their quality of life
- ensuring that opportunities that will help maintain or regain their quality of life are available to them, including fresh challenges and new activities
- encouraging and supporting them to take advantage of the opportunities on offer.

## Self-esteem

Many older people lose their quality of life because of a loss of self-esteem or self-respect. This can be because of:

- their changing body image and reduced ability to maintain their personal appearance and hygiene
- the health and care procedures they have to experience, such as being bathed and helped to use the toilet, which wound their dignity
- their real and increasing physical dependence on others, due to, for example, disability and sensory impairment
- their perceived lack of importance or 'invisibility' – you read earlier about the social creation of dependency, which makes older people feel useless and inadequate
- their changing role, from someone who had a part to play in the family and community to someone who is no longer able or needed to play that role.

To promote the self-esteem and quality of life of the people they support, care workers need to have a kind, understanding, interested and complimentary attitude as well as a person-centred approach. A person-centred approach reassures the individuals needing support that they matter and involves:

- respecting their privacy and dignity
- letting their preferences, wishes and needs shape the way they are supported
- ensuring that their support is focused on their needs and not on the needs of the care worker or organisation providing the care
- encouraging them to make informed choices about their care and the way they behave so that they can remain in control of their own lives.

You will read about informed choice shortly.

## Independence

Becoming independent is a normal part of human development, and staying as independent as possible is important because it helps us maintain our quality of life. Many people lose their **independence** as they get older, because of poor health, disability, diminishing mental agility and so on. As a result they lose the ability to make choices, exercise control over their lives and be responsible for themselves. A loss of independence brings with it a loss confidence, self-worth and wellbeing.

Like quality of life, independence has different definitions for different people and varies according to their situation. However, care workers have a responsibility to help older people maintain or regain their independence, for example by:

- encouraging them to make choices about how they want to live and be supported
- respecting what independence they already have, by allowing them to do as much for themselves as possible
- encouraging them to accept help when needed, particularly if assistance promotes safety. But remember – over-protection can knock people's confidence and self-esteem
- encouraging them to remain physically, mentally and socially active. You read earlier that the activity theory of ageing suggests that the more activities and social contacts an individual has, the better their quality of life
- ensuring that they have access to aids, adaptations, modes of transport and **assistive technologies** that meet their needs for independence
- encouraging a sense of interdependence for the purpose of looking after each other and raising morale, for example by assisting them to attend self-help groups and clubs and to maintain relationships with friends and family
- providing up-to-date information on services that offer advice on how to stay fit and healthy
- challenging negative attitudes to ageing. Exposure to negative attitudes which describe older people as being frail and dependent can cause them to become increasingly dependent.

## Planning for change

The recognition that life is coming to an end can be distressing, and age-related degenerative diseases that predict chronic ill health, memory problems, sensory impairments, mobility difficulties and increasing dependence on others can cause anxieties about the future. Successful ageing is about planning for change so that the experiences of ageing and being old are positive. Care workers have a responsibility to help older people plan for their future in such a way that expected changes are addressed and seen in as positive a light as possible.

**remember**

Success is shaped by good planning. Successful ageing depends on planning for inevitable age-related changes by putting into place a course of action that takes them into account.

Figure 28.13 Successful
ageing

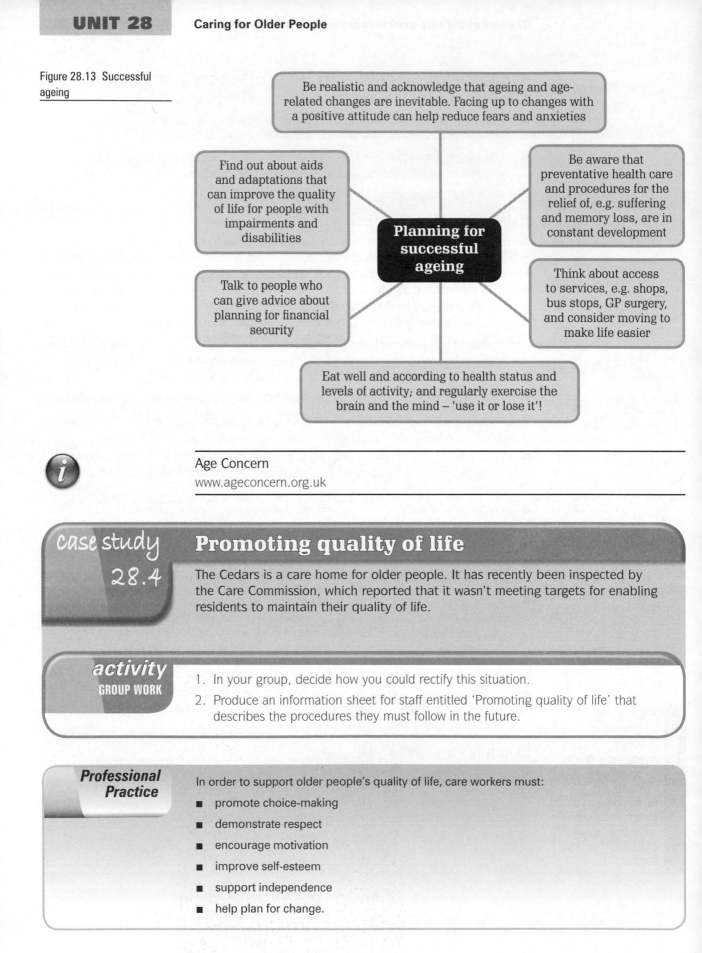

Be realistic and acknowledge that ageing and age-
related changes are inevitable. Facing up to changes with
a positive attitude can help reduce fears and anxieties

Find out about aids
and adaptations that
can improve the quality
of life for people with
impairments and
disabilities

**Planning for
successful
ageing**

Be aware that
preventative health care
and procedures for the
relief of, e.g. suffering
and memory loss, are in
constant development

Talk to people who
can give advice about
planning for financial
security

Think about access
to services, e.g. shops,
bus stops, GP surgery,
and consider moving to
make life easier

Eat well and according to health status and
levels of activity; and regularly exercise the
brain and the mind – 'use it or lose it'!

Age Concern
www.ageconcern.org.uk

## case study 28.4 Promoting quality of life

The Cedars is a care home for older people. It has recently been inspected by
the Care Commission, which reported that it wasn't meeting targets for enabling
residents to maintain their quality of life.

### activity
**GROUP WORK**

1. In your group, decide how you could rectify this situation.
2. Produce an information sheet for staff entitled 'Promoting quality of life' that
   describes the procedures they must follow in the future.

### Professional Practice

In order to support older people's quality of life, care workers must:

- promote choice-making
- demonstrate respect
- encourage motivation
- improve self-esteem
- support independence
- help plan for change.

# Role of the carer in supporting older people's choice and independence

You read in the previous section that choice and independence are crucial for maintaining quality of life. This section seeks to describe how choice and independence can be supported through diet, physical exercise and activities.

To stay healthy and active, we all need to eat a varied and balanced diet. Overweight, for example because of inactivity or eating too much fat and carbohydrate, reduces mobility and increases the risk of heart disease and diabetes. Underweight, for example because of forgetting to eat, eating too little, having a diminished appetite or poorly fitting dentures, can lead to nutritional deficiency diseases and malnutrition.

Ill health and reduced mobility create dependency. To promote independence, care workers should encourage older people to choose to eat well, in particular to choose to eat a diet that incorporates important trace elements and vitamins.

**Link**

You can read about a balanced diet in Unit 24 (Nutrition for Health and Social Care).

Although essential in the diet, trace elements are only needed in very small amounts. Two important trace elements are:

- fluoride, which is associated with strong bones and teeth and helps prevent dental caries. It occurs in drinking water, tea, and seafood, especially fish whose bones are eaten.

- iodine, which is important for the production in the thyroid gland of thyroxine, the hormone that regulates the metabolic rate. Iodine occurs in milk and dairy products, meat and eggs.

Important vitamins for older people include:

- vitamin A (retinol), which occurs in meat and animal products and is needed for night vision

- vitamin C (ascorbic acid), which occurs in fruit and vegetables, particularly fresh varieties, and is needed for maintaining healthy skin and gums and helping wounds to heal

- vitamin D, which occurs in margarine, eggs and fatty fish and is made in the body by the action of sunlight on the skin. Vitamin D maintains bone strength by promoting the absorption of calcium from the intestines and its deposition in the bones.

Figure 28.14  Eating well

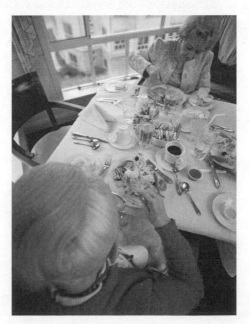

You read earlier that osteoporosis occurs when bones become porous and liable to fracture. The older a person is the less effectively fractures repair, which can lead to a permanent decrease in movement and mobility and an increasing dependence on others. Care workers should encourage older people to choose to exercise by developing an exercise programme to reduce the risk of osteoporosis.

A physical exercise programme that includes weight-bearing exercises, i.e. exercises in which the body supports its own weight, such as brisk walking, stair climbing and dancing, has been shown to reduce the risk of osteoporosis and help maintain movement, mobility and independence. Weight bearing exercises improve:

- bone density and strength, which reduce the risk of fractures
- balance, flexibility and co-ordination, which reduce the risk of falls.

Exercises that are safe for people who have developed osteoporosis include:

- Aquarobics
- Walking
- Line dancing
- Tai Chi.

Exercises that are not recommended for people who have osteoporosis are ones that pose a risk of falling or that require:

- high impact movements, such as aerobics
- sharp, reflex actions, such as badminton
- excessive forward bending, for example touching the toes.

Giving the brain a good workout:

- improves mental agility, such as speed of response and the ability to stay focused and interested
- slows down the mental deterioration associated with ageing, such as memory loss
- provides an opportunity to maintain and develop social contacts.

Maintaining memory and mental agility and having an enjoyable, fulfilling social life provides us with the means to live longer and enjoy a better quality of life. A loss of memory, mental agility and social contacts creates a negative attitude and growing dependency. Care workers should encourage older people to choose to use and develop their brains by developing an activity programme designed to promote and maintain mental abilities, a positive mental attitude and social activities.

Intellectual activities include:

- reading, writing and using the computer and the internet, which can be for pleasure, to promote learning or to maintain contact with family and friends
- listening to music, which promotes learning and interest and can create a positive frame of mind
- doing quizzes and puzzles, for example crosswords, sudoku and jigsaws, which promote problem-solving skills
- playing stimulating games, for example card games, computer games and bingo, which are fun and promote the skills of accuracy and speed of thought
- DIY and repairs about the home and garden, which promote problem-solving skills.

Activities where there is an opportunity to socialise and connect with friends, relatives and the outside world include:

- group discussions, which promote learning and communication skills such as speaking, listening and turn-taking

■ reminiscence therapy, which is where people are encouraged to remember things that happened in their life. It aims to improve memory and thinking skills.

■ visits to, for example, museums, art galleries, theatres, shopping centres, restaurants, pubs, schools, places of worship, which enrich lives and promote interests

■ arts and crafts, which promote learning and interests.

Activities which involve an element of physical exercise are thought to boost mental agility by promoting the growth of new brain cells and getting extra oxygen into the brain. The ones that most successfully promote and maintain mental abilities are those that demand some sort of mental effort, such as:

■ dancing

■ sports and keep fit exercises (see above)

■ doing housework.

As you know, we all have a right to make choices and being able to make choices enables us to stay in control, which builds our self-confidence and self-esteem. Sometimes the choices we make involve taking risks, for example crossing the road, driving a car and using alcohol. On the other hand, we all have a responsibility to protect the health and safety of ourselves and others. It follows that any choices we make that compromise our and other people's safety are irresponsible. We have to balance our right to take risks with our health and safety responsibilities.

The ageing process can reduce people's ability to make choices. As a result they lose their self-confidence and self-esteem. The role of a care worker is to help rebuild this loss by offering them choices and supporting them in making and carrying out their decisions. However, the responsibility to avoid harm remains: there has to be a balance between the loss of confidence/self-esteem and safety. In other words, care workers must ensure that in their efforts to support older people, the choices they offer are safe or carry risks of harm that are manageable.

Figure 28.15 Exercise and activity programmes

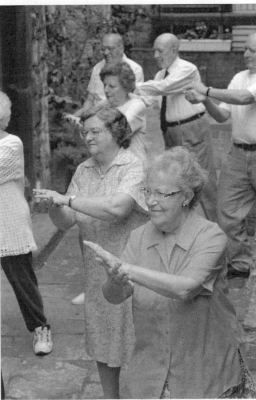
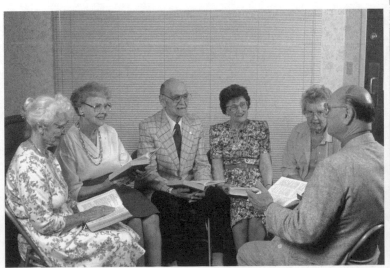

**Professional Practice**

Care workers have a responsibility to support older people's choice and independence by:

■ promoting diets, exercise and activity programmes that meet their individual physical and mental health needs

■ offering alternatives that are enjoyable, safe and only pose risks that are manageable

■ respecting the choices they make

■ supporting them to be as independent as possible without being over-protective.

---

*i*

Food Standards Agency
www.eatwell.gov.uk
Nuffield Orthopaedic Centre
www.noc.nhs.uk
Age Concern
www.ageconcern.org.uk
Help the Aged
www.helptheaged.org.uk

---

**activity**
INDIVIDUAL WORK
28.6

**P5**

**M4**

Research the roles of and dilemmas for care workers in supporting older people. Produce a PowerPoint presentation that:

■ describes these roles

■ explains why the dilemmas exist.

---

**activity**
INDIVIDUAL WORK
28.7

**D2**

Using examples, evaluate the role of the care worker in supporting older people, for example in promoting choice and independence, and dealing with change.

---

## Quality and choice at the end of life

Although much of the practical caring for dying people is carried out by relatives and social care workers, dying and death are usually seen as medical events, for example:

■ we rely on medical professionals to prescribe care for people who are old, infirm, terminally ill or dying

■ we contact medical professionals as soon as we think someone has died

■ medical professionals have the power to declare a person dead

■ medical professionals have the power to say what has caused the person to die

■ causes of death are always based on physical signs described by medical terminology

■ medical professionals have to sign a death certificate before a body can be removed and prepared for burial or cremation

■ medical professionals prepare bodies for burial or cremation.

This medicalisation of death and the end of life implies that death is a disease or failure of life which needs treatment, as opposed to a natural and expected end to life. This can be a problem to people:

■ who have spiritual needs and feel that death and dying have a spiritual meaning

■ whose cultural and religious beliefs welcome death, because it takes them closer to their God; and for their family, who consider it an honour to take part in the ritual of preparing the body for burial or cremation

■ who feel that their quality of life would be improved by a more holistic approach to their care. A holistic approach is one that treats all of an individual's needs – physical, social, emotional, intellectual and spiritual, as opposed to just their physical needs

■ who see dying as a peaceful, natural event, a time to reflect on their lives, to come to terms with their achievements and to prepare to take their leave.

Care workers have a responsibility to find out the beliefs and holistic needs of the people they support so that they can help them maintain quality and choice at the end of their lives.

To make informed choices, people must have access to full and up-to-date information. To enable people who are dying to maintain choice and quality of life, they must be given full, up-to-date information on, for example:

■ their condition and its **prognosis**

■ the range of options available to manage their condition, control their pain, etc., and the benefits, risks and side-effects of each option

■ the support available to them to live in a dignified manner and as independently as possible

■ the range of options available to them as regards place of care at the end of life and place of death

■ the positive experiences of other people in their situation.

Information must always be given in a sensitive manner, and receiving it allows individuals to play an active role in decision-making about their care, to choose how and where they wish to live during their final days and to explore issues about dying and death, including their own ideas and feelings.

Figure 28.16 Making informed choices

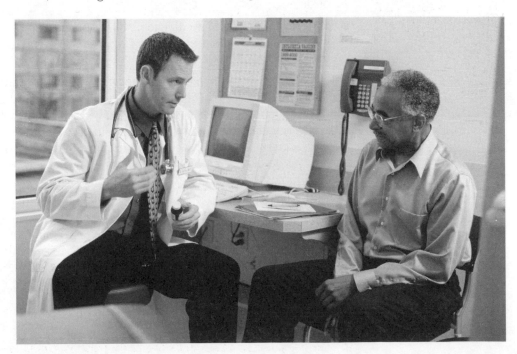

Mentally competent adults can't be given medical treatment without their consent. But if they are not able to discuss and understand treatment options, for example because they are unconscious due to an accident or a stroke, or if they are unable to communicate, for example because of dementia, they are said to 'lack mental capacity'.

Doctors have a legal and ethical obligation to act in the best interests of people who lack mental capacity and they should consult relatives when deciding on treatment. However relatives don't have a legal right to be consulted or to make decisions on a loved one's behalf. In such a situation, it helps doctors if they know the person's wishes. One way of making this information known is through a living will, also known as an advance directive.

A living will allows adults who are mentally competent to describe their future wishes to *refuse* medical treatment, even if it leads to their death, and it can only be used once they lack mental capacity. A signed, dated and witnessed (witnesses must not be a spouse, partner, relative or anyone who would benefit from an ordinary will) written document is the most useful way for the person to describe their wishes but living wills don't have to be in writing. And whilst casual remarks about treatment are not sufficient, witnessed verbal instructions have to be respected.

Living wills cannot be used to ask for assisted suicide and euthanasia. Euthanasia is defined as the painless killing of a patient suffering from an incurable disease or in an irreversible coma. Assisted suicide is where doctors don't kill a person themselves but provide the means for them to take their own life.

Current UK law regards euthanasia as murder, and therefore illegal; and assisted suicide is illegal under the Suicide Act 1961. In addition, the British Medical Association (BMA), which represents doctors from all over the UK and whose policies are decided by doctors, opposes euthanasia and assisted suicide on the grounds that they fly in the face of the traditional ethics and morals of medicine which are enshrined in the Hippocratic Oath. Most doctors when they qualify swear on the Hippocratic Oath, which prohibits them from assisting in suicide or euthanasia.

Euthanasia and assisted suicide continue to be at the forefront of public debate. Arguments for and against euthanasia and assisted suicide include:

- Against. They are both forms of murder and very often, because of pain or coma, the people concerned are unable to make decisions for themselves about whether to live or die.

- For. People shouldn't have to endure incredible pain and suffering, especially if they have no chance of recovery; and forcing them to live prolongs the agony for them, their family and friends.

Erik Erikson was a developmental psychologist who put forward the theory that personality development continues during eight life stages. At each stage, a conflict is experienced, for example in adolescence (stage 5) young people go through an identity crisis in which their role, for example that of the child who is responsible to parents and teachers, conflicts with their identity, for example that they are young, independent adults. Our developing personalities are shaped by the way we deal with these conflicts, which in turn is based on our experiences.

Erikson's eighth personality development stage, the final stage, which occurs from mature adulthood onwards, is to do with the conflict between ego-integrity and despair, in other words the discrepancy between what the person wants to continue to be or do and what they find they can no longer be or do. This stage is introspective – the person spends a great deal of time examining their own thoughts, feelings and memories, and many of them find it difficult to accept what has changed and to move on. As a result they spend their final days in despair.

Care workers can help older people deal with these conflicts, by encouraging them to dwell on happy memories, to embrace their achievements, to search for a positive meaning in their lives and to accept what can't be changed. It's not always possible to delete all of the bad times but an objective evaluation of the past can help to 'reframe' their present.

## Legislation, regulations and conventions

There are a number of laws, regulations and conventions that apply to older people, some of which are described below.

### The Human Rights Act 1998

The Human Rights Act 1998 incorporates the European Convention for the protection of Human Rights and Fundamental Freedoms 1950. Various articles within the Act impact on issues relating to the care of older people.

### The Data Protection Act 1998

The Data Protection Act 1998 is in place to make sure that personal, sensitive information asked of people who need support is protected. As a rule of thumb, no-one should be allowed access to anyone else's personal information unless they have:

- been given permission by the person themselves
- a right or a need to know the information, for example health professionals.

### The Care Standards Act 2000

The Care Standards Act 2000 protects vulnerable people's right to the highest possible standard of care. It ensures that care providers provide care in ways that meet the National Care Standards and that people who work in care are suitable and trained to do their jobs.

Figure 28.17 The impact of the Human Rights Act on the care of older people

Article 2 – the right to life, which means that e.g. life-support mechanisms cannot be withdrawn unless the person is beyond doubt clinically dead

Article 3 – the right to protection from inhuman and degrading treatment, which means that e.g. someone who is competent can refuse to accept the withdrawal of life-prolonging treatment which is thought to be necessary

**The impact of the Human Rights Act on the care of older people**

Article 14 – prohibits discrimination, which means that people must not be discriminated against with regard to e.g. access to particular types of service or levels of care on the basis of their age

Article 8 – the right to respect for private and family life, which means that peoples' choices for e.g. place of care must be respected

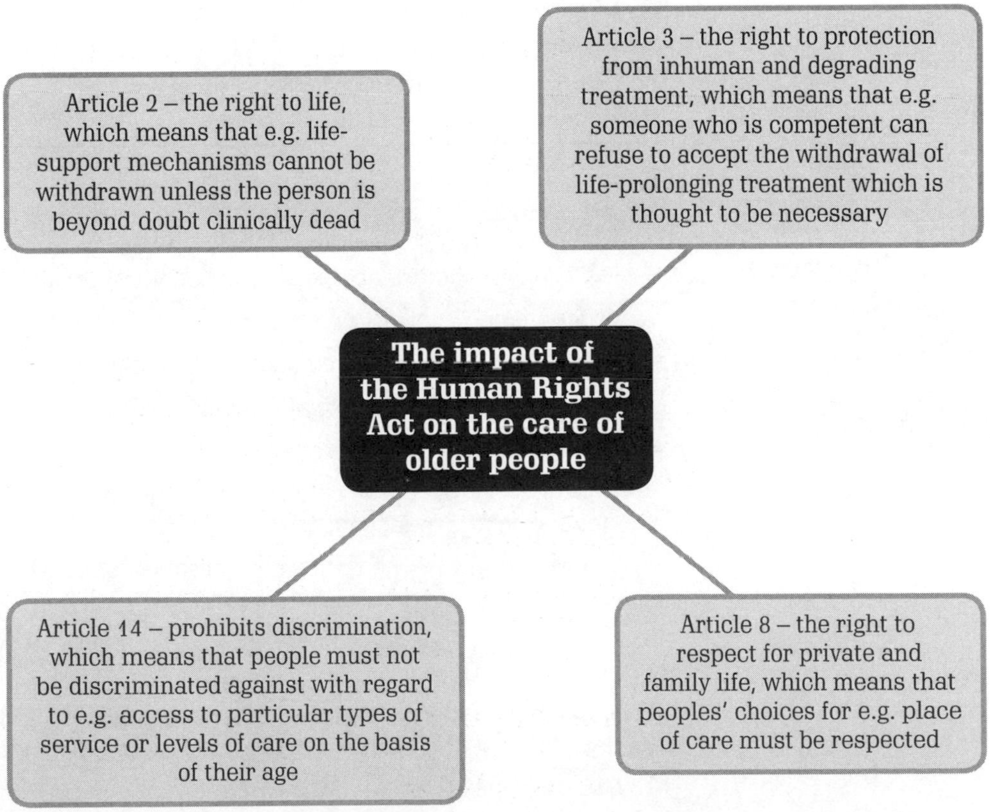

## The Residential Care and Nursing Homes Regulations 2002

The Residential Care and Nursing Homes Regulations 2002 protect the right of older people who live in care homes to be protected from danger and harm.

## The Age Discrimination Act 2006

The Age Discrimination Act 2006 promotes employment for older people by:

- banning restricted employment prospects for older people, for example rigid retirement and redundancy policies that are based on age

- ensuring that employers take older workers' abilities, potential and experiences into consideration when allocating them jobs so that they can do them as well as possible

- ensuring that older workers have access to vocational training.

---

**activity**

**INDIVIDUAL WORK 28.8**

**P6**

**M5**

Write a case study which talks about someone at the end of their life. In your case study:

- describe two aspects of quality and choice for the individual

- analyse, i.e. examine in more detail, the two aspects of quality and choice.

---

British Medical Association
www.bma.org.uk
Age Concern England
www.ace.org.uk
The Liberty Guide to Human rights
www.yourrights.org.uk

---

**Progress Check**

1. Give three definitions of the term 'older people'.
2. Explain why there is no one simple definition of ageing.
3. Compare and contrast two theories of ageing.
4. Explain the impact of three demographic changes on elderly people.
5. Use three examples to explain why life expectancy is increasing.
6. Describe three age-related degenerative diseases.
7. Describe the role of the care worker in supporting older people's quality of life, choice and independence.
8. What is meant by the terms medicalisation of death, informed choice, living will, assisted suicide and euthanasia?
9. What can be done to promote choice and quality of life for people nearing the end of their days?
10. How would understanding Ericson's theory regarding the final personality development stage help care workers support elderly people in their last days?
11. Use examples to explain why caring for older people can be challenging.
12. Describe the legislation, regulations and conventions that are in place to support and protect older people.

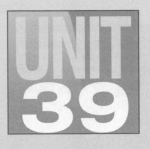

# Infection Prevention and Control

## This unit covers:

- The cause and spread of infection
- How to prevent and control the spread of infection
- Legislation relevant to infection prevention and control
- The roles, responsibilities and boundaries in relation to infection control

Patients and people who use social care services (service users) are particularly vulnerable to infection. For this reason it is crucial that everyone who works in health and social care settings has an understanding of infectious agents and the principles of infection prevention and control. This unit gives you an opportunity to develop a knowledge and understanding of the cause and spread of infection, how such spread can be prevented and controlled, and the roles and responsibilities of organisations and people in relation to the spread of infection. It also looks at the legislation and guidelines aimed at preventing and controlling infection in health and social care settings.

| **grading criteria** | To achieve a **Pass** grade the evidence must show that the learner is able to: | To achieve a **Merit** grade the evidence must show that, in addition to the pass criteria, the learner is able to: | To achieve a **Distinction** grade the evidence must show that, in addition to the pass and merit criteria, the learner is able to: |
|---|---|---|---|
| | **P1** describe the causes of infection. Pg 282 | | |
| | **P2** describe how named examples of a viral, a bacterial and a fungal infection may be spread. Pg 282 | | |
| | **P3** describe standard precautions for the prevention and control of infection in a health or social care workplace. Pg 296 | | |

## grading criteria

| To achieve a **Pass** grade the evidence must show that the learner is able to: | To achieve a **Merit** grade the evidence must show that, in addition to the pass criteria, the learner is able to: | To achieve a **Distinction** grade the evidence must show that, in addition to the pass and merit criteria, the learner is able to: |
| --- | --- | --- |
| **P4** identify key legislation and guidelines relevant to infection prevention and control in a health or social care workplace. Pg 301 | **M1** explain the role of organisational procedures in the prevention and control of infection. Pg 301 | **D1** explain how legal requirements influence infection prevention and control procedures in a health or social care workplace. Pg 301 |
| **P5** describe the roles and responsibilities of staff in relation to infection prevention and control in a **health or social care workplace**. Pg 307 | **M2** report on a risk assessment undertaken at a health or social care work placement. Pg 308 | **D2** explain how risk assessment can contribute to improving infection prevention and control in a health or social care workplace. Pg 308 |

# The cause and spread of infection

## Infection and colonisation

Infection occurs when body tissues are invaded by an infectious agent. Infectious agents include micro-organisms i.e. organisms that are too small to be seen with the naked eye and require a microscope for them to become visible, such as a bacteria, viruses and fungi; and **parasitic** organisms such as lice and mites. Infectious agents that are capable of causing disease are known as pathogens. They or the toxins they produce cause the signs and symptoms that we associate with an infectious illness, for example pain, swelling, discharge and fever.

A localised infection is the term used to describe an infection in which the infectious agent is confined or restricted to a particular site, thereby affecting a specific part of the body only. An abscess is a localised infection, as is Herpes zoster (shingles).

A systemic infection is the term used to describe an infection in which the infectious agent has spread from the site of initial infection throughout several body organs and systems. Systemic infections include respiratory and urinary infections.

Colonisation is the term used to describe the situation where micro-organisms live in or on the body but cause no harm. However, if they invade the skin or migrate to areas where they don't normally reside, or they are introduced into the body during an invasive procedure such as surgery or the insertion of an **indwelling medical device** such as a catheter or intravenous drip, they can cause a localised or systemic infection. For example, *Staphylococcus aureus* is a bacterium that colonises areas of the skin without causing infection, but its migration into the body can cause **septicaemia**.

## Cause of infection

Not all infectious agents cause illness. Normal flora is the term used to describe non-pathogenic micro-organisms that reside normally in or on the body. They are often known as 'friendly micro-organisms' because they help maintain good health and form part of the body's normal defence mechanisms, protecting it from invasion by more harmful micro-organisms. For example, vitamin K-producing bacteria exist in the intestines, and *Lactobacillus acidophilus*, which is found in the intestines, mouth and

**remember**

Many micro-organisms live in or on the body doing no harm but will cause infection if allowed to migrate into areas where they don't normally reside.

vagina, produces lactic acid that maintains acidity at levels that have an inhibitory effect on invading micro-organisms.

There are certain circumstances and conditions in which normal flora can cause infection, for example:

- the use of antibiotics can destroy normal flora. Their destruction makes way for other organisms to invade and cause an infection, for example thrush, which is caused by the yeast-like fungus candida.

- skin and tissue damage, such as exposed wounds and surgical lesions, allow normal flora to invade areas where they don't normally reside

- circumstances such as the use of infected in-dwelling medical devices provide opportunities for normal flora to migrate to areas where they don't normally reside.

Transient flora is the term used to describe micro-organisms that are transient (temporary) residents of surfaces from which they are easily removed. For example, many transient flora live temporarily on the surface of the skin. Their easy removal means they are easily spread by contact with, for example, other parts of the body, other people, clothing and equipment. Transient flora are usually pathogenic.

The skin is just one example of a reservoir, i.e. an environment in or on which an infectious agent can live, and contact is just one method of spread of infection. The chain of infection is a **model** that is used to explain how an infectious agent is spread to and from a reservoir. Infection prevention and control is based on breaking the chain in some way.

Figure 39.1 The chain of infection

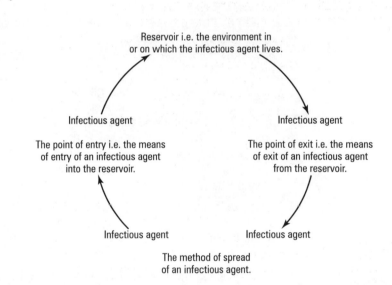

You will read about reservoirs, points of exit and entry, and methods of spread of infection shortly.

## Pathogenic micro-organisms and disease

You read earlier that infectious agents include bacteria, viruses, fungi and parasites, and that those that are capable of causing disease are known as pathogens. This section aims to introduce you to a number of pathogens and the diseases they cause.

### Bacteria

Bacteria are single celled micro-organisms that are found almost everywhere.

Figure 39.2 Structure of a typical bacterial cell

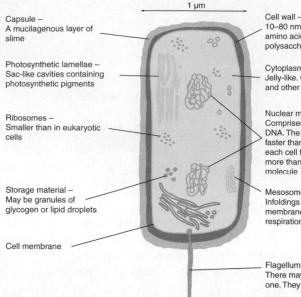

1 μm

Capsule –
A mucilagenous layer of slime

Photosynthetic lamellae –
Sac-like cavities containing photosynthetic pigments

Ribosomes –
Smaller than in eukaryotic cells

Storage material –
May be granules of glycogen or lipid droplets

Cell membrane

Cell wall –
10–80 nm thick. Made of amino acids and polysaccharides

Cytoplasm –
Jelly-like. Contains enzymes and other soluble material

Nuclear material –
Comprises a large circle of DNA. The DNA replicates faster than the cells and so each cell typically contains more than one DNA molecule

Mesosome –
Infoldings of the cell membrane important in respiration

Flagellum –
There may be more than one. They lack microtubules

Pathogenic bacteria include:

■ MRSA (methicillin resistant *Staphylococcus aureus*). *Staphylococcus aureus* (*S aureus*) colonises areas of the skin such as the nostrils, the hairline, the umbilicus (navel) and the perineum (the area between the anus and the scrotum or vulva). MRSA is a **strain** of *S aureus*, so called because it is resistant to commonly used antibiotics. Like *S aureus*, MRSA does not cause infection unless it migrates into the body.

MRSA is usually acquired through contact with a person colonised with MRSA or with MRSA-contaminated environments or equipment. MRSA infections are most common in people in hospital who have a surgical wound or an in-dwelling device. If MRSA enters the body through a break in the skin it can cause infections such as boils, abscesses and impetigo. If it gets into the bloodstream it can cause more serious infections, such as septicaemia, septic arthritis, osteomyelitis, meningitis, pneumonia and endocarditis.

■ *Mycobacterium tuberculosis*, which causes tuberculosis (TB). *M tuberculosis* is usually acquired from an infected person who coughs and sneezes into the air around them. It can also be transmitted in milk from cows that are infected with Bovine Tuberculosis.

*M tuberculosis* most commonly affects the lungs, causing pulmonary TB, but it can affect parts of the body such as the lymph nodes, the skin and the bones. Signs and symptoms of pulmonary TB include fever, fatigue, weight loss, night sweats, a persistent cough that brings up blood-streaked phlegm, and pleurisy, which is an accumulation of fluid in the pleural cavity and partial collapse of the lung.

■ *Legionella pneumophila*, which causes Legionnaire's disease. *L pneumophila* lives in water, especially stagnant water such as in hot water supplies and air conditioning systems that re-circulate water. It can be acquired by healthy people staying in buildings in which the showers and air conditioning systems have become contaminated. However, elderly people, smokers and people with chest problems are especially at risk.

Legionnaire's disease is a pneumonia-type lung infection that causes fever, sweating, severe headache, shortness of breath, a cough that brings up thick, green, sometimes blood-streaked phlegm, chest pain, joint pain and muscle weakness. It can affect other organs and body systems but death is usually due to lung infection.

- *Clostridium tetani*, which produces a toxin that causes tetanus (lockjaw). The **spores** of *C tetani* are present in the soil and in the intestines and faeces of horses and other animals, and usually invade the body through a bite, cut or wound in the skin.

  Tetanus is muscle spasm, of, for example, the chewing muscles, making it hard to open the mouth (hence 'lockjaw'); the throat muscles, making it difficult to swallow; and the neck, chest, back and limb muscles. It can also cause fever, sore throat, rapid heartbeat, breathing difficulties, headache and bleeding into the bowels. Death is usually due to blood poisoning, asphyxia, cardiac arrest or kidney failure.

## Viruses

Viruses are ultramicroscopic infectious agents that are not alive but which can **replicate** themselves within the cells of living organisms.

Figure 39.3 Structure of a typical virus

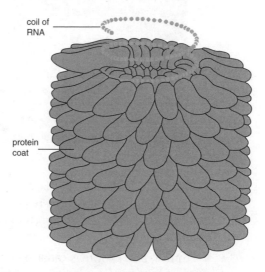

coil of RNA

protein coat

Pathogenic viruses include:

- Human Immunodeficiency Virus (HIV), which attacks cells of the immune system with the result that the body becomes immuno-deficient i.e. unable to defend against a range of infectious diseases. The condition of being unable to defend against a range of diseases is known as Acquired Immunodeficiency Syndrome (AIDS).

  HIV is carried in blood, semen, vaginal secretions and breast milk but not in tears, sweat, and saliva. People with AIDS initially experience flu-like symptoms, followed by any number of infectious diseases, including oral thrush, mouth ulcers, herpes zoster, skin infections, pneumonia, TB, infections of the brain, eyes and intestines, and severe body wasting.

- Hepatitis B Virus (HBV) or hep B is the virus that causes the disease hepatitis B. It is 50 to 100 times more infectious than HIV and is carried in body fluids such as blood, saliva, semen and vaginal secretions. The symptoms of hepatitis B are similar to severe flu, for example headache, fever, fatigue, aching limbs, loss of appetite, nausea and vomiting, stomach-ache and diarrhoea. Jaundice can develop, as can liver failure.

- Paramyxovirus, which causes measles (rubeola) and mumps. Once inside the body, this virus targets cells in the nose, throat and lungs, and then is carried in the blood throughout the body, including to the skin and the parotid salivary glands, which are located just below and in front of the ears. Signs and symptoms of measles include a runny nose, sneezing, watery eyes and swollen eyelids, red eyes and sensitivity to light, a mild to severe temperature, tiny greyish-white spots (Koplik's spots) in the mouth and throat, fatigue, aches and pains, a poor appetite and a dry cough. A red-brown spotty rash usually starts behind the ears, spreads around the head and neck, to the legs and around the rest of the body. The spots are small initially but grow and often join up together.

Signs and symptoms of mumps include a raised body temperature, swollen parotid glands which make the earlobes stick out, and pain when opening the mouth.

Figure 39.4 Mumps

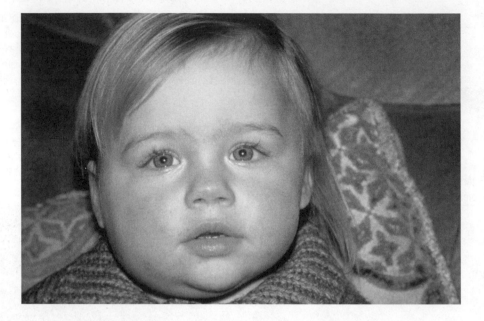

## Fungi

Fungi are plant-like organisms that feed off other organisms in order to survive. They include moulds and yeasts and cause infections such as thrush, athlete's foot and tinea (ringworm).

■ Thrush, also known as candida or candidosis, is a yeast-like fungal infection caused by the fungus *Candida albicans*. In women it can cause itching, irritation, soreness and swelling of the vagina and vulva as well as a thick white vaginal discharge; in men it can cause irritation and redness on the head of the penis; and in babies, signs include nappy rash and creamy yellow or white spots in and around the mouth that make the mouth sore.

Figure 39.5 Structure of typical moulds and yeasts

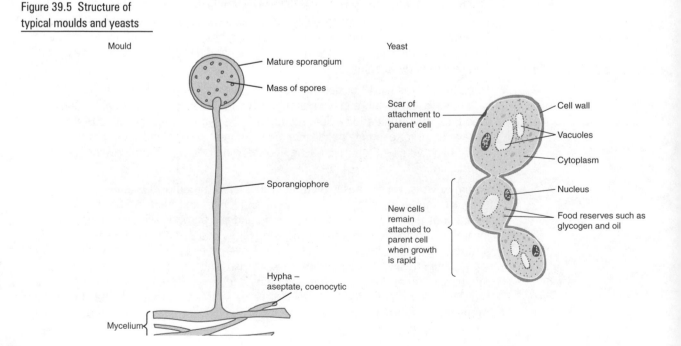

- Dermatophytosis, also known as tinea or ringworm is an infection of the skin, hair and nails caused by fungi called dermatophytes.

    - Tinea pedis or **athlete's foot** occurs when the fungus invades the dead outer layers of the skin, particularly between the toes where conditions are airless, warm and moist. Signs include cracked, sore, blistered skin and an itchy, scaly rash, which migrates from between the toes along the toes and to the soles.

    - Tinea capitis occurs on the scalp, where the fungus causes round, bald, itchy, scaly patches, with small, spreading papules (bumps) that can become inflamed and filled with pus.

    - Tinea corporis occurs on the body, where the fungus causes round or oval sores that are red, scaly and itchy. The patches gradually grow to about 1 inch across, when the central area heals, leaving a red ring on the skin. Sometimes one patch of infection occurs, sometimes there are several patches over the body.

Figure 39.6  Ringworm

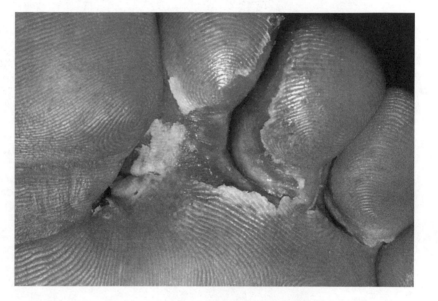

## Parasitic organisms and disease

Parasites are plants or animals that live, grow and feed on or in other living organisms.

Figure 39.7  Parasites

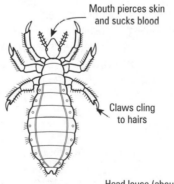
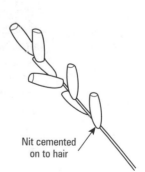

Mouth pierces skin and sucks blood

Claws cling to hairs

Head louse (about 3mm long)

Nit cemented on to hair

- Scabies is caused by a tiny mite called *Sarcoptes scabiei*. It is highly infectious and is spread where people live closely together. The female mite burrows into the outer layer of skin to lay its eggs, and as the **larvae** hatch and grow into mites, an allergic reaction sets in and the skin becomes blotchy and extremely itchy. The burrows appear as thin wavy lines about 2–10 mm long, usually between the fingers, on the wrists and elbows, in the armpits, under the breasts and on the male genitals. However, the blotches and itching are widespread over the body.

  Crusted scabies is where the skin thickens to form a crust, which can contain thousands of mites. It affects in particular older people and people with a deficient immune system.

- Head lice are tiny grey/brown insects that cling to hair close to the scalp from which they feed. Females lay eggs that hatch after 7–10 days, leaving empty white egg shells called nits that attach strongly to hair. Head lice can cause itching but this is due to an allergic reaction, not to biting.

- Pubic lice, sometimes known as crabs, are also tiny grey/brown insects. They attach strongly to pubic hair but can also attach to hair around the anus, in the armpits, and on the face, chest and legs. Females lay eggs which hatch into lice after about seven days. The main signs of pubic lice are itching in the affected areas, faint blue spots on nearby skin, and, if the eyelashes are affected, eye inflammation.

  Like scabies, both head and pubic lice are highly infectious and spread where people live closely together.

You can read more about infectious disease in Unit 12 (Public Health).

**Professional Practice**

When working with patients and service users it is important that you:

- are able to recognise the signs and symptoms of infectious disease

- let someone in authority know immediately you suspect the presence of an infectious disease.

## Growth of micro-organisms

Bacteria, fungi and parasites need a suitable environment in which to reside, and food, moisture, warmth and time to grow and reproduce. Because viruses aren't living organisms, they have no need for food, moisture and warmth, but they do need time and a suitable environment in which to replicate.

The reservoir of infection is the environment in or on which an infectious agent resides or which, if changed in some way, provides the right conditions for growth and reproduction of an invading micro-organism. Changes that encourage growth and reproduction may be brought about by, for example, the use of antibiotics and by fluctuations in acidity and oxygen level. You read about the effects of antibiotics and changes in acidity on the growth of micro-organisms earlier; changes in oxygen level in the intestines have a similar effect, favouring the growth of either **aerobic** or **anaerobic** bacteria.

Reservoirs of infection include:

- the body, particularly that of a susceptible host i.e. someone who is at risk of infection (see fig. 39.8)

- clothing, including uniforms and personal protective clothing such as masks and aprons

- body fluids, including blood, saliva, mucous and tears

- body waste, for example vomit, urine, faeces and menstrual blood

- equipment used in health and social care settings, such as sharps, commodes and protective clothing
- soiled linen, such as bedding and used dressings
- contaminated food and water
- the environment, for example floors, furniture, furnishings, mobility aids, dirt and dust
- animals, including pets and pests, for example ants, cockroaches, rats and mice
- plants and soil.

Figure 39.8  Susceptible hosts

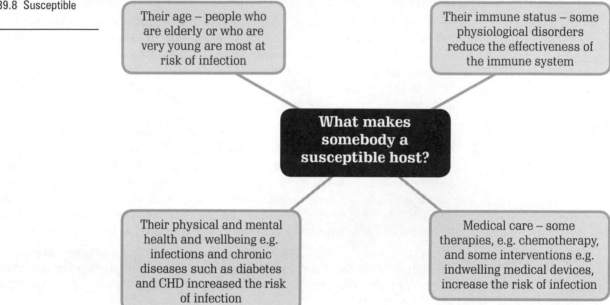

*Their age – people who are elderly or who are very young are most at risk of infection*

*Their immune status – some physiological disorders reduce the effectiveness of the immune system*

**What makes somebody a susceptible host?**

*Their physical and mental health and wellbeing e.g. infections and chronic diseases such as diabetes and CHD increased the risk of infection*

*Medical care – some therapies, e.g. chemotherapy, and some interventions e.g. indwelling medical devices, increase the risk of infection*

As you know, reservoirs have points of entry and exit. The body is the biggest reservoir for pathogenic micro-organisms and the most common source of infection. Different micro-organisms enter and exit the body in different ways.

Points of entry into the body include:

- the nose and mouth. For example, viruses that target the respiratory system such as the bacteria that cause TB and Legionnaire's disease are inhaled through the nose and mouth, and food poisoning bacteria such as salmonella are consumed in food or drink.
- the skin. For example, MRSA can enter the body through a surgical wound, the toxin that causes tetanus usually enters the body via a bite, cut or wound in the skin, and the scabies mite enters the body by burrowing into the skin.
- the site of an invasive procedure. For example, MRSA can enter the urinary tract during insertion of a catheter and the digestive tract during use of an endoscope.

Points of exit from the body include:

- body waste. For example, food poisoning bacteria exit the body in faeces and vomit.
- body fluids. For example, HIV and the hep B virus exit the body in body fluids such as blood and semen.
- the nose and mouth. For example, viruses that cause respiratory infections are exhaled or contained in mucus that is ejected from the nose and mouth.
- the skin. For example, MRSA is easily transferred from the skin to whatever it touches.

## Food

Bacteria, fungi and parasites need a readily available supply of nutrients to grow and reproduce, for example oxygen, carbon, hydrogen, nitrogen, phosphorous, sulphur, calcium and iron. Different organisms obtain their nutrients from different types of food, for example head lice obtain their nutrients from blood, which they get by biting through the scalp; dermatophytes obtain their nutrients from the dead outer layers of the skin; and many bacteria and fungi obtain their nutrients from food used for human consumption, such as meat, eggs and bread. Bacterial growth and toxin production on human food results in it being spoiled and, if consumed, causes food poisoning.

## Moisture

Micro-organisms also need moisture, which is why dehydration and adding sugar or salt to food, each of which makes water less available, are used in food preservation. Bacteria thrive in environments where there is a high moisture content, for example human tissues and air conditioning units, whereas some mould-like fungi can grow on dried foods.

## Temperature

An appropriate temperature is crucial for the growth of micro-organisms. As the temperature rises, they rapidly increase in size and number until it is too hot for survival. Similarly, as the temperature drops, growth and reproduction slow down until it is too cold for survival. Different micro-organisms stop growing and reproducing at different temperatures, but, in general, bacteria cease to grow at -10°C, fungi at about -18°C, and most are killed by temperatures exceeding 63°C. For these reasons, freezers should be maintained at below −18°C and food should be cooked at temperatures above 63°C.

When conditions are unfavourable, such as during a drought and when temperatures are high, bacteria that are not killed either become dormant (inactive) or develop a protective spore. With the return of favourable conditions, they become active again and start to grow.

## Time

In ideal conditions, bacteria reproduce by dividing into two approximately every twenty minutes. This means that after six hours, one bacterium could become over 130,000. When bacteria invade a new environment, they need time to adjust before they start to grow. This time is called the lag phase and lasts about one hour. For this reason, recommended times for, for example, transferring material such as food and specimens from one environment to another, storing, cooking and serving food, and the maintenance of hot water supplies and air conditioning systems must be observed.

| | |
|---|---|
| Health information. | Health factsheets. |
| www.patient.co.uk | hcd2.bupa.co.uk |
| NHS Direct. | Health information. |
| www.nhsdirect.nhs.uk | www.netdoctor.co.uk |
| The Health Protection Agency. | Environmental charity. |
| www.hpa.org.uk | www.encams.org |
| Sexual health information. | The Drinking Water Inspectorate |
| www.thewellproject.org | www.dwi.gov.uk |

# Spread of micro-organisms

Micro-organisms are spread in a number of ways.

Table 39.1 The spread of micro-organisms

| Method of spread | Notes | Examples of diseases |
|---|---|---|
| Contact | Contact includes touch by hand, in particular by the fingers. Touch plays a major part in the spread of infection:<br>■ touching wounds, lesions, rashes, **mucous membranes** and so on can result in the direct transfer of micro-organisms from one person to another.<br>■ touching infected equipment, body fluids and waste and material such as soiled linen can result in the indirect transfer of micro-organisms from one person to another.<br>Close person-to-person contact, for example sexual and head-to-head contact, can also result in the direct transfer of micro-organisms from one person to another. | ■ MRSA, impetigo, TB, HIV/AIDS, hep B.<br><br>■ HIV/AIDS, hep B.<br><br>■ Scabies, lice, fleas, HIV/AIDS, hep B. |
| Droplet | Infectious agents are spread in droplets of liquid that are expelled when an infected person coughs, sneezes and talks. Infectious droplets can be inhaled, in which case they infect the mucous membranes of the respiratory tract; and they can infect the conjunctivae, the membrane that covers the eye. | Viral gastroenteritis, influenza, German measles, mumps and whooping cough. |
| Flies | Flies carry micro-organisms in their mouth parts, their saliva, on their feet and in their faeces. The micro-organisms they carry are spread through biting, ejecting saliva onto a source of food in order to dissolve and suck it up, and when they land. | African trypanosomiasis (sleeping sickness), a parasitic infection which is carried in the saliva of the tsetse fly; and trachoma, a bacterial infection that causes a conjunctivitis-type discharge from the eyes. The discharge attracts flies that subsequently land on other people's skin. |
| Fomites | A fomite is an inanimate object that can become contaminated with infectious micro-organisms and spread them to other people. Fomites include the general environment, furniture, furnishings, bedding, clothing, masks, bedpans, urinals, toilets, manual handling and mobility aids, medical instruments and so on. | Ringworm, influenza, MRSA and *Clostridium difficile*, a bacterial infection that causes mild to severe diarrhoea. Most infections of *C difficile* occur in hospitals and care homes. |
| Faeces | Many micro-organisms, their eggs and spores exit the body in the faeces. Spread of infection carried by faeces usually results from hand-to-mouth transmission following, for example, using the toilet, dealing with a faecal spill and emptying a bedpan.<br><br>Animal faeces can also carry micro-organisms, which are spread through direct faecal contact and contact with contaminated inanimate objects such as the soles of shoes and the wheels of toys. | *Clostridium difficile*, diarrhoeal illnesses and gastroenteritis that are spread by hand-to-mouth; and pinworms and threadworms, the eggs of which are transferred to the mouth after scratching the anal area.<br>    Human toxocariasis, an infection due to hand-to-mouth contact with dog faeces containing the eggs of the parasitic roundworm toxocariasis; and the diarrhoeal condition caused by the bacterium *Campylobacter*. |
| Air | Some micro-organisms and their spores can remain suspended in the air for long periods before they are inhaled. | Diarrhoeal illnesses, TB, chickenpox, diphtheria and measles. |
| Dust | Dust and soil are a reservoir for fungi and bacteria and their spores, and for the eggs of parasites. | The parasitic infection *Toxocariasis* and the bacterial infections Multi-resistant *Acinetobacter* (MRAB), tetanus and anthrax. Also psittacosis, which is a bacterial infection of birds that is spread by the dust in their feathers. |
| Water | Contaminated water can spread micro-organisms when it is drunk, inhaled (as steam) and used for cleaning hands, food, wounds, equipment and so on. | The bacterial infections Legionnaire's disease, dysentery, leptospirosis and pseudomonas, and the parasitic infection cryptosporidiosis. |
| Food | Food becomes contaminated if isn't handled (stored, prepared, cooked and served) safely. Contamination is spread through ingestion. | Hepatitis A and bacterial food poisoning conditions such as those caused by *Campylobacter, E coli, Salmonella, Bacillus cereus, Clostridium perfringens* and *Staphylococcus*. |

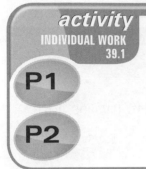

Produce health promotional materials, for example posters or information leaflets, for a target group of your own choice, for example teenagers or elderly people, which describe how a named bacterial, viral and fungal infection is:

■ caused.

■ spread.

# How to prevent and control the spread of infection

## Standard precautions

Standard precautions underpin the prevention and control of infection. By applying standard precautions in their work, people who work with patients and users of social care services minimise the risk of spread of infection.

### Hand hygiene

Hand hygiene or decontamination aims to reduce the risk of the hands being a reservoir of infection and is the single most important activity in reducing the spread of infection. Patients and service users, their visitors and health and social care staff have a responsibility to maintain hand hygiene and to remind each other to do so.

Patients and service users should clean their hands:

■ before eating

■ after they have used the commode or visited the bathroom for any reason, for example to use the toilet, change soiled clothing or replace sanitary wear.

Visitors should clean their hands:

■ when they arrive and when they leave a ward

■ before touching food if they are involved in helping a patient or service user to eat

■ after using the bathroom (see above).

Figure 39.9 Standard precautions

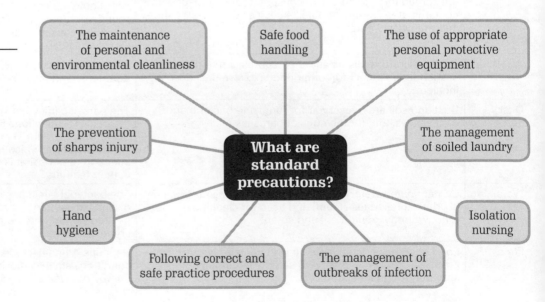

Health and social care staff should clean their hands:

- before and after each work shift and break
- before eating and drinking and before and after serving food and helping patients and service users to eat
- between contact with different patients and service users
- before putting on and after removing protective clothing, including gloves
- after using bathroom facilities and after touching themselves, for example to blow their nose or cover a sneeze
- before and after direct physical contact with a patient
- after any activity that could result in their hands becoming contaminated, for example after contact with body fluids, soiled linen and used equipment such as dressings, sharps, urinals, commodes and urine drainage bags
- before and after smoking.

In addition, staff should keep their nails short and clean, not wear nail polish, artificial nails, wrist watches and jewellery that could harbour infectious agents, and cover any cuts and abrasions with a blue waterproof dressing or plaster.

Hand hygiene can be maintained by using alcohol gels, soap and water, and antiseptics. The use of alcohol gels should be routine but hands that are visibly dirty must be washed with soap and water and dried thoroughly. Antiseptic hand washes are used to disinfect hands in high risk areas, where there is an outbreak of an infection and prior to invasive procedures, such as surgery and insertion of a catheter.

The correct hand washing technique using soap and water is as follows:

1. Wet hands with warm running water and rub some soap between the palms.
2. Rub the right palm over the back of the left hand and then the left palm over the back of the right hand.
3. Rub the palms together again but this time with the fingers interlocked.
4. Rub the back of the fingers of the left hand with the right palm and then the back of the fingers of the right hand with the left palm.
5. Rub around the left thumb with the right palm and then around the right thumb with the left palm.
6. Rub the left fingertips round and round in the right palm then the right fingertips round and round in the left palm.
7. Rub the left wrist with the right hand then the right wrist with the left hand.
8. Rinse hands thoroughly under running water and dry them carefully.

Figure 39.10 The correct hand washing technique

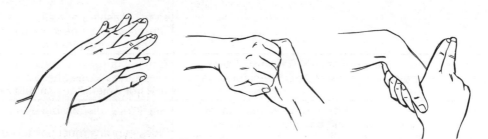

Improper drying can re-contaminate clean hands. The correct technique for effective hand drying depends on the use of good quality disposable paper hand towels to:

1. dry the palms and backs of the hands

2. dry between the fingers

3. dry around and under the nails.

Frequent hand decontamination can dry the skin, and some soaps, alcohol gels and antiseptic hand washes can cause irritation. Skin care can be achieved by:

- using an emollient hand cream, which softens and soothes the skin and protects it from drying – but note that hand creams should not be shared because of the risk of cross infection

- getting advice from the occupational health team in the event of skin irritation or conditions such as eczema or psoriasis.

Facilities for effective hand washing and drying must be available in all areas where infection may be present and should be as close to the 'point of care' as possible i.e. near the place where activities with patient and service users are carried out. Wash hand basins should have mixer taps that can be operated by elbow or wrist levers; there should be wall-mounted liquid soap dispensers and dispensers containing paper hand towels; and there should be foot-operated pedal bins for the disposal of used towels. Everyone has a responsibility to report a lack of or inappropriately placed hand washing and drying facilities to an appropriate person.

> **remember**
>
> Hand hygiene is the single most important activity in reducing the spread of infection.

## Appropriate personal protective equipment

The aim of wearing personal protective equipment is to protect both worker and patient from the risks of cross-infection; and what makes for appropriate personal protective equipment (PPE) depends on the kind of activity being undertaken.

Table 39.2 Appropriate personal protective equipment

| Activity | Appropriate PPE |
| --- | --- |
| Procedures that may cause exposure to blood and body fluids and waste; procedures that involve contact with skin lesions and mucous membranes; and invasive procedures, including surgery. | Single use (one procedure or one **episode of patient care**), well-fitting, disposable gloves, which must be put on immediately before the procedure or episode of care and removed and disposed of as soon as the activity is completed. Non-sterile gloves should be used when there is potential contact with blood, body-fluids or equipment contaminated with body-fluids; sterile gloves should be used where there is contact with skin lesions, mucous membranes and where a procedure is invasive. Note – washing gloves is NOT safe practice, and hands must always be decontaminated before putting on and after removing gloves. |
| Cleaning instruments prior to sterilisation and during contact with potentially contaminated items or surfaces. | General-purpose rubber household gloves. Unlike single use gloves, these can be washed with detergent and hot water. They should be disposed of weekly. |
| Direct patient/service user care; procedures that may cause exposure to blood and body fluids and waste; procedures that involve contact with skin lesions and mucous membranes; invasive procedures; contact with patients and service users who have an infection; bed-making; decontaminating equipment. | Single use, disposable plastic aprons. Note – aprons must be stored in such a way that they don't accumulate dust that can act as a reservoir, and hands must always be decontaminated before putting on and after removing aprons. |
| Procedures where there is a risk of extensive splashing of blood or body fluids or waste onto the worker's skin or clothing. | Full-body-fluid-repellent gowns. Note – hands must always be decontaminated before putting on and after removing full-body gowns. |

| Activity | Appropriate PPE |
|----------|-----------------|
| Procedures that may splash the face, eyes or mouth with blood or body fluids or waste, including when equipment is being manually decontaminated; procedures that involve contact with patients and service users who have an infection or when an infection is suspected. | Face masks and eye protection, which must fit correctly, be handled as little as possible and be changed between patients and service users or procedures.<br><br>Note – masks must be disposed of immediately after use and hands must always be decontaminated before putting on and after removing masks and eye protection. |
| Procedures that involve contact with a patient who has an air-borne infection, for example multi drug resistant tuberculosis (MDRTB) and severe acute respiratory syndrome (SARS). | Respiratory protective equipment, which should be cleaned and disposed of according to the manufacturer's instructions. |

## General cleanliness

The general cleanliness of health and social care settings is dependent on the effective decontamination of the environment, materials and equipment, and also on the personal cleanliness of patients, service users, their visitors and health and social care workers. Although different individuals have different ideas about what makes for good personal hygiene, dirt of any description on the body and on and in clothing can be a reservoir for infection. Because of this, very high standards of personal cleanliness must be maintained in health and social care settings at all times.

Figure 39.11 Maintaining personal cleanliness

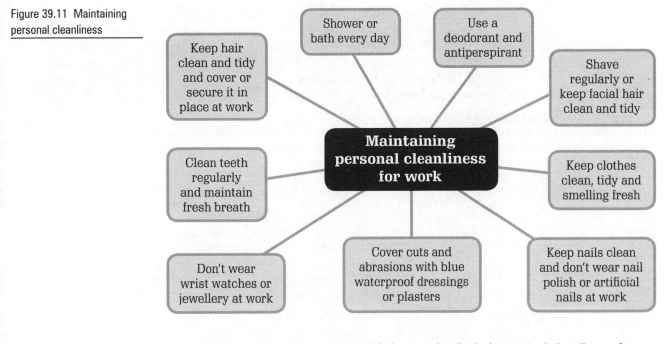

Many patients and service users need help to maintain their personal cleanliness, for example, people with limited movement or mobility may need help to shower or bath, shave, dress, wash their hair and clean themselves after using the toilet; people with a sight impairment may need help to maintain cleanliness when eating; and people who are ill or confined to bed may need help to empty a catheter bag or change an incontinence pad. Health and social care workers who support people with their personal care have a responsibility to do so in such a way that promotes their dignity and upholds their privacy.

## Green Gables

Green Gables is a residential care home for young men and women with profound learning difficulties. Many have sensory impairments and some have physiological conditions that make movement and mobility difficult. All of the residents have problems maintaining personal cleanliness.

- What sort of help do the residents of Green Gables need in order to maintain their personal cleanliness?
- How might this help be given such that their right to dignity and privacy is upheld?

Dirty, dusty health and social care environments are also reservoirs for infection and so must be kept clean to the highest possible standard. The *NHS Healthcare Cleaning Manual* (NHS Estates) describes the correct way to maintain the **general cleanliness of the environment**, including cleaning kitchens, washrooms, toilets, isolation rooms, floors, walls, glass, furniture and so on. Whilst the Cleaning Manual has been written with hospitals in mind, the methods can be applied to social care settings as well.

There are three categories of cleaning or decontamination:

1. cleaning, which physically removes but doesn't necessarily destroy micro-organisms. Manual cleaning materials and equipment include chemicals such as detergent and bleach, dusters, cloths, mops, buckets, aprons and gloves. Automatic and mechanical equipment used for cleaning includes floor polishers, vacuum cleaners, washing machines and **autoclaves**. Automatic and mechanical cleaning methods are more effective and efficient than manual methods and should be used in preference where possible.

2. disinfection, which reduces the number of **viable** micro-organisms but doesn't necessarily **inactivate** certain viruses and bacterial spores

3. sterilisation, which destroys all micro-organisms, including viruses and spores.

You will read about disinfection and sterilisation techniques shortly.

Cleaning, disinfection and sterilisation can be hazardous activities, for example some chemicals used for cleaning present slip hazards if spilled; and some are toxic (poisonous), flammable, caustic or irritant, and as a result can cause respiratory problems such as asthma and skin conditions such as dermatitis and burns. Electrical equipment can cause electric shocks, fires and burns; and trailing flexes are a trip hazard, as are pieces of equipment such as mops and buckets if left lying around.

The following Five Top Tips sum up how health and social care workers can help maintain the highest standards of cleanliness in their workplace as well as support the health and safety of everyone concerned.

Five Top Tips for maintaining the cleanliness of a health and social care setting:

1. Observe and monitor the general cleanliness of the environment and report any concerns about the level of cleanliness to an appropriate person. Also encourage patients, service users and their visitors to observe and monitor environmental cleanliness and report their concerns.

2. Carry out cleaning according to the 'cleaning frequency schedule' (or as requested), using the correct materials and equipment for the task. Good practice dictates the use of colour coding, which links cleaning materials and equipment with specific areas, such as:

- red for bathroom and toilet facilities and floors
- blue for general areas
- green for catering areas
- white for isolation areas and operating theatres
- yellow for wash basins and washroom surfaces.

This ensures that materials and equipment are not used in multiple areas, which in turn helps reduce the risk of cross-infection. Workers who are colour blind should be given alternative methods of linking cleaning materials and equipment with specific areas.

3. Before starting a cleaning activity, identify any risks that prevent the activity from being carried out, including those to do with the cleaning materials and equipment; report any new risks to an appropriate person; if safe to do so, adapt the cleaning method, otherwise restrict access to the risk area until it has been made safe.

4. When carrying out cleaning activities, always follow workplace safe practice procedures. For example, work from the cleanest area to the dirtiest area; always use cleaning materials according to the manufacturer's instructions; use appropriate PPE, which protects against injury from hazardous materials as well as reducing cross-infection; keep the area in which you are working as safe and free from hazards as possible; and put up hazard warning signs when the cleaning activity or cleaned surfaces are likely to cause a risk to people.

5. When the cleaning activity is complete, follow workplace safe practice procedures. For example, return all materials and equipment in good working order and in a clean condition to the appropriate storage place; report any equipment defects or failures to an appropriate person; and remove and dispose of PPE as appropriate.

Figure 39.12 Follow safe practice procedures

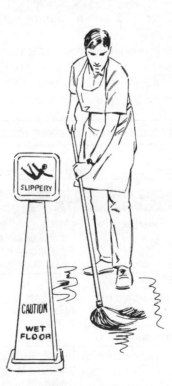

## Isolation nursing

Some infections, such as those spread by droplets and contaminated food or water, spread very readily. Others, such as MRSA, have developed resistance to some of the antibiotics used to help prevent their spread. In order to contain the spread of infection, infected individuals and those who are at particular risk of infection need to be isolated. Isolation nursing is the practice whereby individuals are cared for, usually in a single room where the door can be closed, or, if a number of people are involved, together in one area of the care setting.

The principles of isolation nursing require the following safe practice procedures to be followed:

- Workers must wear appropriate PPE such as plastic aprons, disposable gloves and masks.

- Hand hygiene facilities must be available at the point of care, with a wall-mounted anti-bacterial hand-cleaning gel dispenser for the use of workers and of visitors when they enter and leave the room or area.

- En-suite facilities must include a toilet; and, where patients have infectious diarrhoea, they must have sole use of the toilet, which must be thoroughly cleaned after each use.

- A notice must be placed at the entrance to the patient's room or by their bed, listing the special precautions being taken and treatment being given.

- An assessment must be made of who may visit. For example, pregnant women should be asked to stay away if the patient has chicken pox or shingles; and babies, elderly people and visitors who are sick themselves should not visit as they are susceptible hosts.

## Immunisation and occupational health

Because of the susceptible host nature of patients and service users, the unknown state of health of visitors, and the nature of the work carried out in health and social care settings, all health and social care organisations should have policies in place to protect everyone involved against cross infection through immunisation. They should also have policies in place that enable workers access to occupational health services, for example, for advice regarding the vaccinations they need and when they should receive them, and screening for the presence of an infectious disease.

You can read more about immunisation and screening in Unit 12 (Public health).

Table 39.3  Immunisation and important diseases

| Disease | Who should be immunised? |
| --- | --- |
| Influenza | Health and social care staff, especially those who work with older people; everyone living in long-stay care settings where a rapid spread of infection is likely; everyone over 65 years; everyone with a chronic medical condition such as heart or respiratory disease. |
| Pneumococcal infections, e.g. pneumonia, septicaemia and meningitis | Everyone over 65 years; everyone under 65 years who is in a medical risk group, e.g. those who have a weak immune system, a heart or lung condition, liver disease or diabetes mellitus. |
| Hepatitis B | Health and social care staff who have contact with patients'/service users' blood, blood stained body fluids and body tissues; people who receive blood or blood products, and their carers; patients with chronic renal failure or liver disease; people who work or live with people with learning difficulties. |
| Tuberculosis (BCG vaccine) | Health and social care workers who have contact with TB patients; people who live with people who have TB; people under 35 years who are tuberculin-negative following **Mantoux testing**. |

| Disease | Who should be immunised? |
|---|---|
| Tetanus | Older health and social care workers and older residents of care homes who may not have been immunised against tetanus in childhood or received booster doses. |
| Rubella (German measles) | All women of child-bearing age. |
| Measles | All health and social care workers. |
| Poliomyelitis | All health and social care workers. |
| Chicken pox | Non-immune health and social care workers who have direct contact with patients/service users. |

## Prevention of sharps injury

Sharp instruments (sharps) include needles, scalpel blades, stitch cutters and glass ampoules. A sharps accident happens when blood or body fluids are transferred from a sharp instrument onto, for example, an open cut, skin abrasion or mucous membrane. Sharps accidents are very common but prevention of sharps injury relies on the use of:

- safe practice procedures when handling and storing sharp instruments
- the correct procedure for their disposal.

You will read about procedures for handling, storage and disposal of sharps shortly.

## Management of outbreaks of infection

Despite having appropriate preventative and safety measures in place, outbreaks of infection can and do occur. Management of outbreaks of infection necessitates strict observation of the standard precautions used to prevent and control further spread of the disease, including:

- isolating infected individuals and restricting visitors as appropriate
- using good hand hygiene and appropriate PPE
- taking care with sharps and their disposal
- immunising non-immune health and social care workers who have direct contact with infected individuals.

In addition, GPs should be informed; specimens and secretions should be sent to the pathology laboratory in appropriate, leak-proof containers enclosed in a sealed polythene bag, with a form that identifies the patient and the test required; infected individuals should be admitted to hospital if appropriate; and, in the event of an outbreak of:

- certain infectious diseases in the community or residential care homes, the local authority's Health Protection Unit (HPU), Environmental Health Officer (EHO) or Consultant in Communicable Disease Control (CCDC) should be notified (Public Health (Control of Disease) Act 1984 and the Public Health (Infectious Diseases) Regulations 1988).
- a health care associated infection (HCAI) in hospital, the Health Protection Agency (HPA) should be informed (The Health Act 2006).

You will read about notifiable diseases, HCAIs, and the procedures for their notification and reporting shortly.

## Food handling

As you know, food and water can be a reservoir of infection, and incorrect storage, preparation and cooking can encourage the bacterial growth and toxin production that result in food poisoning. For this reason, safe food handling is crucial for the prevention and control of the spread of infection. Some foods pose more of a risk than others, for example:

- raw eggs, as some are infected with the food poisoning bacterium *Salmonella*. Eggs served to susceptible hosts should be thoroughly cooked.

- pâté, soft cheese and cook-chill foods, which can be a breeding ground for listeria, a bacterium that grows at low temperatures and which can damage a developing foetus and cause septicaemia, meningitis and encephalitis

- unpasteurised milk, which may contain the food poisoning bacteria *verocytotoxin-producing E-coli* (VTEC), *Salmonella* and *Campylobacter*

- undercooked or raw food, which may contain food poisoning bacteria and parasites such as *Cryptosporidium parvuum*

- shellfish, which can trigger life-threatening allergic reactions as well as cause food poisoning

- fruit and vegetables, the skin of which can be contaminated with, for example, fertilisers and pesticides.

Mains supply tap water in the UK is generally of a very high quality. However, to reduce the risk of contamination, mains-fed water coolers and ice-making machines should be regularly maintained and cleaned.

Health and social care workers who are involved in food handling are required to undergo training.

Figure 39.13 Food handling training

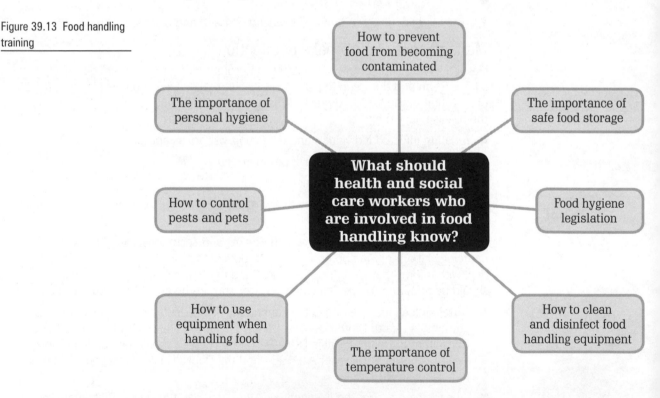

Food can become contaminated biologically, by bacteria and their toxins; physically, for example, by jewellery and pens falling into food as it is being handled; and chemically, for example by washing up liquid and bleach if they are not used carefully. For these reasons, everyone handling food has a duty to ensure that they maintain a high standard of personal hygiene, that they dress appropriately and that they follow safe practice procedures when using chemicals in food handling areas.

Prevention of food contamination and spread of infection is assured by storing and cooking food at the right temperature and, if appropriate, according to the instructions on the packet. In brief:

- Always store food according to the instructions on the packet, for example in a cool, dry place; and throw food away as soon it is past its 'use by' date.

- Ensure that freezers are kept at less than -18°C and that frozen food is defrosted in the fridge.

- Ensure that fridges are kept at less than 5°C, and that raw and cooked foods are covered and stored in different fridges. If there is only one fridge, store raw foods on lower shelves than cooked foods.

- Use a food thermometer or a clean skewer to check that food is thoroughly cooked and piping hot before serving. If food has to be cooked in advance, keep it covered and at 63°C and above until it's time to eat.

> **remember**
>
> 5°C to 63°C is the Temperature Danger Zone! Most bacteria thrive in the Temperature Danger Zone so store food below 5°C or above 63°C.

Prevention of food contamination and spread of infection is also ensured by using different equipment for raw and cooked foods, keeping equipment thoroughly clean, ensuring that food and drink are served onto clean crockery using clean utensils; and by controlling pets and pests in food storage and handling areas by:

- maintaining high standards of cleanliness – sweep floors, wipe up spills, wash and store equipment properly

- keeping doors and windows closed or using fly screens

- keeping food and waste covered

- emptying waste bins regularly.

Should there be any signs of infestation, inform the local authority Environmental Health Department straightaway and throw out any food that might have been spoiled.

Food Safety legislation is in place to ensure that food contamination and spread of infection are minimised; and workplace safe practice procedures, which are based on legislation, tell food handlers how to do their job in ways that comply with the law and that promote health and safety. You will read about food safety legislation in the next section.

## Soiled laundry management

Because soiled linen can also be a reservoir of infection, every care setting should have safe practice procedures for soiled linen management. In general, when dealing with soiled linen:

- use appropriate, disposable PPE

- remove PPE and linen from the individual or their bed carefully and place it in the correct colour-coded bag to be taken away for decontamination. Colour coding of bags for differently soiled linen enables segregation and thus prevents the spread of infection, for example:

  - lightly soiled linen and clothing should go into a white cotton sack

  - heavily soiled and infected linen should go into a red cotton sack.

Never put soiled linen on the floor.

- take the bags to the laundry via the 'dirty' entrance

- place the inner, water-soluble bags in the washing machine and launder with detergent at the highest temperature possible for the item

- use an industrial dryer and a hot iron if appropriate

- store clean linen above floor level in a designated area.

Uniforms, which should be changed daily, must be washed at 65°C for at least ten minutes.

Standard precautions underpin the prevention and control of infection, and health and social care workers have a responsibility to apply the following standard precautions in their work:

- maintain hand hygiene
- use appropriate PPE
- ensure the maintenance of personal and environmental cleanliness
- use the services of occupational health personnel
- follow correct and safe practice procedures in order to prevent sharps injuries and when handling food, dealing with soiled laundry and managing outbreaks of infection.

## Procedures for handling, storage and disposal of waste

### Sharps

Whilst back injuries are the most common cause of occupational injury amongst health and social care workers, sharps injuries run a close second, the main hazards being hepatitis B and C, and HIV. To reduce the risk of injury, sharps must be handled, stored and disposed of safely and carefully.

10 top tips for the safe handling, storage and disposal of sharps:

1. Know and follow safe practice procedures at all times.
2. Know what to do in the event of a sharps injury.
3. Store unused sharps safely, away from the public and out of reach of children.
4. Use your common sense and take responsibility for the way you use and dispose of sharps – be careful, pay attention, don't hurry.
5. Keep sharps handling to a minimum and avoid any actions that are likely to cause an injury, such as pointing a sharp towards the hand or passing one from hand-to-hand.
6. Don't dismantle sharps such as syringes by hand, and never re-sheathe or bend needles.
7. Dispose of used sharps as single units and at the point of use.
8. Dispose of used sharps straight away into the correct colour-coded bin, which should be a yellow, puncture-resistant, leakproof container that conforms to UN standard 3291 and British Standard 7320 and that is clearly marked with the words 'Danger', 'Contaminated sharps' and 'Destroy by **incineration**' or 'To be incinerated'.
9. Don't fill sharps containers more than three quarters full, and drop sharps in carefully – don't push them down.
10. Store sharps containers away from the public.

If you notice that safe practice procedures are not being followed properly, inform an appropriate individual such as a member of the infection control team, whose role is to provide training on the safe handling, storage and disposal of sharps.

### Household waste

Everyone involved with the disposal of household waste i.e. non-clinical, non-contaminated waste, such as non-contaminated food waste, paper, flowers, packaging, cans, bottles, plastic and stationery has a responsibility to handle waste safely, store waste securely and ensure that waste is passed on to a registered carrier (waste collection organisation).

General household waste should be disposed of in the correct colour-coded bag i.e. black plastic bags, which should be stored in spill-proof, lidded, labelled containers in a secure place to await removal by the registered carrier. Broken glass, other breakages and aerosols should be put in heavy duty clear plastic bags in boxes labelled 'Glass and breakages only' and 'Aerosols only' respectively.

## Clinical/hazardous waste

Clinical/hazardous waste is defined as any material that has the potential to put health at risk. Good practice dictates that:

- safe practice procedures must be followed when handling, storing and disposing of clinical/hazardous waste

- foot-operated bag holders should be available in areas where waste is likely to be produced

- areas where waste is produced should display a wall chart that shows the correct colour-coded bag to be used for different types of waste (see Table 39.4). Workers who are colour blind should be given alternative methods of identifying the correct bags to be used for different types of waste.

Table 39.4  The disposal of clinical waste

| Type of waste | Method of disposal |
|---|---|
| Soiled surgical dressings; contaminated waste from treatment areas; material other than linen where an infectious disease has been diagnosed; human tissues, swabs and dressings from laboratories. | Yellow bags, which *must* be **incinerated**. |
| Used tampons and sanitary towels. | If available, dedicated sanibins that are emptied by registered carriers; otherwise yellow bags for incineration. |
| Incontinence pads; used but empty disposable bed-pans, bed-pan liners, incontinence aids, stoma and colostomy bags. | **Maceration** if available; otherwise, if the risk to health is high, yellow bags for incineration; if the risk to health is lower, orange bags, which are taken by a registered carrier for treatment. |
| Non-infected waste. | Yellow bags with black stripes (tiger bags), which can be sent to landfill sites. |

To ensure the prevention and control of spread of infection, yellow and orange bags must be kept separate from black bags, and storage areas must not be accessible to unauthorised people and animals. Storage areas must be fully cleaned and disinfected weekly, although accidental spillages must be cleaned up immediately.

## Biological spillages

Blood and body fluids and waste are potential reservoirs of infection, thus any accidental spillages must be cleaned up straightaway. Health and social care workers should have an awareness of the hazards associated with blood and body fluids and waste as these shape the safe practice procedures they must follow when dealing with a spill. In general, when dealing with biological spillages:

- use appropriate PPE

- use the correct cleaning materials and equipment for the type of spill and the surface on which the spill has happened, for example, carpet or mattress

- use the correct cleaning technique for decontaminating the materials and equipment used for dealing with a spill

- use the correct method of disposal for the cleaning materials and equipment used for dealing with a spill.

Contamination injuries are caused by spillages of high-risk body fluids into the skin, eyes or mouth, for example when the skin is punctured by a bite or a used sharps, and when there is a splash of body fluids. High risk body fluids include blood, blood stained body fluids, amniotic fluid, vaginal secretions, semen, breast milk and saliva, and the main hazards are the viral infections Hepatitis B and C, and HIV. Like biological spillages, contamination injuries must be dealt with straightaway.

A biological spill and any first aid measures must be reported and recorded and occupational health personnel asked for advice regarding the need for vaccination. You will learn about record keeping in relation to infection shortly.

Figure 39.14 Dealing with contamination injuries

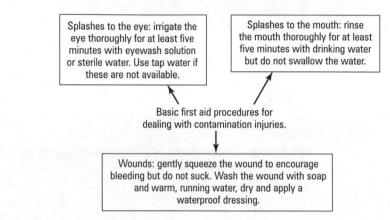

Splashes to the eye: irrigate the eye thoroughly for at least five minutes with eyewash solution or sterile water. Use tap water if these are not available.

Splashes to the mouth: rinse the mouth thoroughly for at least five minutes with drinking water but do not swallow the water.

Basic first aid procedures for dealing with contamination injuries.

Wounds: gently squeeze the wound to encourage bleeding but do not suck. Wash the wound with soap and warm, running water, dry and apply a waterproof dressing.

## Decontamination techniques

You read earlier that there are three categories of cleaning or decontamination – cleaning, disinfection and sterilisation. This section looks more closely at the different decontamination techniques used for low risk, medium risk and high risk equipment and medical devices.

### Cleaning

Cleaning uses hot water and enzyme-containing detergent to physically remove visible contamination. It doesn't necessarily destroy micro-organisms and so is used to decontaminate low risk equipment i.e. equipment that does not touch broken skin or mucous membranes, such as floors and furniture, and mobility aids such as hoists, wheelchairs and walking frames.

Low risk equipment must be thoroughly cleaned and dried after each use and individuals responsible for ensuring cleanliness must follow safe practice procedures at all times.

### Disinfection

Disinfection is used to decontaminate medium-risk equipment i.e. equipment that touches intact skin or mucous membranes, such as bedpans, urinals and commodes. It uses heat or chemicals to reduce the number of viable micro-organisms but doesn't necessarily inactivate all viruses and bacterial spores.

Heat is a more effective disinfectant than chemicals and is used in ultra-sonic cleaners and washer disinfectors, which combine high temperatures and detergents to clean and disinfect, for example, instruments that may be damaged by chemicals. Chemical disinfection is used when equipment can not be heat-disinfected and cleaning alone is not sufficient. Chemicals used as disinfectants include formaldehyde, peroxide, iodine- and ammonium-containing products, sodium hypochlorite, chlorhexidine, phenol and alcohol. Because they are hazardous, the use of chemical disinfectants is regulated by the Control of Substances Hazardous to Health (COSHH) 2002 regulations, which you will read about shortly.

Medium risk equipment must be cleaned and disinfected between each use and everyone who uses disinfectants must be trained in their use and follow safe practice procedures and the manufacturer's instructions at all times.

## Sterilisation

Sterilisation destroys all micro-organisms, including viruses and spores, and is therefore the chosen method for decontaminating high risk equipment, for example instruments that are used for invasive techniques such as touching a break in the skin or mucous membranes, penetrating the skin or entering the body. Sterilisation is often carried out by local Sterile Services Departments (SSD) but where SSD are not available, pre-sterilised, single-use, disposable items should be used or alternatives such as autoclaves and bench top steam sterilisers.

High risk equipment must be cleaned and sterilised after each use and left in a sterile state for subsequent use. Everyone using sterilisers must be trained in their use and follow safe practice procedures and the manufacturer's instructions at all times.

Organisations that provide health and social care services are obliged to have a cleaning, disinfection and sterilisation policy, the aim of which is to provide guidance on decontamination techniques, thereby ensuring that all re-usable equipment is properly decontaminated and that the risks associated with decontamination are properly managed.

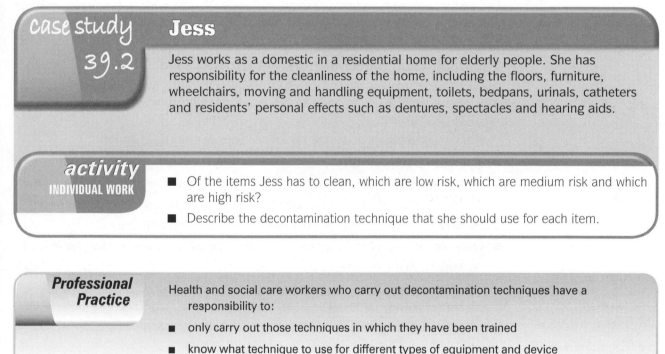

**case study 39.2**

### Jess

Jess works as a domestic in a residential home for elderly people. She has responsibility for the cleanliness of the home, including the floors, furniture, wheelchairs, moving and handling equipment, toilets, bedpans, urinals, catheters and residents' personal effects such as dentures, spectacles and hearing aids.

**activity**
**INDIVIDUAL WORK**

- Of the items Jess has to clean, which are low risk, which are medium risk and which are high risk?
- Describe the decontamination technique that she should use for each item.

**Professional Practice**

Health and social care workers who carry out decontamination techniques have a responsibility to:

- only carry out those techniques in which they have been trained
- know what technique to use for different types of equipment and device
- follow safe practice procedures and manufacturer's instructions at all times.

Royal College of Nursing
www.rcn.org.uk
National Patient Safety Agency
www.npsa.nhs.uk
Health Protection Agency
www.hpa.org.uk
Department of Health
www.dh.gov.uk

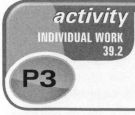

activity
INDIVIDUAL WORK
39.2

**P3**

Produce an information leaflet to be available to either nursing or social care staff that describes the standard precautions for the prevention and control of infection in a health or social care workplace.

# Legislation relevant to infection prevention and control

## Legislation, regulations and guidance that govern infection prevention and control

There is a wealth of legislation designed to prevent and control the spread of infection. This section aims to introduce you to the key points of various legislative regulations and guidelines and to develop your understanding of how they are applied in organisational safe practice policies and procedures.

### The Health and Safety at Work Act (HSWA) 1974

The Health and Safety at Work Act (HSWA) 1974 is the basis of British health and safety law. It requires employers to take sensible measures to ensure the health and safety of its employees and visiting members of the public.

Workers' responsibilities under the Health and Safety at Work Act are to:

- take care of everyone who may be affected by their work, for example by
  - only doing work they have been trained to do, for example managing soiled laundry
  - using and storing equipment and materials properly, for example cleaning materials
  - working safely at all times, for example when working with sharps.
- report health and safety hazards to an appropriate person without delay, for example
  - faulty equipment, such as washing machines
  - safety signs that have been tampered with, such as wall charts that show the correct colour-coded bag to be used for different types of waste
  - infectious diseases, accidents such as biological spills, and injuries such as sharps injuries.
- helping their employer carry out their health and safety responsibilities by
  - following workplace safe practice procedures at all times
  - not tampering with anything provided for their health and safety
  - knowing what to do in an emergency, such as a contamination injury
  - using PPE correctly.

### The Management of Health and Safety at Work Regulations 1999

The Management of Health and Safety at Work Regulations 1999 requires employers to:

- carry out risk assessments (which you will read about later) and write safe practice procedures that are based on risk assessments
- provide workers with health and safety information, such as information on effective hand washing technique, colour coding for waste disposal and soiled laundry management, and immunisation requirements
- provide workers with training in, for example, infection prevention and control, safe food handling, the correct use of equipment, how to work with hazardous materials,

and first aid. Training is essential in that it tells workers what activities they are required to do, and how, when and why they are required to do them.

## The Public Health (Control of Diseases) Act 1984 and the Public Health (Infectious Diseases) Regulations 1988

Under the Public Health (Control of Diseases) Act 1984 and the Public Health (Infectious Diseases) Regulations 1988, doctors in England and Wales have a legal duty to notify an appropriate person at the local authority if they are aware that, or have cause to suspect that, a patient is suffering from a notifiable disease (see next section).

Figure 39.15 Putting the law into practice – training

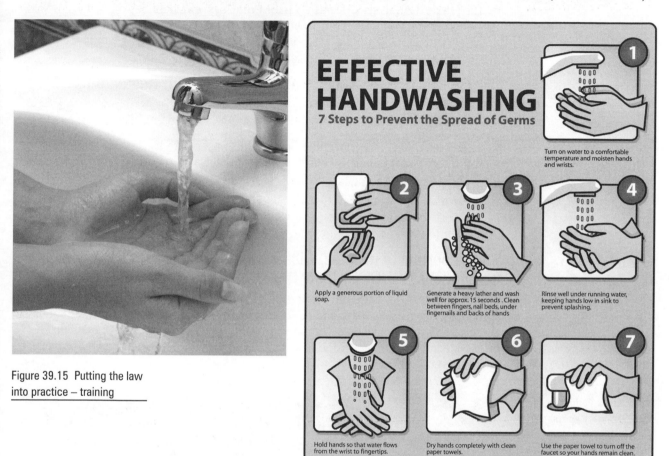

**EFFECTIVE HANDWASHING**
**7 Steps to Prevent the Spread of Germs**

1. Turn on water to a comfortable temperature and moisten hands and wrists.

2. Apply a generous portion of liquid soap.

3. Generate a heavy lather and wash well for approx. 15 seconds. Clean between fingers, nail beds, under fingernails and backs of hands

4. Rinse well under running water, keeping hands low in sink to prevent splashing.

5. Hold hands so that water flows from the wrist to fingertips.

6. Dry hands completely with clean paper towels.

7. Use the paper towel to turn off the faucet so your hands remain clean.

The doctor must complete a certificate stating:

- the patient's name, age and sex
- the address of the premises where the patient is
- the notifiable disease from which the patient is, or is suspected to be, suffering
- the date, or approximate date, of the onset of the disease
- if the premises are a hospital, the day on which the patient was admitted, the address of the premises from which they came, and whether or not they think the disease from which the patient is, or is suspected to be, suffering was contracted in hospital.

## Food safety legislation

Food safety legislation aims to ensure the maintenance of a high standard of:

- personal hygiene in food handlers
- environmental hygiene in areas where food is stored, prepared, cooked and served.

In addition:

- The **Food Safety Act 1990** ensures that the food we buy is safe to eat, that it reaches quality expectations and that it is not misleadingly sold.

- The **Food Hygiene Regulations 2006** aim to improve food safety and reduce the incidence of food poisoning by outlining the hazards associated with food preparation and appropriate methods to ensure food safety.

- The **Food Safety (Temperature Control) Regulations 1995** identify the temperatures required to ensure food safety during storage, preparation and serving.

- The **Hazard Analysis Critical Control Point system** identifies the 'critical points' in food production, processing, manufacturing and preparation where food safety hazards can occur, and puts steps in place to prevent things going wrong. This is sometimes referred to as 'controlling hazards'.

## The Control of Substances Hazardous to Health Regulations (COSHH) 2002

These requires employers to:

- assess the risks from handling hazardous substances such as cleaning materials, blood, body fluids, sharps, household and clinical waste

- manage the risks from handling hazardous substances by writing safe practice procedures. These are usually stored in a COSHH file and it is each worker's responsibility to read the file, get to know the procedures and follow them to the letter.

## The Reporting of Injuries, Diseases and Dangerous Occurrences Regulations (RIDDOR) 1995

These require employers to have procedures for recording and reporting to the relevant authorities any injury, disease and dangerous occurrence or event that has the potential to cause and spread infection, such as sharps and contamination injuries, notifiable diseases and biological spills. The responsibility of workers is to know and follow the relevant procedures.

Figure 39.16 Putting the law into practice – disposing of waste

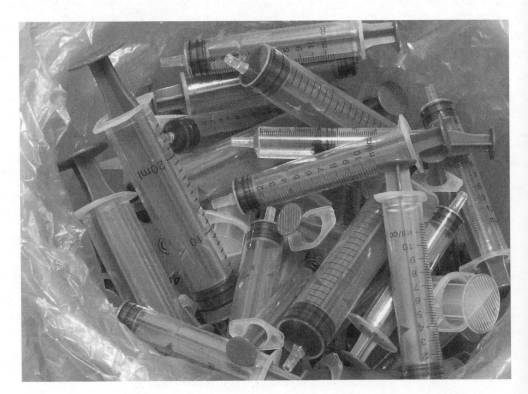

## The Environmental Protection (Duty of Care) Regulations 1991

The Environmental Protection (Duty of Care) Regulations 1991 apply to organisations that produce and store waste, for example household waste, used disposable equipment and contaminated material. Employers have a responsibility or a 'duty of care' to ensure a safe and healthy environment by:

- making sure that there is no unauthorised, harmful treatment or disposal of the waste
- containing the waste i.e. preventing its escape
- ensuring that the waste is transferred to an authorised person
- making sure that a transfer note describing all aspects of the waste is given to the authorised person
- keeping records of waste transfers and associated transfer notes for two years.

## The Hazardous Waste Regulations 2005

The Hazardous Waste Regulations 2005 set out to ensure that waste is dealt with without putting human health at risk and without using methods that could harm the environment or cause a nuisance through noise or odours.

## The Health Protection Agency (HPA)

The Health Protection Agency (HPA) was set up in 2003 as a Special Health Authority (SHA). Its functions included responding to and co-ordinating control measures in the event of outbreak of an infectious disease, providing training and expert advice to those responsible for controlling infectious disease, and working with other organisations to deliver protection against infection.

The Health Protection Agency Bill 2004 changed the HPA from an SHA to a **non-departmental public body**. As a result, the HPA is now able to provide an improved health protection system with a wide range of functions, including working with Primary Care Trusts, NHS hospital trusts and local authorities in each part of the UK.

## NICE Guideline June 2003

As you know, hand hygiene is possibly the most important factor in preventing the spread of infection in both health and social care settings, including in service users' own homes. NICE (the National Institute for Clinical Excellence) Clinical Guideline 2, June 2003 recommends that hands be decontaminated immediately before every episode of direct patient contact or care, and after any activity or contact that could result in the hands becoming contaminated.

In patients' own homes, the method of hand decontamination used will depend on what is practical, available and appropriate for the care or treatment being undertaken. However, NICE recommends that:

- visibly soiled or potentially contaminated hands must be washed with liquid soap and water
- unless visibly soiled, hands must be decontaminated, preferably with an alcohol-based hand-rub, between caring for different patients and between different care activities for the same patient.

*remember*

Health and social care workers have a responsibility to understand legislation relevant to infection prevention and control.

*Link*

You can read about NICE and the Health Protection Agency in Unit 12 (Public Health).

# Organisational policies and procedures

Legislation, regulations and guidelines are written into organisational policies, which set out the organisation's responsibilities in ensuring that the law is obeyed. They are also written into organisational procedures, which are the methods that workers have to use when carrying out their activities.

All organisations that provide health and social care services are legally required to have infection control policies and procedures.

- An Infection Control policy describes the roles and responsibilities of everyone concerned in making sure that infection prevention and control legislation, regulations and guidelines are obeyed.

- Infection Control procedures describe the methods that workers must follow in order to control and prevent the spread of infection. For example, the Safe Handling of Equipment procedure describes the methods that workers must follow in order to prevent the spread of infection when carrying out an activity that involves the use of, for example, sharps.

**Professional Practice**

It is imperative that health and social care workers know their organisation's policies and follow procedures, for the following reasons:

- to maintain safe practice that protects everyone concerned

- to obey the law. Workers have a responsibility to know what the law says. If they are found to be disobeying the law, they can lose their job and the organisation they work for can be closed down.

The following table highlights some important organisational policies and procedures relevant to the prevention and control of spread of infection.

Table 39.6 Policies and procedures relevant to the prevention and spread of infection

| Policies | Examples of related procedures |
|---|---|
| Health and safety | ■ Procedures for the correct use of equipment and materials.<br>■ Procedures for reporting hazards.<br>■ First aid procedures in the event of an accident or injury. |
| Food hygiene | ■ Procedures for ensuring personal and environmental hygiene.<br>■ Procedures for the safe storage, preparation, cooking and serving of food. |
| Infection control | ■ Procedures for standard precautions.<br>■ Procedures for handling, storing and disposal of waste.<br>■ Procedures for decontamination. |
| Control of Substances Hazardous to Health (COSHH) | ■ Procedures for storing, working with and disposal of hazardous material.<br>■ Procedures for the administration of medication and the return of unused and out-of-date medication to the pharmacist. |
| Management of sharps injuries | ■ Procedures for managing injuries in workers and members of the public.<br>■ Procedures for controlling spread of infection subsequent to a sharps injury. |
| Management of infectious diseases | ■ Procedures for standard precautions.<br>■ Procedures for handling, storing and disposal of waste.<br>■ Procedures for decontamination.<br>■ Procedures for managing the outbreak of an infectious disease. |
| Management of spillages | ■ Procedures for dealing with spillages, including biological spills.<br>■ Procedures for disposal of materials and equipment used for dealing with named spillages. |
| Decontamination and waste management | ■ Procedures for decontamination.<br>■ Procedures for dealing with waste.<br>■ Procedures for dealing with an accident involving waste. |
| Challenging behaviour | ■ Procedures for dealing with individuals who have behaviours such as biting and scratching. |
| First aid | ■ Procedures for ensuring there are named, qualified first aiders in the workplace and that the first aid box is maintained.<br>■ Procedures for sending for the emergency health services.<br>■ Procedures for recording accidents and injuries.<br>■ Procedures for ensuring that first aid training takes place. |
| Maintenance of records and reports | ■ Procedures for reporting and recording/notifying a suspected/confirmed outbreak of an infectious disease to the appropriate organisation or individuals.<br>■ Procedures for reporting and recording injuries, diseases and dangerous occurrences or events that have the potential to cause and spread infection. |

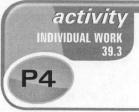

**activity**
**INDIVIDUAL WORK**
**39.3**

**P4**

Interview the individual responsible for infection control and prevention at a health or social care service provider of your choice about the laws, regulations and guidelines that are relevant to the work activities carried out by their colleagues.

Use your findings to create a display entitled 'Infection prevention and control – key legislation'.

**activity**
**INDIVIDUAL WORK**
**39.4**

**M1**

**D1**

Interview the individual responsible for infection control and prevention at a health or social care service provider of your choice about the infection prevention and control procedures that their colleagues have to follow and use your findings to write a report that:

1. explains the role of each procedure in the prevention and control of infection.

2. explains how legal requirements influence infection prevention and control in the workplace.

## Understand roles, responsibilities and boundaries in relation to infection control

### Roles and responsibilities of personnel in relation to infection control

Figure 39.17 Roles and responsibilities of personnel in relation to infection control

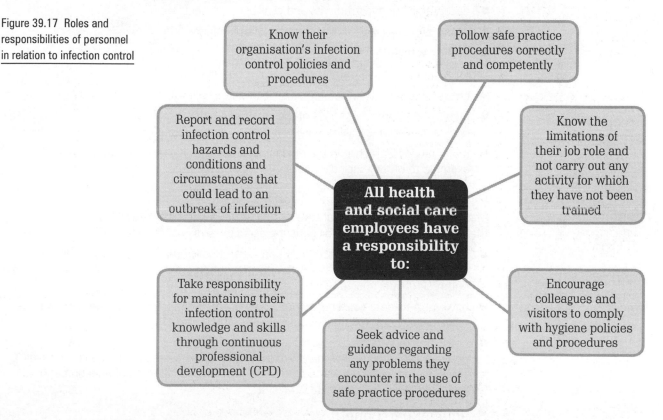

All health and social care employees have a responsibility to:

- Know their organisation's infection control policies and procedures
- Follow safe practice procedures correctly and competently
- Report and record infection control hazards and conditions and circumstances that could lead to an outbreak of infection
- Know the limitations of their job role and not carry out any activity for which they have not been trained
- Take responsibility for maintaining their infection control knowledge and skills through continuous professional development (CPD)
- Seek advice and guidance regarding any problems they encounter in the use of safe practice procedures
- Encourage colleagues and visitors to comply with hygiene policies and procedures

## Care workers

Social care assistants have a particular responsibility to remain aware of and report changes in the health status of the people they support and to follow safe practice procedures when, for example:

- helping service users maintain their personal hygiene, for example, when giving oral care, helping them bathe, use the toilet, change incontinence pads and remove and dispose of soiled clothing
- handling food, for example, when preparing refreshments, cutting and serving food, and helping service users eat and drink
- carrying out general household duties, such as cleaning and making and changing beds
- segregating and disposing of waste
- dealing with spillages.

Health care assistants also have a particular responsibility to remain aware of and report changes in the health status of the people they support. In addition, they have a responsibility to help keep clinical work areas clean and free from infection hazards and to follow safe practice procedures when, for example:

- preparing and maintaining environments before, during and after episodes of patient care
- carrying out activities such as demonstrating inhaler techniques, monitoring blood glucose levels and changing dressings
- collecting, handling and storing laboratory specimens, including blood, body fluids, body waste and wound swabs
- segregating and disposing of waste
- decontaminating instruments and clinical equipment
- giving basic first aid such as treating sharps injuries
- dealing with spillages.

Senior health and social care workers have a particular responsibility to:

- ensure that the workplace remains clean and free from infection hazards
- monitor the working methods of their staff and report potential risks to an appropriate person, usually a specialist individual such as an Infection Control Nurse (see below)
- maintain good practice in their own infection control activities, thereby setting an example to others, including colleagues, patients, service users and visitors.

## Managers

Managers of health and social care settings have a particular responsibility to ensure that the care setting is safe for patients, service users, visitors and staff by:

- having an up-to-date written infection control policy that describes the roles and responsibilities of all staff in relation to prevention of infection and in the event of an outbreak of infectious disease
- having up-to-date written safe practice procedures based on regularly reviewed risk assessments. You will read about risk assessments shortly
- producing reports on a regular basis that describe the systems in place for the prevention and control of infection, for example risk assessments that have taken place and the action taken to rectify any problems; incidences of infection and how they were dealt with; and staff training.

## Specialist personnel

Infection Control Nurses (ICNs) work with other members of an Infection Control Team (ICT). They have a particular responsibility to:

- ensure that the organisation's infection control policies are up-to-date
- ensure that up-to-date safe practice procedures are accessible by all staff and followed to the letter
- ensure that the facilities and equipment needed for safe working practices are available and well maintained
- provide all staff with infection prevention and control training
- carry out surveillance to ensure a timely warning of infectious conditions and outbreaks
- give advice and guidance on infection control issues, in particular how to manage an outbreak.

**Link**

You can read more about surveillance in Unit 12 (Public Health).

Doctors have a particular responsibility to:

- diagnose and treat infectious diseases and health care associated infections (HCAIs)
- liaise with relevant organisations, for example Primary Care Trusts (PCTs) and local authorities about infectious disease control
- notify the Environmental Health Officer (EHO), Consultant in Communicable Disease Control (CCDC) or local Health Protection Unit (HPU) about certain infectious diseases and HCAIs as appropriate (see below).

Environmental Health Officers work for local authorities and are responsible for giving advice on food safety, including hygiene, pest control and waste disposal; inspecting food premises and enforcing food safety legislation; and investigating reported outbreaks of food- and water-borne infectious diseases.

## Health protection units

You read earlier that the Health Protection Agency (HPA) is a non-departmental public body set up to protect the health and wellbeing of the population, in particular against

Figure 39.18 Personnel with infection control roles and responsibilities

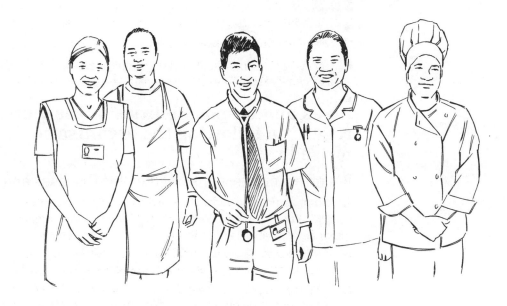

infectious diseases. The HPA works with Primary Care Trusts, NHS trusts and local authorities at regional level, for example, there are HPAs working with trusts and LAs in the Yorkshire and Humber Region, the South East Region and the West Midlands.

Within each region, there are a number of Health Protection Units (HPUs), each serving a different part of the region. For example, in the South West region of the HPA, there are three Health Protection Units; and within the London region, there are four. Each Unit has a leader, consultants who are specialists in infectious diseases, nurses and other staff with specialist health protection skills, whose joint responsibility is to support local organisations on all matters of health protection and infection control.

## Non-care workers

Non-care workers also play a key role in relation to infection prevention and control. For example, housekeeping and domestic staff have a particular responsibility to maintain a clean and tidy environment for everyone concerned through activities such as:

- decontamination of the environment, including general cleaning and tidying, cleaning isolation rooms and dealing with refuse and spills
- washing water jugs, glasses, flower vases and so on
- replenishing hand washing facilities and toilet paper
- making beds
- processing laundry, including soiled linen
- reporting concerns about environmental cleanliness, faulty and damaged equipment and pest infestation to an appropriate person.

Cooks have a particular responsibility to ensure food safety for everyone concerned through, for example:

- maintaining a high standard of personal, environmental and food hygiene
- checking food deliveries for temperature and quality
- monitoring 'use-by' dates and food storage and cooking temperatures
- checking that food served is safe and that waste is dealt with appropriately
- checking that kitchen equipment is in working order and reporting faulty or damaged equipment to an appropriate person
- reporting concerns about environmental cleanliness, faulty and damaged equipment and pest infestation to an appropriate person.

## Roles and responsibilities of the worker with regard to following the organisation's policies and procedures

### Reporting of infectious or notifiable diseases and outbreaks

All health and care workers have a responsibility to observe for any changes in the health status of the people they support and to follow organisational procedures for reporting changes to an appropriate person. Significant changes include cough, fever, diarrhoea, vomiting, rash and itchy skin because these can:

- indicate the presence of an infectious disease, including health care associated infections (HCAI). HCAIs are infections that are acquired by patients as a result of health care treatment or by health care workers in the course of their duties. They include the antibiotic-resistant infections caused by the bacteria MRSA and Clostridium difficile.
- warn of the possibility of an outbreak of an infectious disease.

Prompt reporting of a change in health status enables a prompt diagnosis and action, such as isolation nursing, to be taken quickly. In the event of an HCAI or a suspected outbreak of an infectious disease, an appropriate person, usually a manager, must report their suspicions to the local HPU, which will investigate the situation and co-ordinate any action necessary to control the spread of infection.

According to the Public Health (Control of Diseases) Act 1984 and Public Health (Infectious Diseases) Regulations 1988, the following infectious diseases must be notified by the doctor making the diagnosis to the local authority CCDC.

Table 39.6  Notifiable diseases

| | | | | |
|---|---|---|---|---|
| Acute Encephalitis | Food Poisoning | Meningococcal Septicaemia (Without Meningitis) | Relapsing Fever | Typhoid Fever |
| Acute Poliomyelitis | Leprosy | Mumps | Rubella | Typhus |
| Anthrax | Leptospirosis | Ophthalmia Neonatorum | Scarlet Fever | Viral Haemorrhagic Fever |
| Cholera | Malaria | Paratyphoid Fever | Smallpox | Viral Hepatitis |
| Diphtheria | Measles | Plague | Tetanus | Whooping Cough |
| Dysentery | Meningitis | Rabies | Tuberculosis | Yellow Fever |

## Seeking advice and guidance

All health and social care workers are accountable for the quality of their work and are responsible for maintaining and improving their knowledge and skills. This means that they must inform an appropriate person in the event of any difficulties that might affect their ability to do their job competently and safely; and they must seek advice and guidance if they do not feel able to carry out or are not sure about how to carry out their work activities. As you read earlier, workers can lose their jobs if their actions, omissions, errors or blunders result in things going wrong at work.

Health and social care organisations are obliged to provide supervision for workers. One purpose of supervision is to support workers in identifying and meeting their learning and skills needs, through, for example, training and work shadowing.

## Admissions, transfers and discharges of individuals

If a patient with a highly infectious disease is admitted to hospital, the person in charge of admissions must inform a member of the Infection Control Team, who in turn should inform other members of the ICT, the Occupational Health Department, specialist consultants, the Hospital Chief Executive and the local HPU. This enables special infection control measures to be put in place, such as isolation nursing and screening of staff and patients for immunity.

If the patient needs to be transferred to another department, the department should be told in advance so that special infection control procedures can be put in place. Transport personnel, such as drivers and porters, should ensure that the patient is not left to wait in communal areas and, if the infectious disease is spread by droplets, the patient should be given a mask to wear.

When a patient who continues to be infected is due to be discharged from hospital, a discharge letter should be sent to their GP informing them of the diagnosis. On discharge, family members and health and social care workers who are involved in the patient's care should be told about the infection and how to help prevent and control its spread. Information about the patient should be given to, for example, the EHO, so that the health status of the everyone involved with the patient can be monitored; and thorough decontamination should take place.

## Documentation and record keeping in relation to infection

In addition to using organisational procedures for reporting infectious and notifiable diseases and outbreaks, health and care workers have a responsibility to maintain clear and accurate records of any injury, disease and dangerous event, such as a sharps injury, breach of hygiene and biological spill that has the potential to cause and spread infection.

Organisational procedures describe how records should be made, for example on a workplace Infectious Disease Surveillance Form or a Dangerous Incident Report Form. They also describe how to process a completed record, for example who to send it to; and where and how it should be stored to maintain confidentiality.

## Procedures following the death of an individual

Dead bodies should be treated with respect and dignity and according to the deceased person's religious and cultural background. They are not usually infectious but organisational standard precaution procedures, such as hand hygiene, using appropriate PPE, soiled laundry management, disposal of waste and decontamination must be followed when:

■ washing the body and packing leaking orifices with cotton wool

■ removing dressings, drainage tubes etc.

■ applying and securing clean dressings

■ removing the body to a cool environment.

If the deceased was known to be suffering from an infectious disease, the body should be put in a shroud within a plastic body bag before it is taken to the undertaker; and if the infection is spread by droplet, a mask should be placed over the deceased's mouth. As usual, standard infection control procedures must be followed, and the type of precautions to be taken by the undertaker should be noted on the label attached to the body bag.

## Collection, handling and storing of specimens

Specimens such as wound swabs, blood, sputum, vomit, urine (**MSU** or **CSU**) and faeces are potentially infectious, therefore safe practice infection control procedures must be followed when they are collected, stored and handled.

Eight top tips for collecting, handling and storing specimens:

1. Consent must be obtained from the individual prior to collecting a specimen from them.

2. Hands must be washed before and after collecting, handling and storing a specimen.

3. Appropriate PPE must be used when collecting, handling and storing specimens.

4. Equipment used for collecting specimens must be disposed of correctly.

5. Specimen bottles or containers must be specific to the type of specimen being collected, be clean, have well fitting lids, not be over-filled and be enclosed in a sealed plastic bag.

6. Specimen bottles or containers must be labelled with the patient's name, date of birth, unit number, the date and time when the sample was taken, details of any known or suspected infectious agent and any additional information that may be useful, such as medication being taken and recent holiday location.

7. For accurate results, specimens should be received by the laboratory within 24 hours. Specimens that cannot be taken to the lab straightaway should be stored in a refrigerator within one to two hours of being taken.

8. Specimens should be transported to the lab within a sealed and labelled rigid, leak-proof container in, for example, the boot of a car; and a notice stating that the vehicle is transporting specimens should be visibly placed in the event of an accident. Any spillages should be dealt with according to organisational procedures.

Visitors to health and social care settings also have a responsibility to help prevent the spread of infection, and health and social care workers should encourage them to comply with hygiene policies and procedures.

Figure 39.19 How visitors can help prevent the spread of infection in health and social care settings

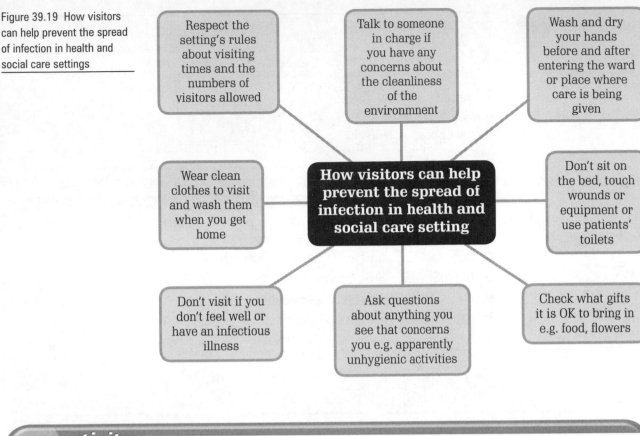

| | | |
|---|---|---|
| Respect the setting's rules about visiting times and the numbers of visitors allowed | Talk to someone in charge if you have any concerns about the cleanliness of the environmnent | Wash and dry your hands before and after entering the ward or place where care is being given |

Wear clean clothes to visit and wash them when you get home

**How visitors can help prevent the spread of infection in health and social care setting**

Don't sit on the bed, touch wounds or equipment or use patients' toilets

Don't visit if you don't feel well or have an infectious illness

Ask questions about anything you see that concerns you e.g. apparently unhygienic activities

Check what gifts it is OK to bring in e.g. food, flowers

**activity**
**INDIVIDUAL WORK**
**39.5**

**P5**

Read the job descriptions for employees at a health or social care provider of your choice, and use your findings to produce an information leaflet for patients or service users which describes the roles and responsibilities of health and social care workers relevant to infection prevention and control.

## Risk assessment

As you read earlier, the Management of Health and Safety at Work Regulations 1999 and the Control of Substances Hazardous to Health Regulations (COSHH) 2002 require employers to carry out assessments of the risks posed by different work activities. Assessing the risks associated with activities involving infectious materials enables safe practice procedures to be written, thereby helping to prevent and control the spread of infection.

The following six steps describe how to carry out a risk assessment.

1. Identify hazardous work activities, for example cleaning up a spill of faeces.

2. Assess the risks associated with each activity – who might be harmed and how?

3. Identify what precautions are currently taken, for example standard precautions, decontamination techniques, waste disposal.

4. Decide whether current precautions are adequate; if they aren't, decide how they can be improved.

5. Write the new precautions into safe practice procedures which everyone can understand and follow, and to which everyone has easy access.

6. Plan a date to review hazardous work activities and the adequacy of both current and new precautions.

Health Protection Agency
www.hpa.org.uk
National Institute for Clinical Excellence
www.nice.org.uk
General Social Care Council
www.gscc.org.uk
Royal College of Nursing
www.rcn.org.uk

---

## *activity*
### INDIVIDUAL WORK 39.6

**M2**

**D2**

Carry out and write a report on a risk assessment for three different work activities at a health or social care provider of your choice.

- Describe the hazards associated with each activity.
- Describe who might be harmed and how.
- Describe what precautions are currently in use.
- Assess whether the current precautions are sufficient or could be improved.
- Where improvement is necessary, write safe practice procedures to ensure that risks are either removed or minimised.

Conclude your report with an explanation of how risk assessment can contribute to improving infection prevention and control in a health or social care workplace.

---

### *Progress Check*

1. Define the following terms: localised infection, systemic infection, colonisation, normal flora, transient flora, pathogen.
2. Describe the chain of infection and its significance in infection prevention and control.
3. Compare and contrast bacteria, viruses, fungi and parasites, and describe one disease caused by each.
4. Describe the factors that influence the growth of micro-organisms.
5. Describe how micro-organisms spread.
6. Describe standard precautions and how they help prevent the spread of infection.
7. Describe how to deal with used sharps, household waste, clinical waste and biological spills.
8. Name a low, medium and high risk item or piece of equipment and describe the decontamination technique for each.
9. Identify five pieces of legislation that are relevant to infection prevention and control.
10. Explain how five organisational procedures promote infection prevention and control.
11. Describe the roles and responsibilities of three health and social care workers in promoting infection prevention and control.
12. Describe the role of visitors to health and social care settings in promoting infection prevention and control.
13. Describe how you would carry out an infection prevention and control risk assessment and why such risk assessments are important.

# Glossary

## Unit 12

**Bacteria** Member of large group of unicellular micro-organisms which can be disease producing

**Communicable disease** A disease that can be passed on from human to human or animal/insect to human

**Cyanosis** Describes a lack of colour (or blueness) due to insufficient oxygenation of tissues

**Demographic** Relating to statistic information about populations and areas

**Epidemic** Spread of disease in surrounding area

**Epidemiology** The study of disease incidence and spread

**Fungal** Spore producing micro-organism that thrives in warm moist conditions

**Gestalt** Form, pattern; organised whole

**Immunisation** Protection from disease by making immune or resistant, e.g. injection to prevent measles

**Immunology** The study of how the body's immune system fights disease and illness

**Incidence** The number of times that something occurs

**Incubation** The period of time when the disease is infectious and multiplying before signs and symptoms are felt

**Inequality** Unequal balance in sharing resources

**Morbidity** The cause of death

**Mortality** The number of deaths in a given period; the state of being subject to death

**Mortality** The number of deaths in a given time

**Pandemic** Disease spread across a wide area, e.g. worldwide

**Parasite** An organism living in or on another

**Pathogen** A disease producing organism

**Pathogen** Micro-organism that causes disease

**Pesticide** Chemical substance used for destroying weeds, insects and organisms harmful to cultivated plants or animals

**Virus** A sub microscopic infective agent that can multiply only within the living cells of a host

**Zymotic disease** disease regarded as caused by the multiplication of germs introduced from outside

## Unit 14

**Allergens** Things that cause an allergic reaction

**Alveoli** Thin walled microscopic elastic air sacs which form the lungs

**Auto-immune** The process by which a person's immune system attacks their body's own tissues

**Care setting** A setting in which caring services are provided

**Critical care** Intensive care given to patients in a critical or unstable condition

**Data** Information

**Decentralisation** The spread of control of services from central Government to local government

**Detoxification** Removal of poisons

**Elective** Chosen

**Enzyme** A protein that triggers chemical reactions in the body.

**Ethical** Moral, right, fair, decent

**Expert witness** Someone who has a knowledge and understanding of a situation

**Orthoses** Special mechanical devices used to support weak or abnormal joints and limbs

**Palpation** Touching or feeling something

**Prognosis** The forecast of the course of a disease

**Relapse** Reappearance of a disease after a period of improvement

**Remission** Period of time when the signs and symptoms of a disease are reduced

**Service user** Someone who uses health or social care services

**Stem cells** Cells at the earliest stage of their development, which have not yet begun to specialize and so can grow into any kind of cell

**Stimuli** Things that cause a reaction or something to happen

**Subjects** The name given to the individuals used in research

**Triage** A system that sorts medical cases in order of urgency to determine how quickly patients receive treatment, for instance in accident and emergency departments

## Unit 20

**Alma-Ata declaration** A WHO initiative setting out a declaration on the importance of primary care as a method of attaining Health for All by the year 2000

**Community development** Working with people to allow them to identify their own health concerns and the solutions for them

**Empowerment model** A model of health education where the individual isn't always seen as responsible for his or her own health. Empowering individuals to take control of their own health is seen as key

**Health belief model** Using analysis of psychological factors affecting beliefs about potential costs and beliefs of health behaviour

**Health education** Any activity that promotes health related learning and therefore brings about some relatively permanent changes in thinking or behaviour of individuals

**Health for All by the year 2000** A WHO initiative setting out health targets for all by the year 2000

**Health promotion** Activities undertaken to promote health; usually includes health education, prevention and health promotion

**Holistic** The 'whole'

**Mass media** Umbrella term for all the different formats of media that can be accessed by the 'masses'

**Needs led** Projects that are determined by the needs of individuals as opposed to the needs of the service

**Ottowa Charter for Health Promotion** A WHO initiative setting a charter for the use of health promotion as a method of attaining Health for All by the year 2000

**Peer educators** The use of peers to educate on health issues

**Public health** Services covering a large population ensuring that their health is not adversely affected by their shared environment

**Root causes of ill health** Examining the 'real' cause of ill health by examining the cause of the behaviour

**Social learning theory** The theory that individuals learn from the way others behave

**Social marketing** The application of marketing themes health education messages

**Stages of change model** Using analysis of stages an individual will go through when changing behaviour, to understand health behaviour

**Theory of planned behaviour** Using analysis through attitudes, subjective norms and perceptions of belief over control, to understand health behaviour

**Theory of reasoned action** Using analysis of intentions through attitudes and subjective norms to understand health behaviour

**Two-way communication** Dialogue between individuals of groups to educate on health.

**'Victim-blaming' model** A model of health education where the individual is seen as responsible for his or her own health

# Unit 21

**Compounds (as in a chemical compound)** A substance containing 2 or more elements or molecules

**Developed world** The industrialised, first world countries

**Diuretics** Drugs that increase the production of urine and are used to remove excess fluid from the body

**Endorphins** Hormones that reduce the sensation of pain and affect the emotions

**Enzymes** Proteins that trigger a chemical reaction in the body

**Essential fatty acids** Fatty acids that the body can't make itself

**Fat** Lipids that are solid at room temperature

**Hydrogenation** Treat with hydrogen

**Kilocalories (kcal)** A unit of energy in food which is equal to the amount of energy needed to raise the temperature of 1 kilogram of water by 1 degree Centigrade

**mg** Milligram, which is one thousandth of a gram

**Oils** Lipids that are liquid at room temperature

**Processing (as in food processing)** Preparing and preserving food

**Socio-economic** The interaction of social and economic factors

**Vegetarians** People who don't eat meat

# Unit 22

**Bias** Having a particular viewpoint or perspective; not being neutral

**Confidentiality** Only allowing limited, if any, access to any other people

**Ethics** Rules or guidance governing good practice in research to ensure minimal disruption or hurt. Usually based on what is deemed morally right by a society

**Hypothesis** A statement which needs proving or disproving

**Mean** The traditional 'average', calculated by adding all numbers up and then dividing by the number of numbers

**Median** An 'average' represented by the number which falls in the 'middle', when all the numbers are organised into numerical order

**Methodology** The type of research method chosen to collect raw data

**Mode** An 'average' represented by the number occurring most frequently

**Primary research** Data that is collected for the first time by the researcher

**Qualitative** Data based on opinions/behaviour/values

**Quantitative** Numerical data

**Reliability** The likelihood of the same results occurring if the same research was repeated

**Research question** A question which the researcher hopes to answer through research

**Sample** The selected population who will participate in the research

**Secondary research** Data that has been collected already by another researcher

**Sources of error** Potential ways that research could have been affected, swayed or manipulated

**Triangulation** Choosing 2 or more (usually 3) sources of data to improve validity

**Validity** How 'true' the results are to reality

# Unit 26

**Acute** Sudden on-set, may require immediate intervention if serious, short in duration

**Chronic illness or condition** Longer term on-going illness or condition

**Codes of practice** A set of principles and guidance

**Self advocacy** An individual speaking up and speaking out in order to make choices about their lives. Self advocacy is all about choices and influencing the services

**Self-esteem** Feeling good about yourself; self-worth and value, confidence and self-belief

**Social construct** Something (a view or a social structure) within a society which has been developed by the society

**Standard precautions** Protection against the transmission of infection in the work place by wearing PPE and treating all bodily fluids and tissues as potentially infectious. This approach protects both the worker and the service user

**Whistle blowing** When a person within an organisation informs authorities/press/external organisations regarding bad practice or areas of concern

# Unit 28

**Angioplasty** Use of a sausage-shaped balloon, which is inflated in an artery to open it up

**Assistive technologies** Technological equipment designed for people with, e.g. communication and mobility needs

**Auditory nerve** The nerve that carries nervous impulses from the ear to the brain

**Biological** Relating to the body

**Cochlea** The inner ear

**Disorientation** Confused as to time or place or personal identity

**DNA** Deoxyribonucleac acid – the substance from which genetic material is made

**Dysphasia** The inability to find the right words to use

**Empty calories** Calories that have no nutritional content

**Gender** Femininity and masculinity, which are defined by the culture in which one lives

**Gene** A distinct section of DNA that determines a specific characteristic

**Genetic predisposition** Having genes which make one liable or inclined to have a particular condition

**Hair cells** Cells in the cochlea that are sensitive to sound waves

**Human resources** Workers, staff, people

**Identity** The way we see ourselves

**Median** The middle number in a sequence of increasing or decreasing numbers

**Mutation** A change in structure

**Paranoia** A feeling of being persecuted

**Peripheral vision** Vision in the top, bottom and sides of the field of view

**Prognosis** The likely course of a disease

**Psychological** Relating to the mind

**Retina** The nerve tissue that lines the back of the eye and which is sensitive to light and colour

**Social exclusion** Marginalisation or exclusion from society and an adequate quality of life

**Socially constructed concept** A view, idea or belief that is formulated and held by a social or cultural group

**Sociological** Relating to society

**Somatic cells** Body cells as opposed to reproductive cells

**Vertebrae** Bones of the spine

# Unit 39

**Aerobic** Living only in the presence of oxygen

**Anaerobic** An organism that can live in the absence of oxygen

**Autoclave** A container used for processes that require high pressure and temperature

**CSU** Catheter specimen urine, which is a specimen of urine collected from a catheter bag

**Episode of care** Care that starts with a referral or admission and ends with discharge e.g. an inpatient episode, an outpatient episode, a day case episode

**Inactivate** To make inactive or put out of action

**Incineration** Destroy by burning

**Indwelling medical device** A device that is situated within the body, such as a catheter

**Larvae** The newly hatched, wingless, often wormlike form of an insect

**Maceration** Destroy by soaking in water

**Mantoux testing** The skin test for TB. A positive result indicates natural immunity whereas a negative result means the person is susceptible to infection

**Model** An idea or example that is used to describe or explain a theory or phenomenon.

**MSU** Mid stream urine specimen, which is collected after urine has flowed for a short while and terminated before the flow ceases

**Mucous membrane** The skin that lines internal passages such as the digestive and respiratory tracts and the vagina and which contains glands that secrete mucous

**Non-departmental public body** A body that has a role in the processes of national government but is not a government department. Instead it makes day-to-day decisions at national, regional and local level independently of Government ministers and Civil Servants

**Parasitic** An organism that lives in or on another organism and contributes nothing to the survival of its host

**Replicate** To reproduce or make an exact copy or copies of, for example, a cell

**Septicaemia** Blood poisoning

**Spore** The resistant form of a bacterium, which enables it to survive adverse conditions

**Strain** A group of organisms of the same species, having distinctive characteristics but not usually considered a separate breed or variety

**Viable** Capable of surviving

# Bibliography and suggested further reading

## Unit 12

Babb P., Butcher H., Church J., Zealey L. (eds), National Trends Social Statistics, Office for Social Trends No. 36, Office for National Statistics, New York: Palgrave Macmillan, 2006.

Carstairs V. and Morris R., *Deprivation and health in Scotland*. Aberdeen: Aberdeen University Press, 1991.

Department of Health, *Choosing Health: Making Healthier Choices Easier* (Public Health White Paper), London: DH, 2004.

Ewles. L. and Simnett I., *Promoting health: a practical guide*, 4th ed. London: Bailliere Tindal, 1995.

Jarman B., Identification of underprivileged areas. British Medical Journal 28 May 1983, 286 (6379): 1705–9.

*Measuring Multiple Deprivation at the Small Area Level: The Indices of Deprivation 2000*, Indices of Deprivation 2000.54DETR: London, 2000.

Noble M., Smith G.A.N., Penhale B., Wright G., Dibben C., Owen T. and Lloyd M., The health of children and young people, Chapter 8, Social Inequalities Office for National Statistics, March 2004 500.

Overview of Communicable Diseases 1999, Health Protection Agency http://www.hpa.org.uk/infections/publications/1999_2000_review/index.htm

Social Inequalities Office for National Statistics, March 2004 Alison Macfarlane (City University, London), Mai Stafford (University College London) and Kath Moser (London School of Hygiene and Tropical Medicine).

## Unit 14

Clancy, J. and McVicar, A., *Physiology and Anatomy: A Homeostatic Approach*, Second Edition, (London: Hodder Arnold, 2002).

Hubbard, J. and Meehan D., *The Physiology of Health and Illness with Related Anatomy*, (Cheltenham: Stanley Thornes, 1997).

Nield, C., What is MS?, The Multiple Sclerosis Society, 2006.

Ross, J. R. et al., *Ross and Wilson's Anatomy and Physiology in Health and Illness*, (Edinburgh: Churchill Livingstone, 2001).

Toole, G. and Toole S., *Advanced Human and Social Biology*, (Cheltenham: Nelson Thornes, 1997).

Tortora, G. and Grabowski S., *Principles of Anatomy and Physiology*, (New York: John Wiley and Sons, 2000).

Ward, J., Clarke R. W. and Linden R., *Physiology at a Glance*, (Oxford: Blackwell Publishing, 2005).

Biological Science

New Scientist

Nursing Times

## Unit 20

Alma Ata declaration – www.who.int/hpr/NPH/docs/declaration_ almaata.pdf

Choosing Health – www.dh.gov.uk

Department of Health – www.dh.gov.uk

Donaldson, R. J. and Donaldson, L. J., *Essential Public Health Medicine*, (Lancaster: Kulwer Academic, 1993).

Ewles, L. and Simnett, I., *Promoting Health, A Practical Guide*, (London: Balliere Tindall Publishers, 2003).

Health Protection Agency – www.hpa.org.uk

Hubley, Initial., *Communicating Health: An Action Guide to Health Education and Health Promotion*, (London: MacMillan, 1993).

Institute for Social Marketing – www.ism.stir.ac.uk

National Commission for Health Education Credentialing – www.nchec.org/index.htm

NHS Breast Screening Programme – www.cancerscreening.nhs.uk/breastscreen

NHS Immunisations – www.immunisation.nhs.uk

Ottawa Charter for Health Promotion – www.who.int/hpr/NPH/docs/ottawa_charter_hp.pdf
Oxford Dictionary – www.AskOxford.com
Regional Public Health Groups – www.gos.gov.uk/publichealth/?a=42496
Saving Lives: Our healthier nation – www.archive.official-documents.co.uk
Society for Public Health Education – www.sophe.org/index.asp
Tannahill, A., 'What is health promotion?', *Health Education Journal*, (Sage, 1985), 44:167–168.
Townsend, Davison and Whitehead, *Inequalities in Health: The Black Report and The Health Divide*, (London: Penguin, 1998).
WHO – www.who.int/en

# Unit 21

Arnold, E. and Bender, D. A., *Food Tables and Labelling: Combined School Edition*, (Oxford: Oxford University Press, 1999).
Barasi, M., *Human Nutrition: A Health Perspective*, (London: Hodder Arnold, 2002).
Bender, D. A., *An Introduction to Nutrition and Metabolism*, (London: Taylor and Francis, 2002).
Byrom, S. E., *Pocket Guide to Nutrition and Dietetics*, (Edinburgh: Churchill Livingstone, 2002).
Disabled Living Foundation, (DLF 2005), *Choosing eating and drinking equipment*.
Fox, B. A. and Cameron, G. A., *Food Science, Nutrition and Health*, (London: Hodder Arnold, 1995).
Garrow, J. S. and James, W. P. T. (Editors), *Human Nutrition and Dietetics*, (Edinburgh: Churchill Livingstone, 1999).
Gibney, M. J., Voster, H. H. and Kok, F. J., *Introduction to Human Nutrition*, (Oxford: Blackwell Publishing, 2002).
*Health Service Journal*.
*Human Nutrition and Dietetics*.
MAFF – *The Manual of Nutrition* (1995 HMSO).
Mann, J. and Truswell, S. (Editors), *Essentials of Human Nutrition*, (Oxford: Oxford University Press, 2002).
National Diet and Nutrition Survey 4–18 years.
National Diet and Nutrition Survey Adults 19–64 years – www.statistics.gov.uk/ssd.
Nutrient Databank Data Files – available from Her Majesty's Stationery Office, St Clements House, 2-16 Colegate. Norwich NR3 1BQ.
*Public Health Nutrition*.
Thomas, B. (Editor), *Manual of Dietetic Practice*, (London: Blackwell Science, 2001).
Truswell, S. A., *ABC of Nutrition*, (London: BMJ Books, 2003).
Tull, A., *Food and Nutrition*, (Oxford: Oxford University Press, 1997).
Webb, G. P., *Nutrition: A Health Promotion Approach*, (London: Arnold, 2002).

# Unit 22

Bailey et al., *Essential Research Skills*, (London: Collins Educational, 1995).
Bandolier – www.jr2.ox.ac.uk/bandolier/index.html.
Bland, M., *An Introduction to Medical Statistics*, (Oxford: Oxford University Press, 1995).
British Journal of Nursing – www.info.britishjournalofnursing.com.
British Journal of Social Work – www.bjsw.oxfordjournals.org.
British Medical Journal – www.bmj.com.
British Psychological Society – www.bps.org.uk.
British Sociological Association – www.britsoc.co.uk.
Department of Children, Schools and Families – www.dfes.gov.uk.
Department of Health – www.dh.gov.uk.
ERIC – www.eric.ed.gov.
GCSE bitesize – www.bbc.co.uk/schools/gcsebitesize/maths/datahandlingh.
Green, S., *Research Methods in Health, Social and Early Years Care*, (Cheltenham: Nelson Thornes, 2000).
Joseph Rowntree Foundation – www.jrf.org.uk.
National Institute of Clinical Excellence – www.nice.org.uk.
Office of Public Sector Information – www.opsi.gov.uk.
Oxford Dictionary – www.AskOxford.com.
Social Care Institute for Excellence – www.scie.org.uk/index.asp.
Sociology central – www.sociology.org.uk/index.htm.
Sociology online – www.sociologyonline.net.
SPSS – www.spss.com.
Twain, Mark., *Autobiography*, (London: Harper Collins, 1924).
Wikipedia – www.wikipedia.org.

# Unit 26

Barnes, C., Mercer, G., *Disability*, (Cambridge: Polity Press, 2003).
Barnes, C., Mercer, G., Shakespeare, T., *Exploring Disability*, (London: Polity Press, 1999)
Chappell A., L., (1997) Disability Studies: Past Present and Future Edited by Barton L. and Oliver M. (Leeds: Disability Press, 1997).
Christie, I, Mensah-Coker, G., *An Inclusive Future Disability, Social Change and Opportunities for Greater Inclusion by 2010*, (London: Demos, 1999).
The Data Protection Registrar, *The Data Protection Act 1998*, (The Data Protection Registrar, 1998).
DoH, *Choosing Health: Making Healthier Choice easier*, (London: Department of Health, 2004).
DoH, *Our Health, Our Care, Our Say: A new direction for community services*, White Paper, (London: Department of Health, 2006).
DoH, *The Expert Patient*, (London: Department of Health, 2006).
DoH, *Valuing People A New Strategy for Learning Disability for the 21st Century*, (London: Department of Health, 2001).
DRC, *Equal Treatment: Closing the Gap*, (Disability Rights Commission, 2000).
Lindsey, M., Russell, O., *Once a Day Good Practice*, (NHS Executive, 1999).
Morris, J., Pride Against Prejudice Transforming Attitudes to Disability, (London Womens press 1991)
Nursing and Midwifery Council (NMC 2004) *The NMC code of professional conduct: standards for conduct*, performance and ethics.
Philpot T., and Ward L., (eds), *Values and Visions* (Oxford: Butterworth Heinman, 1995).
Rogers, A., 5 March 2007 The National Primary Care Research and Development Centre
Thornton, P., Tozer, R., *Having a say in change – older people and community care*, (Joseph Rowntree Foundation, 1995).
UPIAS, *Fundamental Principles of Disability*, (London: Union of the Physically Impaired Against Segregation, 1976).
WHO, *International Classification of Impairments, Disabilities and Handicaps*, (World Health Organization Geneva, 1980).
WHO, *International Classification of Functioning and Disability*, (World Health Organization ICIDH-2, 1999).
www.who.int/classifications

# Unit 28

'Ageing can we stop the clock?', (Wellcome Trust, 2006).
Bernard, M., *New lifestyles in old age: health, identity and wellbeing in Berryhill Retirement Village Bristol*, (Bristol: Policy Press, 2004).
Bernard, M., *Promoting Health in Old Age*, (Milton Keynes: Open University Press, 2000).
Joseph, J., *Warning When I am old I shall wear purple*, (London: Souvenir Press, 1997).
Kirkwood, T., *Time of Our Lives,* (London: Phoenix Paperbacks, 2000).
Woolham, J., *Assistive Technology in Dementia Care*, (London: Hawker Publications, 2006).
*Care and Health*
*Community Care*
*Nursing Times*

# Unit 39

A Matron's Charter: An Action Plan for Cleaner Hospitals, (NHS Estates: Department of Health, 2004).
Ayling, P., Knowledge Sets: Infection Prevention and Control, (London: Heinemann, 2007).
Damani, N., Manual of Infection Control Procedures, (Greenwich Medical Media, 2003).
Essential steps to safe, clean care: Preventing the spread of infection, (Department of Health, 2006).
Good Practice in infection prevention and control, (Royal College of Nursing, 2005).
Infection Control Guidance for Care Homes, (Department of Health, 2006).
Kennamer, M., Basic Infection Control for the Health Care Professional, (New York: Delmar, 2001).
MRSA and other health care associated Infections: Information for visitors – www.rcn.org.uk.
*NHS healthcare cleaning manual* (NHS Estates, 2004c)
Owen, G. A., HACCP Works, (Doncaster: Highfield Publications, 2005).
Richards, J., Complete A-Z Health and Social Care Handbook, (Hodder Arnold, 2003).
Sprenger, R., The Foundation HACCP Handbook, (Doncaster: Highfield Publications, 2007).
Sprenger, R. and Fisher, I., The Essentials of Health and Safety (Carers), (Doncaster: Highfield Publications, Year).
The Health Care Act 2006: Code of Practice For the Prevention and Control of Health care Associated Infections (Department of Health, 2006).

# Index

# Index